The Creative Age

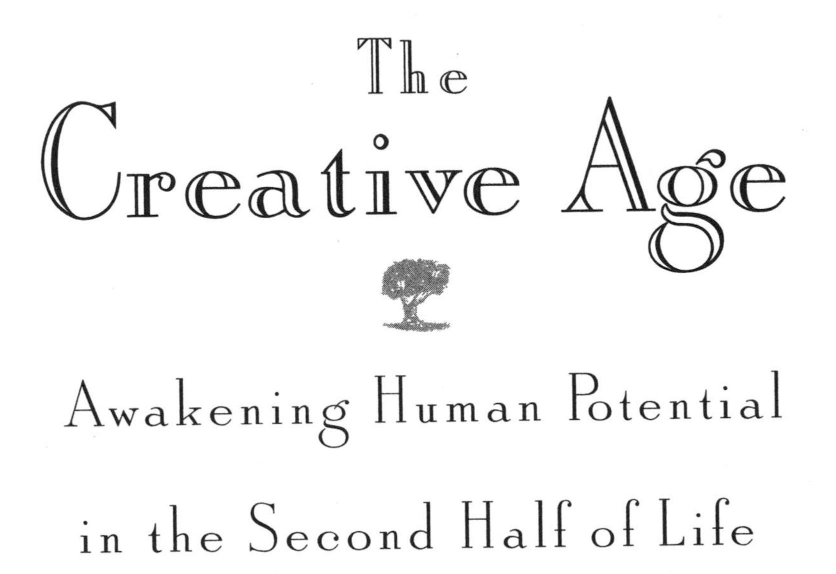

Gene D. Cohen, M.D., Ph.D.

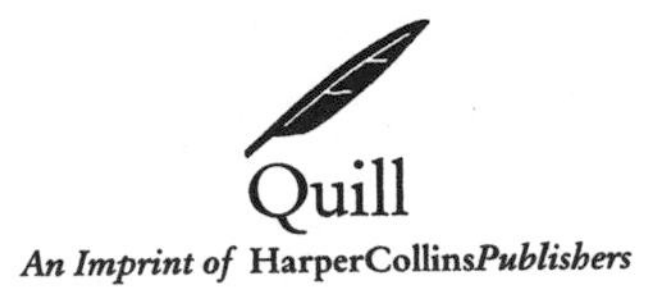

A hardcover edition of this book was published in 2000 by Avon Books Inc., an imprint of HarperCollins Publishers.

HarperCollins books may be purchased for educational, business, or sales promotional use. For information please write: Special Markets Department, HarperCollins Publishers Inc., 10 East 53rd Street, New York, NY 10022.

First Quill edition published 2001.

Designed by Richard Oriolo

The Library of Congress has catalogued the hardcover edition as follows:

Cohen, Gene D.
The creative age : awakening human potential in the second half of life / Gene D.
Cohen.—1st ed.
p. cm.
ISBN 0-380-97684-6
1. Middle age—Psychological aspects. 2. Creativity in old age. I. Title.
HQ1059.4.C58 2000
305.244—dc21 99-058721

ISBN 0-380-80071-3 (pbk.)

08 09 10 QW 10 9 8 7 6

To the memory of my father, Ben Cohen,

the greatest fan a son could ever have,

and a dedicated keeper of the culture

of family life, values, and fun.

Acknowledgments

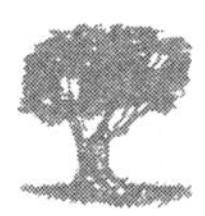

FIRST, I WOULD LIKE to acknowledge the great support and patience my family provided me while I wrote this book. My wife Wendy Miller made numerous suggestions about important source material from the arts and healing literature. My son Alex helped in researching biographical information and critiquing ideas. My little daughter Eliana shared the big screen computer with me at home, waiting patiently to put in her *Madeline* disk. All of my family members were very understanding and tolerant of the reduction in valuable time we had together during the writing of the book.

I especially want to acknowledge the invaluable contributions of Teresa Barker, who assisted me in the writing of the book. Her pen is like a magic wand, wondrously elevating the quality and flow of writing. It was an absolute delight working with her, an ideal collaborator who pushed me ever so artfully and effectively to a higher level for a far better product. I am extremely grateful to her. I appreciate, too, the support of Teresa's family, including her mother Maxine Barker.

I also want to express my deep appreciation to my agent, Gail Ross, for her successful efforts in connecting me with Avon Books and for her ongoing assistance in keeping things on course. And many thanks to Howard Yoon who worked with Gail in this process.

Much gratitude is due as well to Jennifer Brehl, my editor at Avon Books, who always promptly and helpfully worked closely with me in attempting to answer questions, solve problems, and move things along.

Finally, numerous friends and colleagues were very supportive with their encouragement, enthusiasm, and advice about the book, particularly Marsha Weiner and David Kennard with whom I am working on complementary projects.

Contents

Introduction

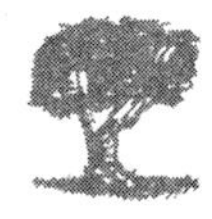

NOT SO LONG AGO, old people were considered a dead-end career choice for a young doctor. It was that way in 1973 when I announced to my mentors and colleagues that I planned to build my career around the study of aging and the treatment of older adults. Gerontology? They thought I was nuts.

"You're throwing away your career!"

"You're a Harvard graduate—you should know better!"

"You need to have your head examined!"

In 1973, I had just entered the United States Public Health Service (PHS), in the last group of physicians drafted during the war in

Vietnam. I was very fortunate, though, in that my draft assignment was at the National Institute of Mental Health (NIMH), part of the National Institutes of Health (NIH). I had already become interested in the field of aging, though I did not initially seek out work in this area. It happened by circumstance, at least in part. In 1971 I was a resident—a physician-in-training—in psychiatry at the Georgetown University Medical Center in Washington, D.C. One of my clinical rotations that year was supposed to involve community consultation.

The program called for me to be available to a community-based agency to consult about clients' behavioral problems. Typically, as a consultant, a resident physician was expected to work with the patient's case on paper only, reviewing the file and making treatment recommendations, all without ever seeing the client. This "blind" doctoring bothered me, because, although I knew the agency staff was competent and would carry out my treatment plan, it bothered me that I would never get to see how my intervention ultimately worked out. I believe in medicine, not magic, and I wanted the feedback, even if my consultation proved worthless. If it worked, I wanted to know why; if it didn't, I still wanted to know why.

To get that feedback, I knew I had to work in a system that would allow me to follow up on my patients. I wondered where, other than in a small town, I might find that kind of arrangement. Then it hit me: a senior citizens' building was like a small town. I could consult to the resident manager of the building and because anyone discussed would be living in that building, I could learn the outcome of my efforts. The public housing programs were particularly interested in consultation at that time, because they typically had a number of residents who had been discharged from state hospitals.

I found the public housing high-rise that needed me, but can admit now that at the time, I hesitated to enter the building, myself affected then by negative stereotypes about aging that were at their zenith in America in the late 1960s and early 1970s. But once in the building I was stunned by what I found and experienced. It was not at all like the stereotypes predicted. This was not a morbid, immutable lot. Nor were they looking for miracle cures.

These older individuals were quite realistic in their expectations and savored greatly any improvements through medical treatments or therapy. In fact, many got much better once there was a program in place to diagnose and treat their problems.

Instead of what others warned would be the most depressing of patients, these elderly women and men proved to be among the most alert, attentive, and responsive—a satisfying kind of patient for a doctor who cares. These were men and women with some history, medical and otherwise; a past, to be sure; but also a future still rich with potential. As a result of my motivation and their surprising responsiveness, I fell in love: with the people, with the work, and with the potential I saw to make a difference. I was hooked.

The next step in the medical resident program required that I find a supervisor to guide and oversee me on my work. I was informed that there weren't any: In all of this distinguished faculty there was no expert on mental health and aging. Gerontology was not a new experience for me alone, as a young psychiatrist. It was a new frontier for my profession, and I was thrilled by the thought. I liked being there.

The teachers and colleagues who questioned my sanity and career choice had good reason to do so. Where I saw a field of pioneering discovery, they saw no field at all. They saw a wasteland. Influenced by the myriad negative myths and stereotypes that painted hopeless and depressing pictures about work with elderly patients, they wondered whether I had some morbid fascination about working with dying and decrepit old folks. My view couldn't have been more different; quite apart from what can be done to help those who are dying, these individuals were in fact *living*, and I was certain that many could be living better—much better. I didn't see them as decrepit; those who struggled with a high level of disease and disability were inspiring to me. I knew we could be doing more for them.

I am as much a product of my culture as the next person, and as I thought more about my career choice, I concluded that my feelings reflected a positive stirring in our culture and its attitude toward aging. I just happened to be at the front end of this emerging and positive curve. This fueled my excitement about seeing aging as a new field even more. That there was so little there, as my colleagues pointed out, only added to my sense of challenge and opportunity in a realm that was so wide open scientifically.

My obligation from the draft was to serve two years. Nearing the end of my two years in 1974, at the age of twenty-nine, I asked for an appointment with the director of NIMH, Bertram Brown. With some combination of inspiration, arrogance, and naïveté, I argued before Dr. Brown that aging was going to be the field of the 1980s, and now was a great time to seize the opportunity to proactively prepare for it.

I then confessed that though it would be self-serving, I nonetheless would be proud, excited, and ready to head a new center addressing issues of mental health and aging. He smiled, and said I might be right, but the timing unfortunately was not right for NIMH. My bubble burst, and I was disappointed; but I felt I had given it my best shot. Soon it would be time to leave the Public Health Service and return to academic life.

Two months later, just as I was about to sign papers to set in motion my resignation from the PHS, Bert Brown called me back to his office to say that I made a good case and that NIMH should launch such a program. He was very supportive. I was appointed to head what became the first federal research program on mental health and aging established in any country.

My main concern was that I felt and looked very young to occupy such a leadership position on aging. So I grew a beard and donned a bow tie, both of which I still wear today. Two decades later, after fifteen years at that post and another five at the National Institute on Aging (NIA)—where during my last three years I served as acting director—I realized that the gods had "punished" me by granting my wishes. It had been a challenge and a labor of love, watching and helping a new field become established and move forward. I felt very privileged.

As I think back—even further back—I can see that my interest in aging began much earlier than my years of formal medical training. It was actually 1961, the year Yuri Gagarin from the Soviet Union became the first man to enter space and John F. Kennedy became President. I was a junior in high school. That year I won a first prize in the Massachusetts State Science Fair held at MIT. It was only when I thought back over the years that I remembered what had been so long forgotten—that my project was one on aging and oceanography. Only much later I realized that my science project reflected an approach to aging that I adopted when I was at NIH—that is, by focusing on aging we have a chance to learn something new about broader issues in science and life. Research on aging provides a new pathway for finding additional pieces to science's many puzzles, independent of age.

That science project also gave me my first painful experience of the power of fixed ideas against new ideas, even in science and even when the new idea was supported by data. For an idealistic young scientist it was a deeply disturbing clash with the world of adult power.

My science project involved calculating the age of fish using a previously abandoned method in an improved way. The goal was to establish normal growth curves for fish at different ages. Then, if a fish was found not to be as large as it should be at a given age, the discrepancy might suggest that its habitat was not healthy. A focus on age enabled a new way of assessing the status of the ecology; research on aging was providing answers to broader questions.

As it turned out, I won a first prize at the fair, but only after a confrontation with one of the judges that left me believing I had been eliminated from the running. My data showed that unlike humans, who for the most part reach maximum growth by the end of their teen years, the fish I was studying seemed to keep growing. The age/growth curve didn't curve the way that it did with humans and most other living things.

One of the judges gave me a terrible time about this. He said living creatures follow typical biological age/growth curves, but my curves were quite inconsistent with what we knew. He actually reprimanded me, but I showed him how my technique had been validated and that my curves reflected the actual data based on the study of a large—not a small—sample of fish. He left, grousing.

For years that encounter bothered me. Some fifteen years later, after having become a gerontologist, I learned that extraordinary data from research on aging revealed that various fish not only keep growing, they don't even age. The judge had reprimanded me for a controversial presentation that was "inconsistent with what we knew." I find it so ironic since science is based on confronting what we don't know. I am deeply satisfied that findings from aging research are building upon that tradition of exploration and openness to new ideas and information. At least the judge must have respected that I was being true to my data, given the positive outcome for me at the fair.

When I joined NIH in the early 1970s, less than $50 million a year was going into federally supported research on aging. When I left NIH in 1994, that number had passed well beyond $500 million. My bold prediction that aging would become a hot field of interest for the 1980s basically rang true—it was definitely one of the most exciting and rapidly growing research areas of that decade, a golden era for studies on aging.

I feel now that the field of aging is at a new juncture. Much of the important research that was supported during my twenty-year career at NIH focused on distinguishing normal aging changes from deficits that reflected the impact of disease and disability in later life. The guiding questions were "What is aging?" and "What are the disorders that occur in association with aging?" In the past, many views of aging were influenced by those who were ill rather than those who were healthy, a discrepancy that made this research even more important. Then, as understanding of later life disorders progressed, considerable research focused on their treatment. It was only in the late 1980s and 1990s that studies on normal or healthy aging were mounted.

The new juncture we have reached is one in which we move beyond studies of *what aging is* to *what is possible with aging*. We have moved from a time not that long ago when aging was seen as synonymous with senility, to one in which a glimpse of human potential has opened up for cultural consideration. Finally, we are ready to talk about what is possible, not despite aging, but *because* of it. There is no denying the problems that accompany aging. But what has been universally denied is the potential. The ultimate expression of that potential is creativity. Creativity has always been there with aging, but many have not recognized or searched for it in themselves in later life because society has so denied, trivialized, or maligned it with advancing years.

The importance of understanding creativity in relation to aging is profound, because doing so will not only enable older people to have access to their potential in later life, but it will also challenge younger age groups to think about what is possible in their later years in a different way. If potential in later life is denied, then we do not plan or prepare for it. With awareness of it, our sense of opportunity, challenge, and responsibility to ourselves is altered in a positive way.

We already see this change in relation to physical exercise. As we have begun to notice people who are aging well physically, we have grown more interested in physical fitness as younger adults. In the past, when we were more influenced by negative stereotypes of aging, we focused on the disease and disability of older adults. This contributed to our negative views of aging and a denial of it. In denying aging, people didn't prepare for it. But with the changing image of what is possible as we age, we have a growing sense that we can and should do something to help make that possibility even more likely. Today we recognize the benefit of exercise at all ages for long-term health gains.

In the same way, now that we recognize that preventive health strategies can help keep us healthier longer and make us more resilient in the face of illness, we seek those options and find a growing array of choices in the marketplace. Now that we see how attention to emotional distress can save lives and lead to more productive and satisfying years of life, counseling and other forms of therapy are becoming increasingly common choices for families and individuals.

I believe we are on the cusp of a similar phenomenon relating to human potential in later life. Focus on the baby boomers for a moment. There are approximately 75 million boomers in the United States who were born between 1946 and 1964. Most social observers emphasize the boomers' potential influence in terms of their numbers, their potential political impact, and at times their sense of entitlement.

But I feel there is a larger psychological issue at work here. The boomers are the first major population to grow up with positive images of aging. Many of their parents have aged well physically, mentally, socially, and financially. They are the first major population group that has looked beyond stereotypes to glimpse what is possible in later life. Much of this point of view is unconscious, but it is real and it is powerful.

They are not denying the existence of old age; instead, they are experiencing a new awareness of what can and should be in later life. If it can be good, people are more motivated to give it every chance to be so. Again, this awareness fundamentally affects our sense of personal opportunity and empowerment. But the boomers aren't going to just want later life to be okay; like the rest of their experiences, they are going to want it to be special. More and more older adult models out there are showing it can be just that—particularly in relation to the expression of human potential.

We live in a creative age. The focus on creativity and the use of the term is entering more and more spheres of our lives. We are told we need to be creative in problem solving, in urban planning, in social policy, in our relationships, in marriage, with childcare, at our work, with our finances, in recreation, with our backyard, and so forth. But the full scope of our creative potential from a life cycle perspective has been minimally appreciated. What gerontology is increasingly showing us is that later life can be an especially creative age.

Moreover, studies of aging are showing that the potential for creative expression in the second half of life is not the exception but the rule. It is remarkably universal in possibility. Creativity is not just for geniuses and it is not found just among the young. In this book, I will share with you the view from the fascinating intersection of aging and creativity that exists in everyday life.

The old negative views of aging stifled individual motivation and short-circuited social policy deliberations that could improve individual and societal access to what is possible with advancing years. We need to peel away all the negative stereotypes that have erected so many obstacles to seeing what we are truly capable of accomplishing in the second half of our lives.

This book, based on my approximately thirty years of research on the problems and potential associated with aging, aims to do just that. Here I will present facts and findings of our remarkable capacity that has previously been trivialized, distorted, or denied as we age. President John F. Kennedy once said, "The great enemy of truth is very often not the lies—deliberate, contrived and dishonest—but the myth—persistent, persuasive and unrealistic."

I want to put the misconceptions to rest, and to help people in the second half of life awaken the partnered powers of age and creativity to find a new sense of possibility.

1

The Flames of Creativity

You see things: and say "Why?"

But I dream things that never were: and say "Why not?"

—GEORGE BERNARD SHAW, *BACK TO METHUSELAH*

THE HUMAN SPIRIT OF creativity is indomitable. It has uplifted lives in every civilization and every era, from dirt play-grounds to marble palaces. It has survived catastrophic acts of inhumanity, ignorance, and apathy, to bloom in the darkest days as well as the brightest hours of human existence. It has illuminated our lives with flashes of singular brilliance in advances in human understanding and in the softer, warmer light of words or deeds that daily enrich the human experience.

"The greatest discovery of my generation is that a human being can change his life by changing his attitude of mind."

—WILLIAM JAMES

Each one of us is endowed with the spirit of creativity, whether we recognize it or not. We see it easily in the young child who turns a bed into a sailing ship and pillows into fortresses. We readily admire it in the brilliant pianist or determined inventor. We celebrate it in the ingenious efforts of survival by those caught in the path of nature's fury or the storms of war and other human cruelty. But we tend to overlook the same creative energy when, transformed by age and experience, it leads a retired chemist to become an education activist, or prompts a once travel-shy homemaker to take her first vacation abroad. Creative potential is there in all of us, an inner resource, renewable and vibrant, no matter how much or how little it is used. This creative spirit has the power to change our lives at every age, and to do so in quite different ways as we get older.

Playwright George Bernard Shaw believed in lifelong creativity. He espoused this belief in his writing, reflected in the chapter's opening quote, and he practiced it throughout his lifetime. Despite adversity in the earlier days of his writing career, Shaw persevered. He wrote *Back to Methuselah* when he was sixty-six, and was awarded the Nobel Prize in Literature in 1925, at the age of sixty-nine. He continued to write for more than two decades and was at work on a comedy when he died at age ninety-four.

Shaw's contribution to literature is of historic measure, and not only for the pleasure of scholars. Like so many products of the creative spirit, his ideas found new expression in the lives of others. Years after the playwright died, when Sen. Robert Kennedy repeated Shaw's urging to "dream things that never were: and say, 'Why not?' " it was to inspire a new generation of creative social and political action that would, itself, earn a prominent place in history.

"If you have built castles in the air, your work need not be lost; that is where they should be. Now put the foundations under them."

—HENRY DAVID THOREAU

As we explore the powerful potential that creativity brings to us as we age, we can begin by posing Shaw's question anew. Each of us, in our own life, needs to dream things that have not happened for us and ask: "Why not?" After all, modern science and medicine have strengthened the foundations of life as we age. Preliminary research and evidence from life around us makes clear that creativity is a catalyst for change of the best kind, with benefits that are immediate, long-lasting, and within the reach of every person. Even more interesting is that as we age, some key ingredients for creativity—life experience and the long view—are only enhanced. In studies of aging people and in my work with them, four aspects of creativity stand out:

1. *Creativity strengthens our morale in later life.* Creativity allows us to alter our experience of problems, and sometimes to transcend them, in later life. Part of the nature of creativity is its engaging and sustaining quality—no matter what our actual physical condition, we *feel better* when we are able to view our circumstances with fresh perspective and express ourselves with some creativity. Creativity makes us more emotionally resilient and better able to cope with life's adversity and losses. Just as exercise improves our muscle tone, when we are creatively engaged, our emotional tone is elevated.

"I do believe it is possible to create, even without ever writing a word or painting a picture, by simply molding one's inner life. And that too is a deed."

—ETTY HILLESUM

2. *Creativity contributes to physical health as we age.* Increasing numbers of preliminary findings from psychoneuroimmunological studies—research that examines the interaction of our emotions, our brain function, and our immune system—suggest that a positive outlook and a sense of well-being have a beneficial effect on the functioning of our immune system and our overall health. These findings are particularly strong among older persons.

Creative expression typically fosters feelings that can improve outlook and a sense of well-being. Just as chronic unrelieved stress has a detrimental effect on the immune system, continuing creativity, by promoting the expression of emotions, promotes an immune function boost.

3. *Creativity enriches relationships.* For young or middle-aged adults, knowing there is a potential for creativity in later life will improve their outlook and expectations of those years. Adult children with optimistic expectations of aging typically are more comfortable discussing issues of aging and other life passages with their parents. The effect is a boon for both generations: the younger adult learns firsthand about achieving a more satisfying aging experience, and the older adult remains engaged in the circle of relationship and emotional intimacy that strengthens connections to others and richness of life.

4. *Creativity is our greatest legacy.* To be creative in later life provides an invaluable model of what is possible as we age, for our chil-

Mother Teresa (1910–1997) was born in Albania, but later she became a citizen of India and an Indian nun. Until she died at age eighty-seven, she vigorously and incessantly worked to establish missions among the needy in several continents, providing compassionate aid to lepers, abandoned children, the elderly, the dying, and others in desperate need. At the age of sixty-nine she received the Nobel Peace Prize.

dren, grandchildren, great grandchildren, and society. As a role model in your family or in the lives of others, you can shape individual thinking and societal policies about aging. Historically, creativity has distinguished elders as "keepers" of the culture, those who pass the history and values of family and community on to the next generation.

Most of us will never win the Nobel Peace Prize or a Presidential election, but we can use creativity to shape our lives and, especially as we age, to unleash new potential for personal growth and self-expression. Before we can fully access our creative potential in aging, we need to clear away the internal and external obstacles to understanding and to individual self-expression. Those obstacles loom in the form of misconceptions about the nature of creativity, negative stereotypes, and falsehoods about aging, and how elements of our individual life experience color the lens through which we view ourselves and our lives.

Changing Our Perceptions: Creativity as an Equal Opportunity Attribute

When we talk about *creativity*, I'm not referring simply to the paint-on-canvas kind of artistic creativity, nor do I mean those visionary thinkers whose imaginative ideas and inventions have shaped or shaken civilizations. Creativity is built into our species, innate to every one of us, whether we are plumbers, professors, short-order cooks, or investment bankers. It is ours whether we are career-oriented or home-centered. It is the flame that heats the human spirit and kindles our desire for inner growth and self-expression. Our creativity may emerge in many different ways, from the realm of art, science, or politics, to the pursuit of an advanced college degree, a new hobby, or public-spirited community activism.

Carl Jung (1875–1961), the pioneering psychiatrist who advanced understanding of the "collective unconscious" and archetypes of man's basic psychological nature, completed his autobiography, Memories, Dreams, and Reflections, *the year he died at age eighty-six.*

Rollo May, in his book *The Courage to Create*, describes creativity as "the process of bringing something new into being"—creating an original idea, perspective, process, or product that has an impact. This idea includes a vast range of creative expression. Creativity and its effects may be a solo experience in which we develop a new attitude or facet of self-understanding, and by doing so, fundamentally alter the way we approach and experience life, relationships, and activities. Our creativity may also alter our thinking, our behavior, or our experience of our community or culture.

In general, discussions of creativity tend to focus more on attempting to explain its nature and origins than on elaborating its meaning to us. Even so, there is considerable cross-cultural recognition of its meaning. For example, Carl Jung, the Swiss psychoanalyst and one of the great psychological theorists of the twentieth century, viewed creativity as part of our unconscious life and rooted in what he called the "collective unconscious," or that part of everyone's inner psychological life that taps into universal human issues and themes.

Creativity in many parts of the Pacific is perceived in relation to *mana*, a word used in Melanesian and Polynesian languages to express special energy concentrated in objects or persons. The concept includes creative energy. Though viewed as having divine origins, creative energy derived from mana is also believed to be available to ordinary people, who can gain access to it through performing appropriate rituals or by studying and acquiring skills. Every individual is considered to have the potential for some form of creativity emanating from mana.

I offer these varied views of creativity not to quibble over definitions, but to illustrate that no matter how you define it, no matter what your gender, race, ethnic heritage, or spiritual view, creativity is universally recognized as a basic human attribute. Just as aging is a journey and not an end, creativity is a process or an outlook, not a product. It is a distinctly human quality that exists independent of age and time, reflecting a deeper dimension of energy capable of transforming our lives at any age.

However we define it, too many of us are blind to the power of creativity to transform our lives and enrich our relationships at work and at home. Even when we recognize the value of creativity, too often we remain blind to the presence and potential of creativity throughout our life span, no less at age eighty-five than at age five. Our vision is clouded most of all by stereotypes, misunderstanding, prejudice, and ignorance about aging, and then muddled more by the stereotype of creativity as belonging only to the artist's domain. But when the falsehoods and

Emily Greene Balch (1867–1961) was an American political scientist, sociologist, economist, social reformer, and pacifist. She was a leader of the women's movement for peace during World War I. She helped establish the Women's International League for Peace and Freedom in 1919 (age fifty-two, and was later its secretary-treasurer, 1934–35 (ages sixty-seven to sixty-eight). She continued promoting peace throughout her life, sharing the Nobel Peace Prize in 1946 (at age seventy-nine) with John Raleigh Mott (age eighty-one) and writing **Toward Human Unity** ***in 1952 (age eighty-five).***

stereotypes are stripped away, we see a remarkable and inspirational reality: Creativity is a powerful inner resource that is not only possible in later life, but common.

Creativity and Aging: Defying Myths and Misconceptions

Since aging is the backdrop for our exploration of creativity, it's important for us to understand how our beliefs and feelings about it shape the way we use creativity in our lives—or may fail to—especially as we age.

Nobody wants to think too much about growing older. If we view old age as a wasteland of "sleepless nights and unamusing days," as English clergyman Syndey Smith concluded in 1842, then surely we dread each year we travel toward that dismal end. Even if getting old "beats the alternative," as comedian George Burns quipped at ninety, aging still has a bad reputation, a grim connotation of mental and physical deterioration in a hopeless downhill slide through major illness and disability, indignities and loss, to death.

The idea that advancing age could offer exciting opportunities for personal growth and profound satisfaction seems foreign to most people. Even as we listen to news of scientific and medical advances that prolong life, we know that the extra time—the quantity of days—can be a burden or a blessing, depending on many things that seem out of our control. We want a promise of something more—quality time.

Sigmund Freud (1856–1939) published his well-known works **The Ego and the Id** *at age sixty-seven and* **The Future of an Illusion** *at age seventy-four.*

Sigmund Freud, considered the "father of psychoanalysis," noted that our most basic human emotional needs are met by work and love; and it is true that our measure of our lives' worth depends largely on the degree to which we can feel productive, loved, and loving as we age. This transcends matters of blood chemistry, heart rate, and bone density. It reflects not just how we feel but how we feel *about our life.* This elusive quality of life is certainly influenced by our physical circumstances but need not be defined or necessarily limited by them.

We hear a lot about "the effects of aging." It's ingrained in our language, from old sayings like "You can't teach an old dog new tricks" to references about an older person being "over the hill" or "in the autumn of life." Most often we hear age blamed for anything undesirable, from facial wrinkles to major clinical depression, from creaky joints to cranky attitudes. It was in the 1960s that we popularized the notion that "you can't trust anyone over thirty." The teenagers of that era, born in the post–World War II baby boom years of the late 1940s, are today's powerful population of middle-aged professionals and consumers. When boomers talk about "the fifties" today, the phrase is just as likely to refer to their age as it is to the nostalgia for yesteryear. By 2000 approximately thirty million men and women were nearing or entering their fifties (45–54), a midlife passage characterized by a desire for greater meaning in life, for new interests and experiences.

This is a particularly exciting prospect, because it marks the first generation with every reason to have high expectations of growing older. Advances in science, medicine, and preventive health are improving the prospects of aging, and all around us are individuals whose lives are models of vibrant living well into old age. Despite all the evidence, however, and despite the intellectual energy and activism apparent in the boomers and other younger adults, the specter of aging remains colored by the historic assumption that aging is defined by difficulty.

So let's talk about those "effects of aging." As a psychiatrist and geriatrician (a specialist in the health concerns of aging), a scientist, and a public policy activist on behalf of older Americans, I have worked with older patients and with colleagues in the field of aging and research for thirty years. I am immersed in the effects of aging, quite literally, and I see the wide range of the effects routinely overlooked in the public perception of older people.

I think of Madeleine Albright, who at age sixty became the first woman to head the State Department—or of Dr. C. Everett Koop, born in 1916, who served as one of the outstanding surgeon generals of the United States, from age sixty-five to age seventy-three, and continued into his eighties as an outstanding spokesperson for improved public health. In the media, I think of Barbara Walters, now in her sixties, easily the "First Lady" of television journalism. Johnny Carson, hosting the *Tonight Show* beyond the age of sixty-five, continued to demonstrate

Elizabeth Garrett Anderson (1836–1917), became the first woman to practice medicine as a physician in England in 1865 (at age twenty-nine). At the age of seventy-two (1908), she became the first woman to be elected a mayor (of Aldeburgh) in England.

legendary personality, wit, humor, charm, and sex appeal, and win a large and loyal following even as he stepped out of the spotlight to pursue a more private life. Maya Angelou, at sixty-five, was asked to compose and present her poem "The Rock Cries Out to Us Today" for President Clinton's 1993 inauguration.

History and literature offer us more remarkable stories that illustrate the potential for intellectual and emotional vitality with age. Sophocles, one of the great ancient Greek dramatists, wrote his noted play *Oedipus at Colonus* when he was ninety. The Russian lyric poet and novelist Boris Pasternak wrote his first novel—*Dr. Zhivago*—at the age of sixty-six. Susan B. Anthony, the famous social reformer and women's suffrage leader and pioneer, remained internationally active into her eighties, founding the International Woman Suffrage Alliance in Berlin at age eighty-four.

These highly visible individuals may be uniquely talented in the realm of their public endeavors, but they are not at all unique in the vitality they bring to life during their advancing years. I think of Darlene, who, following her divorce at age sixty and having to return to the workplace, chose to train as a masseuse, and at age seventy is so highly sought after that clients schedule appointments months in advance. Or Karl, who had never found time to pursue his interest in woodworking until he retired at age sixty-five from a management career and turned to cabinetmaking. In his seventies now, his cabinetry graces a growing number of new community buildings in his town.

Imogen Cunningham (1883–1976) was an accomplished American photographer, still teaching at the Art Institute of San Francisco in her nineties. A monograph of her work, **Imogen! Imogen Cunningham Photographs** *appeared in 1974 when she was ninety-one, and her final photographs were published the year after she died, at age ninety-three, in the book* **After Ninety**.

Charlotte, seventy-six, described herself as a "shrinking violet" in her youth; she never raised her hand in class, she was hardly visible at school dances, and at one point she was diagnosed as "socially phobic"—afraid of social interaction. Following retirement from secretarial work in her mid-sixties, she confronted her social fears and joined a community theater. It was "like having a fear of water, then diving in to get over it," she said. By her early seventies she was not only acting but singing publicly.

Robert, eighty-eight, retired from a career as a government lawyer when he was in his early seventies, and after a five-year stint with his own business, took up photography. Ten years later he had earned a new reputation as a documentary photographer and had produced an extensive international photo series spanning from Alaska to Tahiti, much to the delight of his retirement community, where he is frequently booked as a speaker for community education programs.

Finally, I am reminded of the transformative effect of the creative spirit in easing the tension of day-to-day living when, despite stressful circumstances, we respond with welcome humor, kindness, or enthusiasm. I see this in countless moments between office coworkers and people on the street, between parents and children, teachers and students, clerks and customers. I see it in myself when I'm in a hurry to get somewhere in my car and I hit every red light, or when someone is inconsiderate around me. I can be inflexible and angry, or I can take the setbacks in stride and not allow them to ruin my day.

Clearly then, dreams, desires, ambition, determination, wisdom, and compassion are also among the many effects of aging. There is no denying that health complications are a part of life for many older people, and that the risk of chronic disease or disabilities increases with age. But all around us, throughout history and today, there is evidence that the creative spirit can find expression despite obstacles, grief, and loss, and sometimes even more powerfully in the process.

"In the past few years, I have made a thrilling discovery . . . that until one is over sixty, one can never really learn the secret of living," said Ellen Glasgow, who won the Pulitzer Prize at age sixty-seven (*In This Our Life*). "One can then begin to live, not simply with the intense part of oneself, but with one's entire being."

At age sixty-seven (1959), Archibald Macleish won both the Pulitzer Prize for drama and the Antoinette Perry Award for the best play of the year. The play was* J.B.*, a verse play.

The secret of living with one's entire being to which Glasgow refers is the creative spirit that dwells in each of us. It is the creativity that empowers us, no matter what our demographic markers of gender, age, race, religion, income, or health status; and that enables us to participate in life as a journey of exploration, discovery, and self-expression. It can occur at any age and under any circumstances, but the richness of experience that age provides us magnifies the possibilities tremendously. The unique combination of creativity *and* life experience creates a dynamic dimension for inner growth with aging.

Everyone Has "The Right Stuff" for Creativity

Joan, forty-six, is discouraged about the aging process as she sees her seventy-two-year-old mother, Marie, grow more bitter and mean-spirited with each passing day. Her mother had always had a somewhat critical and inflexible personality, but since the death of Joan's father two years before, Marie has become increasingly intolerant, brazenly insulting her family, friends, and even strangers who have the bad luck to encounter her. Her insensitive, hurtful behavior has alienated everyone who knows her, and it has become the source of escalating tension between mother and daughter as well.

"Maybe creativity is an option for some people, but not my mother," says Joan. "I think that some people just don't have it. They don't respond well to the disappointments in life, and the longer they live, the more they have to be bitter and angry about. My mother is an angry woman—not about any one big thing, about *everything*—and she takes it out on everyone around her. She wasn't always this bad. Aging has changed her into this awful person."

John Bertram Phillips (1906–1982), the English bible translator, was the author of twelve best-sellers, including **The Wounded Healer** *in 1984, at age seventy-eight, which focused on his twenty-three-year battle against depression.*

Is Joan's mother without creative potential that could better her life? How about the other bitter, cranky old people you know, or those you encounter in checkout lines or waiting rooms? Are they, too, the "exceptions to the rule" of creativity as a lifelong inner resource? No, they are not exceptions. They do have creative capacity and the potential to use it in ways that would improve their lives. What they lack is access.

In fact, Marie is trapped in her tough shell of anger and bitterness. Her bitterness is not an effect of aging, however. It is a symptom of individual personality characteristics and emotional consequences that have become internal obstacles to creativity. The mounting bad feelings or "emotional baggage" between her and her family and friends, and her alienation from them and the increased physical isolation that accompanies it, have become external obstacles to creativity. She needs help.

This is no different from someone fifteen or twenty-seven or forty-three years old who might suffer from depression, anxiety disorders, or any other behavioral or medical condition that merits treatment. Mental illness at any age creates obstacles to creativity, and before people can begin to explore their creativity, they have to deal with the issues holding them back. For instance, 15 percent of older adults have clinically significant symptoms of depression—somewhat higher than young adults who have less physical illness, which is a risk factor for depression. The vast majority of them could find relief from depression, as sufferers at any age may, through appropriate diagnosis and treatment. Until they can manage the depression, it will restrict their ability to develop their potential and enjoy the benefits of more creative living. There are, of course, numerous examples of creativity on the part of those with mental illness—independent of age—but their creative accomplishments typically occur during periods when their symptoms are under control.

Whether it is depression, fear, anxiety, dependence, substance abuse, work pressures, or limiting relationships, until we recognize those obstacles and take steps to reduce their grip on our lives, they will continue to obscure our creative resources.

Even in the best of circumstances, creativity is an evolving process; it ebbs and flows, and moves us in different ways at different times. This is no different from many other of life's phenomena in the realms of work life, relationships, and emotions. We all have good years, bad years, and some years that are better than others—they're all part of being human. Creativity doesn't protect us from life, it helps us engage more fully in it and helps us develop the opportunities inherent in life's challenges.

There are other aspects of human nature and human behavior that contribute to underlying creativity; we are always influenced by personality, situation, and life experience. Our creativity is enhanced by certain qualities, including self-motivation; stick-to-it-iveness; resourcefulness; independence; curiosity; attraction to the unknown; a sense of challenge; tolerance of ambiguity; ability to "step outside the lines"; desire to seek something different, if not a new frontier; courage, the ability to imagine things that aren't; and the willingness to take risks, to dream, and to draw inspiration from within oneself.

> ***"Nothing will ever be attempted if all possible objections must be first overcome."***
>
> —SAMUEL JOHNSON

What is critical to keep in mind in this discussion is that none of these aspects are biologically "hard-wired" or off-limits to you by the nature of your genes. In other words, it's not a matter of whether you have or you don't have the "right stuff." The right stuff—those aspects of human nature and human behavior that can make a difference—become activated at different times and under differing circumstances. Until such circumstances or life events occur, you may not even know you had the capacity to mobilize them. This is one of the profound experiences and lessons of aging.

Why do I feel creativity can be stimulated in all of us? Why do I view aging as a unique opportunity for creativity and growth? Because I have seen it. Most of my work has focused on older patients, and I have been a helper and a witness to the creativity that is possible when we are able to unlock our inner and outer barriers to self-expression. I have seen creativity unfold in older persons from all walks of life, from cabinetmakers to cabinet members. They reveal time and time again that it is never too late, even in the face of obstacles, to enjoy a fuller experience of our human potential.

Eleanor Florence Rathbone (1872–1946), the English feminist and social reformer, made an extensive study of widows under the Poor Law in Great Britain and became the leading British advocate for family allowances in her 1940 work, **The Case for Family Allowance,** *written when she was sixty-eight.*

In a study I conducted in the mid-1980s, we examined the ways in which aging individuals met adversity and loss. The study included a group of women—age sixty-five and older—who were part of the generation whose job was the home, and although they were very resourceful in their homes, they had been relatively dependent on their husbands. When they became widows, as painful as it was, the amount of growth they experienced once on their own was staggering. These were everyday people. The nature of the situation was such that they hadn't had a chance—or taken the initiative—to develop their potential. These people did remarkable things in terms of moving in different directions; whether it was writing, volunteering, or becoming involved in the arts, the amount of change and diversity of direction they experienced was eye-opening. It really made a statement about the number of people who go through life letting their circumstances constrain them—men included—and it is inspiring to see how people can blossom in later life and in the face of psychological and social crisis.

Even as I write this book, so much of our attention as individuals and in public policy is focused on the problems of aging that we fail to realize that this limited view—no matter how well intended—interferes with our sense of possibilities and the ways in which our society could approach issues of aging. We need to put the misguided ideas about creativity and aging in their proper place to understand what is possible for each one of us, and for those we love who struggle to transform the challenges of aging into opportunities of a lifetime.

Myths at Work in Public Policy and Private Lives

How can myths and misconceptions about aging and creativity hold the power to shape our expectations with such pessimism? Our willingness to believe the worst about aging—to dwell on the downside and ignore the upside—is a reflection of human history and human nature. Up until right now, most people have dreaded aging because they saw it as a decline into disease and disability. They have tried to deny it and block it out of their minds, paint a pejorative picture of it, as with any group we don't want to be a part of. This is how misconceptions build and endure; this is how facts are distorted to become stereotypes that limit our view of others as well as ourselves. Given today's advances in medicine, technology, and lifestyle options, this is one minority group everybody should aspire to join!

To the extent that the nature, potential, and prevalence of creativity in later life are misunderstood, then research, practice, and policies addressing the needs and potential contributions of older adults will suffer.

To recognize the potential for creative expression independent of age is more likely to bring policy makers to the table not with a sense of skepticism—or worse, cynicism—about what is possible, but with a new sense of opportunity, challenge, and, one hopes, creativity. Again, there is no denying the magnitude of disease and disability associated with aging. But what is considerably underappreciated—even denied—is the opportunity for and frequency of creative growth and expression among aged individuals.

"It is not by muscle, speed, or physical dexterity that great things are achieved, but by reflection, force of character, and judgment; in these qualities old age is usually not only not poorer, but it is even richer."

—CICERO

To think about older adults primarily in terms of decline and disability, or to view them primarily as a national burden, is to overlook their value as a national resource of exceptional potential. When we discount that potential, or view age as an excuse to marginalize those older

Karl von Frisch (1886–1982), an Austrian zoologist, conducted a forty-year study of bees that led to the discovery that they communicate information through dancing. For example, a circling dance means food is within 75 meters; a wagging dance means the distance is longer. This and related research on insect and animal behavior led to his becoming co-recipient of the 1973 Nobel Prize for Physiology at the age of eighty-seven. When he was eighty-eight he wrote his classic work, Animal Architecture.

Antonio Stradivari, also known as Stradivarius (1644–1737), was the legendary violin maker. Estimates are that from age twenty-two up until the year he died at age ninety-three he made more than a thousand violins, violas, and cellos. His methods created the standard for all that followed, as he brought the art of violin

ones among us, we sidestep the challenge and responsibility to support this growth in skills and adaptability in later life. We also ignore the inevitable, that we, too, will grow older. We need to look beyond dismissive stereotypes of the elderly and recognize among us the many inspiring models of older age. We need to learn from them and develop skills of our own for maintaining a satisfying quality of life as we grow older.

Our government leadership offers an excellent example of the power of antiaging fabrications to obscure the truth and distort present-day judgment in harmful ways. How could it be that we have so many older, accomplished members of Congress, in both the House of Representatives and the Senate, who can espouse such unenlightened views of aging? The answer is that these people grew up with negative views of aging. They've denied and disparaged it and are unable to look at it. For them, the negative images endure, unfettered by the reality that older people have decades of potential still available for personal growth and social contribution.

I see this attitude often in the resistance I encounter as an advocate for programs serving older Americans. In one memorable meeting, in my role as acting director of the National Institute on Aging, I was defending the budget request for research studies of aging and diseases of later life. One Congressman was critical of spending money on such studies because he felt it represented an inequitable distribution of dollars for the elderly and the treatment of their health problems. He suggested that we might be better served by adopting a "historical" perspective, which would put greater resources into health care for the young and allow "nature to take its course" in matters of health among the aging. This, he said, would "reestablish the equity" of funding in favor of the younger population.

His suggestion reflected an assumption of a culturally approved policy of benign neglect—the belief that at a certain age it is appropriate for old people to do society a favor and disappear from the landscape, go quietly off to the tundra and be done with. Two destructive ideas were at the heart of his thinking: one was that older people didn't have much to contribute; the other was that earlier societies knew something that we were forgetting, which is that benign neglect of the aging was a tradition as old as humankind itself.

History does, in fact, deserve a place in our discussion of aging, but not as a justification for a policy of benign neglect. In fact, when we examine history closely it offers dramatic evidence of historical traditions of health support for the aging and of cutting-edge advances that point to vast new potential for old age.

If we want to look to past human societies for inspiration, let's consider the Neanderthals, a name that is routinely used to mean brutish or stupid. The Neanderthals were an early form of Homo sapiens that inhabited much of Europe and the Mediterranean during the late Pleistocene, about 100,000 to 30,000 years ago. Neanderthal remains have also been found in the Middle East, North Africa, and western Central Asia. In the study of fossil bones of Neanderthals, scientists have found evidence of osteoarthritis, a disease of advanced age, characterized by bone deterioration and fractures. Some of the bones show no fractures and others show healed osteoarthritic fractures.

This tells us, first, that a significant number of people in the Neanderthal culture achieved old age, and then, that if they had fractures that were healed it is because the injuries weren't ignored, but rather the people received help. If these primitive humans not only rejected the idea of benign neglect but clearly offered concern and care for their older, afflicted members, what should the most affluent and enlightened civilization do with the resources available to enhance older age today?

Returning to the question of dollar equity—that is, how much we spend on whom—to satisfy critics we would need to reestablish an equity of illness distribution, in which dollar distribution would follow illness distribution, which would entail returning to the days when children died of diseases we rarely see anymore and adults typically died in what we now consider middle age.

Today, as in no other time in history, we are witnessing dramatic advances in health, nutrition, and medical care throughout all age groups. Life expectancy didn't pass fifty years until the turn of the twentieth century. Today, as we begin the twenty-first century, life expectancy has passed seventy-five years. That's a *50 percent increase* we've hardly begun to recognize, accept, or understand in a meaningful way. Even so, it is clear that the last thing we'd want to do is reestablish

making to its highest level—what is broadly regarded as perfection. Two of his most famous violins—the "Habeneck" and the "Muntz"—were made when he was ninety-two.

***Mary Leaky (1913–1996), the noted archaeologist, made a number of significant finds of prehuman fossils in Africa, discoveries that helped to support theories that the human species evolved on that continent. At sixty-five she found her most important discovery, hominid footprints preserved in volcanic ash, approximately 3.5 million years old. This find provided evidence that hominids walked in an upright position at a much earlier date than previously believed. At age seventy-one (1984) she published her autobiography,* Disclosing the Past.**

equity of illness distribution. As we come to terms with the impact made by these advances in health and medicine, we must use this new reality to enlighten our ideas about aging.

Creativity: Different Styles

Ernst Alexanderson (1878–1975) was awarded his 321st patent in 1955, when he was seventy-seven, for the color television receiver he developed for RCA.

Thomas Edison took out more than one thousand patents during his career, continuing to invent throughout his life. When he was sixty-five (1912), he produced the first talking motion pictures. During World War I, when he was in his seventies, he headed the Naval Consulting Board and directed research in torpedo mechanisms and antisubmarine devices. He devoted his eighties to efforts to develop from domestic weeds a substance that would resemble rubber.

When we think about creativity as a life force, we often think first of renowned artists, leaders, scientists, or inventors whose works powerfully illustrate creativity as "the process of bringing something new into being," as suggested by author Rollo May. But where does that leave those who live lives of less spectacular achievement, lives of more ordinary interests and activities?

In order to have a better grasp of creativity, we must first understand a simple truth: Creativity is not just for geniuses. You don't have to be born with inherited talent or raised in a special environment to be creative. Silvano Arieti, a renowned psychiatric researcher and author of *Creativity: The Magic Synthesis,* celebrated the importance of what he called "ordinary creativity" that is satisfying and often may eliminate a sense of frustration.

John Cunningham McLennan (1867–1945), the Canadian physicist, succeeded in liquefying helium in 1932, when he was sixty-five.

In a similar vein, Harvard Prof. Howard Gardner, a noted expert on human development, distinguished two types of creativity: Creativity with a "big C" and creativity with a "little c." Creativity with a "big C" applies to the extraordinary accomplishments of unusual people, for example, Albert Einstein's theory of relativity or Georges Braque's Cubist paintings. These forms of creativity not only changed entire fields of thought—in these cases, physics and art—but also influenced other fields of thought and, in some ways, world history.

Creativity with a "little c" is grounded in the various and sundry realities of life. "Every person has certain areas in which he or she has a special interest," Gardner explains. "It could be something they do at work—the way they write memos or their craftsmanship at a factory—or the way they teach a lesson or sell something. After working at it for a while they can get to be pretty good—as good as anybody whom they know in their immediate world." For example, the man from whom I bought my first house began during his retirement to plant and sculpt the backyard garden, creating a beautifully landscaped three-level visual experience, which in his late eighties was photographed for a national magazine featuring houses and gardens.

"The aspects of things that are most important for us are hidden because of their simplicity and familiarity."
—LUDWIG WITTGENSTEIN

Creativity with a "little c" also applies to individuals who set small challenges for themselves, like making a meal a little differently or approaching a problem at work from a new perspective. While these examples would not seem on the level of significance as Einstein's theory of relativity, creativity with a "little c" is no less important in the way we develop our individual potential for highly successful creative lives in our own realms.

My own view of creativity, drawn from my years of research and other work and life experience, is that there is *public* creativity and *personal,* or more private, creativity.

Public creativity represents creative acts that are recognized and celebrated as such by your own community, culture or beyond. We often think of public creativity along the "big C" lines, something widely recognized that is the product of a famous person. Indeed, public creativity can be as obvious as a major sculpture or a cure for a disease. But public creativity also includes something as close to home as a wall mural in your community, or a bulletin board display you might create as a volunteer in the school down the street.

At age eighty-six (1963), sculptor Meta Warrick Fuller created her noted work* The Crucifixion *with the head of Christ raised, honoring the memory of the four young African-American girls killed in the church bombing in Birmingham, Alabama, earlier that year.

Personal creativity depicts something new, perhaps a product or idea, or simply a fresh perspective; something that you have brought into being that has enhanced your life and given you satisfaction. It simply hasn't reached a level of public awareness or impact, and it may never do so. You may not have even intended for it to matter to anyone but you or those close to you.

For instance, through your imagination and inventiveness you may have created a new recipe, a new floral arrangement, a poem you can send via E-mail to your daughter or granddaughter, a new trick you taught your old dog, or a new exercise regimen. These are examples of personal creativity.

Comparing public and personal creativity, your result may seem quite different, but the value of the underlying creative process, the emotional experience of creative expression, is the same. Both dimensions of creativity are valuable and both continue robustly throughout the human life cycle, independent of age.

Personal Creativity and Aging in Action

Arlene Jacobson, seventy-five and widowed, was a participant in a longitudinal study of older persons that I conducted in the early 1980s, which focused in part on the study of change and new strategies in late life. Arlene had enjoyed a long, fulfilling marriage of more than fifty years. She spoke with pride of her life as a wife, mother, and homemaker for her husband and their three children. Upon her husband's retirement, Arlene and her husband enjoyed a new life of leisure until her husband's sudden death three years later. The loss of her husband had been very difficult for Arlene, and she confronted a host of new challenges that forced her to rely on herself. To mitigate these challenges, she moved to a retirement community that provided a wide range of support services.

Arlene had never gone on a major trip without her husband, but one of the new friends she met at the retirement community urged her to come along on a trip to Rome. After much deliberation and procrastination, Arlene finally agreed to go.

Not long after arriving in Italy, which she thoroughly enjoyed, in a routine call back home she learned that a longtime friend had just died. Arlene wanted to return home to attend the funeral. The problem was that it was August. In Italy, the entire country, all of Europe, and much of the rest of the world were on vacation, and there were no empty seats on flights that would get her back home to the United States in time for the funeral. Her only chance was to go to the airport in Rome, wait in the standby line and hope for a seat on the next flight to New York.

Sir George Cayley, an engineer and pioneer of aviation, at the age of eighty-two, constructed the first successful man-carrying glider in 1853.

Unfortunately, she arrived at the airport later than she had planned, and that day the line was very long for the last flight to the States. She patiently waited, but the line moved very slowly, and at some point she realized that she would never get her turn at the counter in time for the flight. An unusual thought entered her mind: The only chance she would have for getting a ticket was to cut in line. She had never in her whole life cut in line. But time was passing quickly. The line still moved slowly. Retelling the story months later, Arlene recalled her heart pounding and sweat forming as the intensity of the situation and her anxiety mounted. Under the heightening pressure, she thought "now or never," and she did this thing she had never done before: she broke rank and stepped ahead in line. People started yelling at her, but her inability to understand Italian spared her the angry details. She stood the pressure, and with an elevated and forceful voice explained her emergency to the ticket attendant. She got her ticket, made the flight, and arrived in time for the funeral.

Michelangelo (1475–1564) at age seventy-two was appointed architect of St. Peters in Rome—the cathedral of the Popes; he devoted himself to his work until his death at age eighty-eight, and during this time designed the dome of St. Peters.

Though totally exhausting for Arlene at one level, the experience proved emotionally exhilarating at another. She discovered a latent part of herself that she did not know existed—a hidden, assertive, brave inner self. The experience triggered the start of a changing self-image for Arlene and provided the jump-start for her to be more active in seeking out interesting new experiences and relationships. It was a creative turning point for her, a creative new strategy that started unleashing much of her untapped potential. It was personal creativity—creativity with a "little c"—but the change in Arlene's self-image and her approach to life loomed monumental.

She reflected with a sense of awe that in the past she had never seemed to have personal goals; her goals had always been in the service of her family, her marriage, her children, her grandchildren, her friends, and even the unexpected but needy stranger, but never specifically for herself. After the airport episode this began to change, as she began to experiment with mostly new interests.

Gertrude Jekyll (1843–1932), the English landcape architect, was the most successful advocate of the natural garden. Her books* Colour in the Flower Garden *and* Garden Ornament *were both published in 1918, when she was seventy-five.

She started gardening, then added volunteer work at the National Gallery of Art, and returned to playing bridge one night a week, more frequently than when she had played with her husband. She then joined a monthly dinner club, followed by a monthly book club, followed by a monthly theater club. She got the travel bug, no longer intimidated by the unknown; she lined up three trips for the next eighteen months. Moreover, while she took on new interests, she maintained most of the others as well. As she told her story, she confessed that her latest interest was a desire to learn how to fly a helicopter, though she thought she probably would take up hiking instead.

Arlene's story also illustrates that the obstacle to change is not aging, but emotional issues and life experiences that over time have colluded to set up barriers to trying or even thinking about something new. In fact, as we will see in Chapter 3, aging often enables us or gives us permission to attempt something different. Change, though, does not occur by itself. Initially, it is often accompanied by anxiety. But the process can be liberating, setting us on a new path like that of Arlene.

Intelligence and Creativity

"Change is always powerful. Let your hook be always cast. In the pool where you least expect it, will be a fish."

—OVID (43 B.C.–17 A.D.)

Even if we distinguish between the public and private forms of creativity, there are other ways to think about creativity, other domains for it, other ways to identify our own inner sources of unique self-expression. The graceful movements of Michael Jordan, the stirring dream and language of Martin Luther King Jr., the mathematical wizardry of physicist Richard Feinman, or the humanitarian and compassionate skills of Mother Teresa—all account for forms of creativity that lie outside the boundaries of the performing and fine arts. If creativity isn't based in the arts, then where does it come from? With what inner voice does our creativity speak?

The answer is that creativity speaks from our emotional landscape and through our particular style of "intelligence" or brain function. If you think about the people you know, and the different ways they approach a vacation or a problem or a crowded room, you'll probably see a variety of different intelligence styles at work. One will plan a vacation meticulously, right down to the number of pencils to pack along, while another picks a destination more on impulse than by plan. One needs a quiet place to work through a problem, another prefers the stimulation of routine background noise. One is anxious entering a room full of strangers, another is eager to meet new people and make new friends.

Howard Gardner, the expert on human development, gave us the theory of "multiple intelligences," which describes how our individual characteristic "strengths" and "weaknesses" are a reflection of our brain function and the ease with which we manage certain kinds of learning and mastery. According to Gardner's theory, independent of how "smart" we are by school-style standards, there are seven styles of intelligence that shape our learning and self-expression. Defined and paired by the kind of brain activity each requires, they are linear and spatial intelligence, evident in analytical thinking; emotional and social intelligence, evident in ease of understanding and relating to other people; body and movement intelligence, evident in sports and dance; and intuitive intelligence, characterized by clear and insightful thought or vision.

Mother Teresa's gifts as a humanitarian are a beautiful example of emotional and social intelligence used as a wellspring of creative vision that shaped her global work on behalf of the poor.

It is reasonable to believe we all have varying levels of each kind of intelligence, and that they evolve with life experience and inner growth. Intelligence is not the same as creativity, because you can be intelligent without bringing something new into being. But creativity can build upon intelligence. That is why each of us, depending upon our inner resources and external influences, has the capacity for unique creative discovery and self-expression.

Emotional intelligence, a concept first introduced by psychologists Peter Salovey at Yale University and John Moyer at the University of New Hampshire, and later popularized by Daniel Goleman in his best-selling book, *Emotional Intelligence,* is especially important to our understanding of creativity because it contributes to what I refer to as *social creativity*.

Social creativity is a form of creative expression that has been especially strong among older members of society throughout the history of civilization. Prior to the technological age, older adults were the keepers of knowledge, the key to transmitting knowledge to younger members of society.

Now, as we have become deluged with data, older adults, through

Albert Schweitzer (1875–1965), known for his remarkable work as a missionary in Africa, for which he received the Nobel Peace Prize in 1952 when he was seventy-seven, was also a theologian, musician, and philosopher who lived to be ninety. He published his work* The Mysticism of Paul the Apostle, *gave recitals, made recordings of his music throughout Europe, and edited a number of Bach's works. He initiated an autobiography,* My Life and Thought, *in 1931, when he was fifty-six, adding a significant postscript in 1949, when he was seventy-four.

their wisdom, help us determine what matters and what doesn't. It is not surprising that so many diplomats and Supreme Court justices are older persons; life experience and developmental gains have enabled them to build social creativity. It is also not surprising that many unique aspects of our cultures, such as indigenous foods, crafts, trade, song, or dance, are passed down from an older generation to a younger one. One of the most important creative roles of older persons is as *keepers of the culture.*

Social Creativity with a Big *C* and with a Little *c*

Indeed, social creativity in older adults is reflected along the entire continuum from creativity with a big *C* to creativity with a little *c*. Let's look at an example of each:

An important dynamic of creativity that comes with age is courage—courage that gives permission to make a decision that may be risky, controversial, and necessary. It is courage reflective of George Bernard Shaw's poetry in later life. "I dream things that never were: and say 'Why not?' " It is courage prompted by an age-related perspective and pressure that, in effect, says, "If not now, when?" A good contemporary example of this was in the 1993 back-door negotiations begun by Israeli Prime Minister Yitzhak Rabin (age seventy-one) and Israeli Foreign Minister Shimon Peres (age seventy) with Palestine Liberation Organization Chairman Yasser Arafat (age sixty-four). These negotiations were notable for a number of reasons. Arafat and Rabin grew up as enemies, and Rabin and Peres had once led offensives against Israel's neighbors, while Arafat's PLO has been Israel's enemy for decades.

American general and statesman George C. Marshall became Secretary of State at the age of sixty-seven (1947), and for the next two years he developed the enormously successful Marshall Plan for the reconstruction of Europe. For this remarkable effort, he was awarded the Nobel Peace Prize at the age of seventy-three.

Despite these initial obstacles, as well as the opposition of many Israelis and Palestinians to a peace settlement, Peres, Rabin, and Arafat pursued these negotiations. They led to the historic and extraordinary Israel/PLO Peace Accord later that year. The next year all three of these courageous, aging leaders received the Nobel Prize "for their efforts to create peace in the Middle East." The prize was also intended "to honor a political act which called for great courage on both sides." The agreement was an extraordinary achievement in global politics, and a recent example of social creativity with a big C.

Yet courage and risk do not have to be on the level of a historic peace accord. They can occur at a more personal, familial level. A friend of mine is the cousin of two brothers who had not spoken to each other in more than twenty years because of a feud that nobody seemed to understand. All three men were now in their late sixties. Their extended family was quite close-knit and deeply pained by the distance between the brothers.

The relationship finally changed when one of the uncles in the family died. The cousin arranged for both brothers to give tributes to their beloved uncle. The brothers did not know that they would be speaking one after the other, and as one left the altar and the other approached, the cousin with utmost grace placed the hand of one brother into that of the other. After a dramatic pause, caught up in the emotions of the circumstances, the brothers embraced. While the cousin's actions were a form of social creativity in a personal—or little c realm—it was, for all involved, a truly important development.

I remember my own encounter with social and personal creativity from a time in my life before I could even spell *creativity*. It was a small moment, but one that etched itself in my mind and today reminds me of the power such small moments have to shape lives.

Grandma Higginson, as everyone called her, was the mother of the principal of the nursery school I attended. Every afternoon at nursery school, all of the children in my four-year-old age group were supposed to take a nap. But one afternoon I was not sleepy, and I asked Grandma Higginson, who was supervising class that day, if I could skip the nap. I'm sure, in retrospect, I put her on the spot, because in other situations at other times children always were out to buck the system.

But Grandma Higginson came up with a clever solution: She whispered that I should lie down with the other children and then, after all of my classmates fell asleep, get up and play quietly at the other end of the room. I'm sure she thought that once my eyes closed, they would stay shut in slumber. But a few minutes after all of my classmates lowered their heads on the mats, I rubbed my eyes, raised my hand, and silently motioned for Grandma Higginson to keep her part of the bargain.

The principal, a stern authoritarian, had returned, however, and was quite upset about this deal her mother had struck with me. She and

Maria Ann Smith (1801–1870), during her sixties, was experimenting in Australia with a hardy French crabapple seedling from which developed the late-ripening Granny Smith apple, which because of its outstanding taste and keeping qualities formed the bulk of Australia's apple exports for many years.

her mother got into a heated argument. They bickered back and forth for several minutes, but in the end, Grandma Higginson was allowed to keep her word and let me play in a quiet section of the room.

I realize now that Grandma Higginson had found a creative way to solve the problem of a little boy who wasn't sleepy at nap time. She was able to look at the situation from a different perspective, while her implacable daughter had only one viewpoint. The memory has stayed with me all these years, and the experience of Grandma Higginson's problem-solving style stands as a good model of creative thinking that can bring change to a system needing it. This is the way creativity empowers us to bring about change in our lives and those around us as we age.

Collaborative Creativity: When Two Heads Are Better

Oscar Hammerstein II was sixty-five when he wrote the lyrics to accompany Richard Rodgers' music for* The Sound of Music *in 1959.

Just as we often mistakenly assume that creativity is for artists only, we also tend to view creativity as a solo act, a highly individualistic demonstration of self-expression. But creativity is more than that. In fact, certain creative endeavors cannot be accomplished without equal collaboration by partners. Examples abound around us. If you have ever been part of a musical ensemble or chorus, a sports team or hiking group, a successful problem-solving team in your workplace, a quilting group or a volunteer effort to help others in need, then you have experienced collaborative creativity.

Of course, the Manhattan Project is a paradigm for the ultimate example of collaborative creativity where the efforts of many talented scientists working together were essential in accomplishing a major scientific goal, on time and in time, to help end World War II.

The Evanston Quilt Project is a wonderful example of collaborative creativity. More than twenty older African-American residents of a Cincinnati public housing community participated in transposing a photo essay of their treasured moments onto a quilt they created by hand. They selected the fabric, and after the images were applied using computer technology, they sewed the quilt together. The product was both a work of art and a documentary of many aspects of African-American life in that community—a true contribution from keepers of the culture.

It doesn't stop there.

You don't have to be a rocket scientist, a team player, or community volunteer to experience the unique satisfaction of collaborative creativity. Do you have a friend? A spouse? A family? The potential for collaborative creativity is infinite in marriage, family, and other relationships. It is also essential if you want your relationship or family to offer a nurturing environment for emotional intimacy, personal discovery, and creative self-expression.

Sigmund Freud and Albert Einstein collaborated to publish* Why War? *in 1933; Freud was seventy-seven, Einstein was fifty-four.

Relationships are, by their very nature, collaborative enterprises. Because they establish both the external setting and the inner emotional context for our lives, relationships have a tremendous impact on our personal creativity, nurturing it or inhibiting it. By the same token, our personal creativity can have a powerful effect on our relationships, making them engaging and vibrant, or triggering tension when the creative energy is not shared, or when it threatens the stability of the relationship (see Chapter 5).

Intergenerational Collaborative Creativity: The Best of Both Worlds

As we age, enormous potential lies in collaborative endeavors, especially of an *intergenerational* nature that brings the energy, experience, and vision of different ages together for problem solving or pure enjoyment. At one level, intergenerational relationships are appealing simply because they bring interesting experiences of sharing time with somebody of a different age, the way a grandparent and a grandchild so often thoroughly enjoy each other's company. And being a different age sometimes means bringing a different perspective into a relationship, thereby enriching it intellectually and emotionally.

Different ages add to the diversity that feeds new possibilities in relationships. For example, several years ago I visited an interesting program in Baltimore called "Magic Me," among whose goals it was to link schoolchildren with nursing-home residents. I went to one of their nursing-home sites that had brought together junior high school students with behavior problems and a group of nursing-home residents in their eighties and nineties (and a few who had passed one hundred!). The children and the older individuals paired off into teams that together produced life histories in words or pictures, then talked about them in the larger group. The smiles on the faces of the nursing-home residents were infectious. And the behavior of the children was exemplary. The interaction clearly influenced the self-image and self-esteem of the young people, almost all of whom went on to improve both socially and scholastically after participating in the program.

Characterizing Creativity: A Dream and the Message of "Me"

"I have a dream that my four little children will one day live in a nation where they will not be judged by the color of their skin but by the content of their character."
—MARTIN LUTHER KING JR.

For many months I had been pondering how to make a cohesive characterization of creativity that took into account the multiple, varied, and interacting factors that influenced its expression. And this was after years of being immersed in the topic of creativity. Then one night I had a dream.

Earlier that day I had gone shopping with my young daughter Eliana. She wanted a new cereal, or at least a new cereal box. The cereal aisle in the grocery store held a dizzying array of choices, but after an exhaustive review of these colorful, cartoon-style attention getters we finally settled on an alphabet variety that looked particularly appealing in its picture, floating in a bowl of milk. That night, as I began to dream, Einstein's $E = mc^2$ equation floated by me, followed by a huge shallow bowl with cereal letters floating about. Suddenly, the dream went dark and the floating letters seemed to light up in brightness and swirl upward like a tornado into the night sky, where they spread out and twinkled like stars. In my dream I was captivated by the imagery and action and tried to see if I could detect a pattern in the sky—like the Big Dipper. I saw the moon. It was a crescent shape and pointed to the right, where I saw a cloud in the shape of an arrow. The cloud pointed to what looked like a bright star or a shining cereal letter in the sky forming the letter *m*. Then, cruelly, my alarm went off. I immediately wrote myself a note about the dream details, and studied the features, looking for meaning. After the months of effort to devise a way to describe creative energy in scientific terms, I wondered if the dream presented a clue, especially since it began with one of the most classic, dramatic, succinct, and elegant solutions ever—Einstein's $E = mc^2$ encapsulation of energy.

There is nothing like a dream to create the future.

—VICTOR HUGO

What particularly stood out to me were these imgaes:

- Einstein's formula
- the letters, in the form of both cereal and stars
- the moon
- the cloud in the shape of an arrow
- the letter *m*

I wrote down as much of the dream as I could before memory of it would start dissipating. I also wanted to diagram the final scene of the dream, since I felt that the sounding of the alarm prevented it from giving me more clarity. I drew the diagram below with my computer:

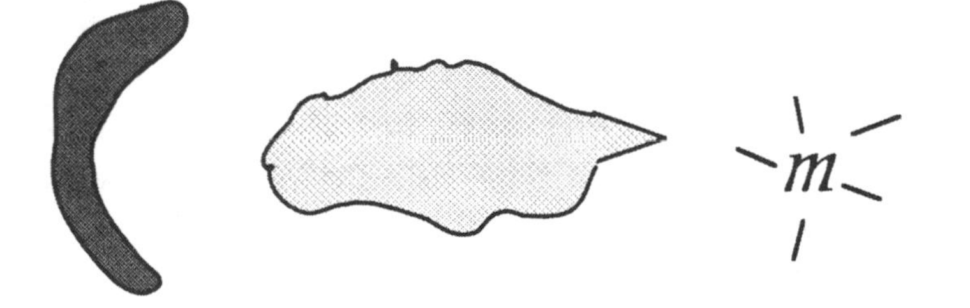

I studied and studied the diagram, moving it back and forth. Just as something at a distance becomes clear as you move closer, as I studied the images of the moon, the cloud, and the *m* star, a new image emerged. The crescent moon became a *c*. The arrow cloud became the mathematical symbol > signifying "greater than." The *m* remained unchanged.

$$c > m$$

Then it hit me again. I was looking at an equation—though one interrupted by the alarm clock. I rewrote it in the format of an equation.

$$c = m$$

Could it be, I wondered further, that the *c* represented *creativity* or creative expression? Reviewing again the elements of the dream, I was now particularly struck by the presence of Einstein's equation. Was it too much of a coincidence, or did the dream present a meaningful play on letters with Einstein's equation? If it did, perhaps the play on letters was incomplete owing to the alarm's short-circuiting the process. What would a complete play on letters look like? I added the remaining *e* and the ^{2} symbol for "squared" from Einstein's equation, and my dream equation took on a wonderful meaning.

Imagination is more important than knowledge.
—ALBERT EINSTEIN

$$C = me^2$$

My first reaction was a good laugh. In fact, the equation captured the everyday truth about creativity at a personal level: Creativity does equal "me" to a greater power. Could the equation offer anything more than humor to our understanding of creativity? I studied it more, elaborating on the meaning of each symbol and its relationship to the others:

- *C* refers to *creative* expression, which could include a creative accomplishment, product, idea, or understanding
- *m* refers to the *mass* of knowledge or experience you must accumulate before *mastering* a particular field, approach, or technique that leads to creative expression
- e^2 represents two dimensions:

1. The first dimension is that of *experience*, which includes external life experience—the accumulated experiences of daily life in the outside world—and internal life experience, which would include qualities of your inner life, such as the nature of your personality and style of your intelligence. Your internal life experience would further include your unique pattern of thinking, including how you look at, interpret, and interact with the outer world; aspects of your nature, such as curiosity and the ability to become motivated; intangible qualities of the human condition, including your capacity for intuition and insight and your ability to become inspired.

2. The second dimension is the *squaring* of the *e*—the way in which our external and internal lives interact to produce new insights and energy for self-expression.

In other words, creative expression (*c*) was to be found in the successful interaction between our mass of knowledge in a particular field or endeavor, our experience in both our outer and inner worlds, and the synergy that this produced. The equation described is a classic example of the whole being considerably more than the sum of its parts.

As we will see in Chapter 3, this understanding of the creative process helps explain why groups of individuals in different fields—mathematicians as opposed to philosophers, for example—may produce their peak creative accomplishments at different average ages. We will see that the underlying dynamics are not caused by age but by other factors relating to the nature of creative development.

My $C = me^2$ formula is meant to describe the nature of creativity—not serve as a prescription for making it happen. Certain pieces of the formula aren't in our power to do or change, while others are a reflection of patterns of choices made throughout our lives, patterns that we can change if we need or want to.

For instance, two major external influences are, first, the material to be mastered, and, second, experience from the outside world. Many of us do not have the time to spend developing an expertise to pursue a dream, at least not until later in life. You may not have been able to take that class on embroidery, woodworking, photography, or writing until your children were in high school or your professional work demanded less of your attention.

Experience from the outside world is a combination of opportunities and avoidance of too many obstacles. If you grow up in a house where people love to work with their hands, you see that work modeled and you learn the language of it, so to speak. It becomes part of your experience, perhaps to be expressed in your later tangible expressions of creativity. If you grow up in a musical household, that culture and language becomes part of you, perhaps to be expressed in the creativity of music. If you grow up in a household of social activists, your life experience may be reflected in how socially creative you become.

John Napier (1550–1617), the Scottish mathematician, described his famous invention of logarithms in* Mirifici Logarithmorum Canonis Description *in 1614 (at age sixty-four) and the calculating apparatus called "Napier's Bones" in* Rabdologiae *(1617), when he was sixty-seven; Napier's Bones is a mathematical device to aid in calculations that was the forerunner of the slide rule. At this time, too, Napier was making original contributions to the development of spherical trigonometry.

This helps explain why some people appear to be "more creative" than others or have an easier time gaining access to their creativity. Some people have had more opportunity and fewer obstacles in acquiring experience or expertise; some have had the good fortune of ample exposure to positive influences and opportunities.

But it is never too late to benefit from new opportunities and positive influences. We can more actively seek them out by taking special-interest classes or meeting new people who affirm our sense of self-worth. Retirement takes on a new and exciting sense of promise when you view it as time to explore and discover. We also can confront our inner obstacles to creativity—depression, anxiety, and fears—and seek help in overcoming them, from informal support or self-help groups to professional counseling, if necessary.

"How do I work? I grope."

—ALBERT EINSTEIN

When we look at all the elements and influences regarding creativity, what seems to matter the most are sufficient knowledge or mastery of an area; motivation and perspiration, or the willingness to *do;* some intangibles that are part of the human condition, such as intuition and insight; and the capacity to become inspired. The good news is that we can all master some area of knowledge; we can all get motivated; we can all get inspired; we can all muster courage to experiment with something new; we can all do something we want to do. Whatever life's variables, $C = me^2$ tells us that you cannot dismiss yourself as a candidate for creative potential. No matter what your age, and especially as you grow older, you do have the capacity for creative expression. The challenge is to recognize it and use it.

In a time when our lives are dictated by demanding schedules and expectations, when days are crammed with organized living, when our vision of ourselves and our future is darkened by distorted media images and cultural messages, then simply to remain open to the possibilities requires a kind of courage born of creativity. It is that inner voice that whispers: "Why not?"

2

Biology and Mystery: The Inside Story of Creativity and Aging

A living thing is distinguished from a dead thing by the multiplicity of changes at any moment taking place in it.

—HERBERT SPENCER, *PRINCIPLES OF BIOLOGY*

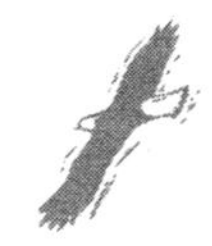

A NUMBER OF YEARS AGO, I was asked to visit an eighty-year-old blind woman who lived by herself in a tidy one-bedroom apartment. Ms. Thompson, I was warned, had quite a bite—an acid personality. A community social services agency had arranged for a homemaker to help with daily chores, but in the past three months, eight different homemakers had come and gone from the assignment. She managed to insult the social workers from the agency every time they went out to evaluate her need for a new homemaker, and I was left with the impression that Ms. Thompson had driven away the homemakers with similar verbal assaults.

I was no exception.

Almost immediately after I introduced myself, Ms. Thompson

At the age of seventy-five (1955), Helen Keller—blind, deaf, and mute since she was nineteen months old—published Teacher, *in honor of her miracle-worker teacher, Annie Sullivan.*

told me she had never met a psychiatrist who knew anything. She was enrolled in an education course on how to become a funeral parlor director and told me she was most looking forward to being the director of *my* funeral. She wasn't laughing when she said it.

Ms. Thompson continued to hurl insults my way as I continued my interview. I wanted to find out why so many homemakers had left their position with her. I needed to understand the source of her mercurial nature, because without a homemaker, Ms. Thompson was in jeopardy of losing her apartment. She would be forced into a nursing home or an assisted living facility.

Leonhard Euler (1707–1783), the Swiss mathematician considered one of the greatest mathematicians of the eighteenth century, was one of the founders of pure mathematics. Already blind in one eye, he lost the vision in his other eye, when he was around fifty-nine, becoming totally blind. One of the many remarkable feats he accomplished following his blindness was to carry out all the intricate calculations in his head for the improved theories of lunar motion when he was sixty-five. His prodigious memory that allowed him to cope with total blindness also enabled him to recite Virgil's Aeneid *in its entirety by heart.*

I knew before my visit that Ms. Thompson had recently suffered detached retinas in both eyes. Surgery was unable to halt the deterioration of her eyesight, so she was left with a sudden onset of blindness. It became clear that Ms. Thompson had always been a fiercely independent individual, but circumstances now forced her to be dependent on a lot of different people. This feeling of dependence, though it was certainly appropriate given her situation, made her anxious, which was the reason she typically resorted to insulting whoever was trying to help her, including me.

Ms. Thompson was a proud and accomplished woman. To her, the sudden blindness was a startling reminder of her mortality. Taking the class on funeral parlor procedures was one way she sought to control her anxiety about death. Keeping her own apartment was another.

When I learned that Ms. Thompson's career began as an information specialist in a large library system, I realized she was using this background in her relationships with the homemakers. She didn't want to be in the position of being helped, so instead, she insisted on "helping" the homemakers—helping them find other jobs, that is. Fighting unfamiliar feelings of dependence, she struggled to reverse roles by assisting these aides in researching career alternatives. During their visits, Ms. Thompson would grill the homemakers with questions about their career interests. Then she would get on the phone to locate the career training programs that most closely reflected their talents and skills. She encouraged, even pressured, each of them to pursue these career opportunities on her time. Her relentless needling either wore out the homemakers or resulted in their new career path.

During my interview, Ms. Thompson used a gentle but mocking tone to make her points, and we fell into a kind of bantering. When I mentioned, for example, that the dress she was wearing looked very nice, she reprimanded me about my lack of gentlemanly etiquette.

"You don't tell a woman her dress looks nice," she quipped, "You tell her *she* looks very nice in her dress!"

She clearly enjoyed this kind of banter, especially when she made a point that underscored her experience and wisdom as a woman, in contrast to mine as a man. As I reflected on Ms. Thompson's behavior and her situation, I realized that all of her previous homemakers had been women. How would she respond to a male? Would she try to find *him* a better job? I suspected not.

My hunch proved right. She preferred the company of men and she did not push her new male homemaker to find another job. He stayed for two years, and during that time she was able to work with me to reduce her anxiety and change her communication style. She came to feel more comfortable about accepting the help of homemakers in general, regardless of gender. She was able to keep her own apartment for another sixteen years, until at age ninety-six she felt it was time to move into an assisted living program.

Along the way, she came to terms with her blindness and dependencies, but she was also able to tap her energy for creative means. She pursued a challenging continuing education program for herself—this time not in funeral planning—and used the latest devices to aid the visually impaired. She sought out a wide variety of audiotapes that ranged from books on tape to formal courses, and accepted visits from volunteers knowledgeable in diverse fields who engaged her in fascinating conversation.

Even in her mid-nineties, she continued to be a character. When I had to reschedule an appointment with her to do a public service message with George Burns, she chatted away: "Oh, George Burns, he's my comic hero. Here's a joke you should give him when you see him in Hollywood: What's the difference between a tire and 365 condoms?"

"I don't know," I replied.

"When you think of a tire," she said, "you think of a *Goodyear,* but when you think of 365 condoms, you think of a *great* year!"

Jack Benny (1894–1974), the comedian, continued to carry on as if he were thirty-nine until he retired from his successful TV show at age seventy-one.

Mae West (1892–1980) was an American stage and film sex symbol, flaunting frank sensuality with a touch of humor. In 1959 when she was sixty-seven, her autobiography, **Goodness Had Nothing to Do with It**, *was published. She maintained her glamorous presence well into later life, starring at age seventy-eight in the film* **Myra Breckenridge**, *and at eighty-five in the film* **Sextette**.

When I met with George Burns, I told him I was working with a ninety-five-year-old blind woman with a sharp wit, and I passed along her risqué riddle. When he heard the punch line, he paused, then nodded with deadpan delight and said: "That's a good joke."

Ms. Thompson may have lost her eyesight, but she never seemed to lose her edgy wit, and she ultimately transformed a negative, downhill period of her life into a personally productive, satisfying time by dint of her creative energy.

Was she an exception to some biological rule of aging? Was George Burns's continuing comic genius in old age a fluke, or was his fresh outlook an affirming source of life itself? How about any of us? How do our brains respond to aging and life experience? How does biology influence our potential for intellectual growth and for creative expression?

The Biology of Aging: A Story of Adventure and Mystery

Whenever I give a lecture on creativity and aging, whether it is before a Congressional body or a student body in a university or community center classroom, I can expect a challenge from at least a few skeptics in the audience. Sometimes they suggest that I'm romanticizing aging as a time of growth, when to so many people, it is quite visibly a time of deterioration. "How can you overlook the fact that biological systems decline over time?" they say. "Just look in the mirror! Look at the human body!"

It is true, of course, that biological systems to varying degrees do decline over time, and the human body certainly offers an excellent illustration of that even in the most fit individuals. But if, as we know, many individuals live emotionally rich and expressive, creative lives despite physical disabilities—chronic disease, blindness, deafness, and even paralysis—then what exactly is the nature of this biological change as it affects biological potential as we age? Specifically, how do the changes in the aging brain uniquely influence the capacity for and nature of creative expression in later life?

The biological process of aging might seem to be a simple case of wear and tear, a kind of inevitable internal erosion that weakens cells, organs, and organ systems from head to toe, limiting their functioning as we age. Yet, scientifically we know this is not universally true. We know that not all living things age alike.

The variation in life spans of living things is remarkable. A common mayfly lives less than a day. The giant sequoia tree in the western United States has an estimated life span of 2,400 years. The family's pet hamster is old at three years, the dog at sixteen.

Some more primitive species don't appear to age at all, but simply continue to add more years of growth. Various fish, including sharks and sturgeons; amphibians such as alligators; certain tortoises; and sea sponges all exhibit this unusual characteristic of adding years, but not aging in the conventional sense. Among those species that do not appear to age, death is more closely associated with increased risks related to time and environment, as opposed to aging in the sense of deterioration or compromising internal biological changes. The longer a fish lives, for example, the greater risk it runs of being caught by a fisherman.

Admittedly, these species are more the exception than the rule. But they offer us an important reminder that "aging" has many different meanings in nature. Advanced age in any species signifies an individual with the strength and smarts to survive.

Unlike alligators and sea sponges, most living things do "show their age" in more apparent, familiar ways. We typically think of old trees as growing thick, with gnarled and pitted bark. We think of aging animals as losing agility and speed. And we think of ourselves, as humans, growing wrinkled and slowing down with advancing years.

With that apparent decline in full view, since the dawn of civilization humans have sought the secret of "eternal youth"—basically a way to avoid or forestall aging—with their efforts recorded everywhere, from the diaries of early explorers and alchemists to today's respected medical journals and tawdry tabloids. The theory, speculation, belief, and dogma vary as widely as the seekers, from the patently absurd to the scientifically plausible.

Yet as we follow the different pathways proposed by different theories, we become increasingly aware of the extraordinary mystery of aging; it is a veritable whodunit with all the suspects, surprises, and slippery clues that one finds in any great mystery. The magnitude of the

Jacques Cousteau (1910–1997), the French oceanographer and filmmaker, popularized the study of the ocean environment through his many books, films, and television productions. The 1953 publication of **The Silent World** *gained him international recognition. The book was subsequently made into a documentary that received an Academy Award. His partly autobiographical final book,* **Man, the Octopus, and the Orchid,** *was published after his death at age eighty-seven.*

Cell biologist and embryologist Ethel Browne Harvey made significant contributions to the study of marine biology. Her work **The American Arbacia and Other Sea Urchins,** *published when she was seventy-one (1956), advanced our understanding of the biology of how cells divide and develop.*

mystery, the great curiosity about it, the glamour that would be associated with cracking it, and the universal interest in aging—since it so profoundly affects each of us—help explain the fervor of the quest. Despite centuries of this impassioned study, however, the truth is that we do not yet have a definitive explanation of the basic biological process of aging. Why does the hamster grow old in three years, when humans can live to be over one hundred, and the giant redwoods more than two thousand years old?

According to the Bible, Abraham lived 175 years. It is probably safe to say he lived to a ripe old age. Though he is typically revered, from reading the Old Testament, as the father of the Hebrew people, he is more broadly regarded as the father of the three great monotheistic religions: Judaism, Christianity, and Islam. By his third wife, Keturah, he had six sons, who became the ancestors of the Arab Tribes.

One of the leading theories on aging suggests that the process of aging is genetically programmed, "hard-wired," or built in. The remarkable consistency in the life span of a species suggests that there is a unique genetic coding for each species. With humans, for example, excluding Biblical references of people like Methuselah, nobody has ever been documented to have aged beyond 130 years. This points to remarkable stability within the human biological system, again suggesting a built-in mechanism that determines the upper limits of our life span.

Gerontologist Leonard Hayflick, an active major contributor to our understanding of underlying mechanisms of aging, notes that aging theories fall into two broad groups: "Those that presume a preexisting master plan, and those based on random events." In other words, we age because we are genetically programmed that way or because of outside factors such as our environment.

This addresses the question of why we age—what prompts us to age—but it doesn't explain the biological process of aging itself, what kind of changes occur and how these biological changes affect our mental processes, our emotional health, and our creative potential.

Historically, people have viewed aging as a process of gradual decline in multiple, if not all, areas of functioning. Vision, hearing, taste, and smell are faculties that typically do diminish with age, just as disease and disability historically imposed on people's lives, in a pattern illustrated by a normal curve (see diagram that follows).*

*James F. Fries, "Aging, Natural Death and the Compression of Morbidity." The concepts I've discussed are drawn from Fries's work.

THE CHANGING PICTURE
OF FUNCTIONING WITH AGE

Historical Curve of Decline in Functioning with Aging

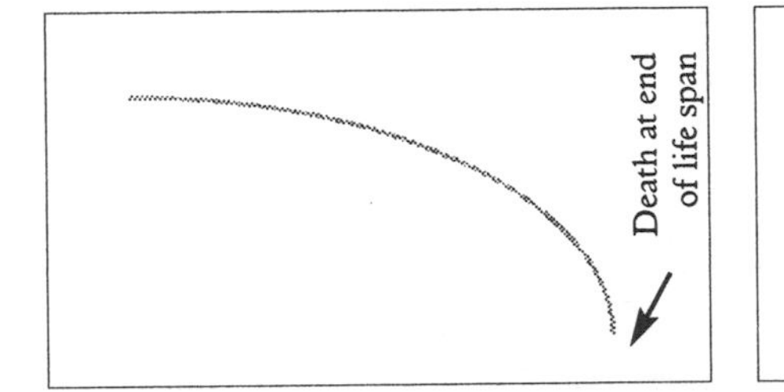

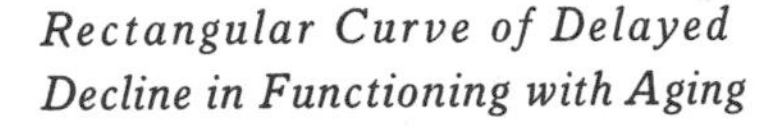

Rectangular Curve of Delayed Decline in Functioning with Aging

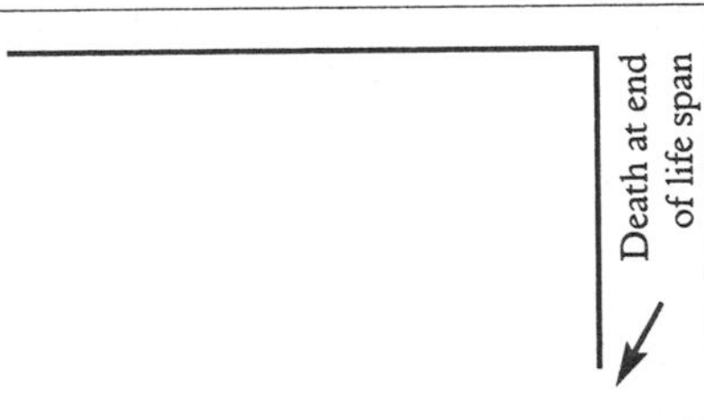

Today, however, expectations and experience of aging are changing because of improved public health practices, better general medical and geriatric care, and more informed personal health habits, such as improvements in diet and exercise along with reduction in smoking, alcohol consumption, and other toxic factors. For a large and increasing number of people, aging is more accurately illustrated by the "rectangular curve" of functioning (see the diagram above), which suggests we can maintain a fairly high level of quality of life right up to the end of it.

This is the goal of modern geriatrics, to maintain the optimal quality of life as long as possible within the boundaries of the human life span. This is also the fervent hope in each of us through middle age and beyond: to maintain our capacity—our brain power—to respond to new ideas or generate "something new," developing our creative potential as we age. All of this is possible if we look beyond the misconceptions around biological decline to discover how the biological processes of aging and of creativity continue to offer opportunities for growth and change.

Genetic Programming at the Cellular Level

Leonard Hayflick's scientific study of aging was groundbreaking when it was published in 1961. In laboratory experiments, typical cells are found to grow, divide, and increase in number. Until Hayflick's research, scientists thought that cells could divide indefinitely. What Hayflick discov-

Geneticist and physician Madge Thurlow Macklin coined the term "medical genetics" and advocated the inclusion of genetics courses in medical curricula. At the age of sixty-six (1959), she was elected president of the American Society for Human Genetics.

ered, though, was something remarkable: After a certain number of divisions—in humans, approximately fifty—cells stop dividing.

He found that cells slowly lose their capacity to function, then stop dividing and die. He concluded that the same general decline we commonly associate with aging in a person was mirrored in the life of individual cells. He did not, however, suggest that people age or die because their cells stop dividing. He suggested, instead, that the mystery force that causes aging also causes cells to stop dividing.

Other theories have attempted to define that mystery force, suggesting a wide variety of culprits, from "death" hormones released on cue by our "biological clocks," to maverick free radical cells or restricting cross-linkages between cells that trigger decline. The number of ways these theories intersect with one another is both confusing and intriguing. Many of them do not appear to be mutually exclusive. For example, hormonal changes are suspected to play a role in aging; cross-linkages can interfere with the efficient production or release of hormones. Free radicals appear to cause faulty protein formation, which can trigger an autoimmune response in which the body doesn't recognize the protein as its own and attacks it. Related genetic mutations can generate free radicals, which can trigger cross-linkages, which can disrupt normal cell life.

Sir Frank Macfarlane Burnet was awarded the Nobel Prize for the discovery of acquired immunological tolerance to tissue transplants. At age seventy-one (1970), he published his important work **Immunological Surveillance.**

It is difficult to determine whether a finding reflects cause or effect. Does the buildup of free radicals cause aging, or is the buildup an effect of some other biological circumstance? Does our immune system weaken with age, or does it diminish for some other reason, increasing our vulnerability? Many of these theories offer valuable clues, but clues are all. Each theory appears to have a smoking gun that implicates a culprit as a cause or contributor to the aging process. But each theory has one or more inconsistencies that keep us from fingering it as the ultimate culprit. (See Appendix A for additional discussion of the theories of aging.)

In this flurry of theories and clues, sturdy studies like Hayflick's bring us closer to a more fundamental understanding of the mechanisms at work that influence the process of aging; and a closer look at the life of cells raises new questions and greater optimism about our creative potential with aging.

Brain Cells: A Different Story of Life and Death

Just as different species age differently, within our own bodies, different kinds of cells age differently. Not all cells divide. Brain cells called *neurons*, in the thinking part of the brain—nerve cells of higher intellectual function—do show changes with age; but they also continue to show adaptive capacity regardless of age. Contrary to popular view, only a relatively small percentage die, more in some parts of the brain, less in others, but still a distinct minority; until we die, the vast majority of the neurons we were born with are still present and performing. But they do not divide.

So the story of aging differs dramatically for brain cells than for skin cells or the cells that line the stomach or form our bones. The biological behavior of neurons determines the way our brain functions as we age, and it is clear that our brain function and creative potential don't diminish as other body systems do.

This simple contrast in the way cells age is one of the most fundamental differences between the aging brain and the aging body, even though they are obviously part of the same organism: *They differ in their potential for ultimate accomplishment with age.* When we compare outstanding performance of different age groups, we can see differences in physical and mental performance. Somebody at age seventy-five may be in great physical shape for his age, and may be a great runner in his age group, but would not be able to compete with an outstanding young runner who was twenty-five.

Yet the same cannot be said in comparing intellectual performance. A seventy-five-year-old historian, for example, could very well run circles around a twenty-five-year-old Rhodes history scholar when it comes to discussing or interpreting history. Arnold Toynbee, the great historian, at age seventy-seven, said, "Every stage of life has its own ordeals and own rewards. My reward for having reached my present age is that this has given me time to carry out more than the whole of my original agenda; and an historian's work is of the kind in which time is a necessary condition for achievement."

Abū Ja'far Muhammad ibn Jarir at-Tabari (839–923), was a noted Arab historian, born in Persia. He made a major contribution in consolidating, condensing, and ultimately preserving the historical thinking of prior generations of Muslim scholars. His major works were* Qur'an Commentary *and the* History of the Prophets and Kings. *He also wrote a history of the world from creation until 915 when he was seventy-six years old.

Brain cells, in other words, hold special potential, because even as they age, the effects of aging present new and unique opportunities for intellectual growth and creativity.

The "Shrinking Brain" Theory

Tilly Edinger, vertebrate paleontologist, was named president of the Society of Vertebrate Paleontology when she was sixty-six. She is considered to have virtually established the field of paleoneurology (the study of fossil brains).

We naturally assume that creativity, or the ability to think about something in a new way, depends on the condition of the brain. The brain is often viewed as a control center, and it is through brain activity—neurobiological actions—that this control center executes major decisions that influence the way our body works. The brain has a series of subcenters that influence a wide range of functions, including hormonal activity, movement, memory, and emotions. If the control center is knocked out, the systems are critically disrupted.

Some experts believe this is exactly what happens when someone with Alzheimer's disease dies. Even if the person appears to die of pneumonia, which is a common recorded cause of death in Alzheimer's patients, some geriatric specialists and neurologists believe the cause is Alzheimer's itself and the way it interferes with the brain's ability to function as a control center. For instance, if the brain is disabled by Alzheimer's, a patient might be less mentally aware of the need to cough up sputum accumulating along the respiratory tract. Even though the subsequent death appears to be a result of pneumonia, the reason for this pneumonia is a disabled brain.

For years, scientists have known that the brain shrinks with age. That physical fact is often presumed to mean that the shrinking brain is equal to brain failure in slow motion, a slower version of the brain debilitation of Alzheimer's. Does normal brain shrinkage over time mean an inevitable decline in mental functioning? Does normal brain cell loss, or even loss caused by injury, necessarily cut into the capacity for creativity?

Neuroscience research offers some very clear conclusions about the link between brain size and brain function as we age. A mature human brain, around age twenty, weighs on the average 1,400 grams—a little more than 3 pounds. By one's ninth decade the brain has reduced in weight by 90 to 100 grams, a little less than 10 percent.

Meanwhile, women's brains on average weigh 10 percent less than men's, though no differences in overall intelligence have been detected; their brain weight differences probably can be attributed to the differences in total body mass between the sexes and their brain weight loss with aging is proportional to that of men. The overall brain/body ratios between men and women are similar.

So the issue is not over loss of brain size, but how much loss makes a difference. Studies find that an adult would have to have a brain weight under 1,000 grams for impaired intellectual function to be predicted on brain size alone. This is far lower than the average 10 percent loss that occurs with normal aging.

Brain studies performed on a number of intellectually gifted individuals upon their deaths show clearly that brilliance is not simply a matter of bigger brains. While the nineteenth-century Russian novelist Ivan Turgenev was reported to have had a brain weighing in excess of 2,000 grams, the equally gifted French novelist Anatole France, who won a Nobel Prize in Literature in 1921 and wrote accomplished works up until the year he died at age eighty, was reported to have had a brain weighing less than 1,200 grams. This means that the average normal eighty-year-old brain has a greater weight than that of a Nobel laureate. Moreover, many people who have had very large brains were no Einsteins; Albert Einstein himself did not have a remarkably large brain and he worked creatively even in his last years.

At age seventy-four, Einstein was still "groping," as reflected in his 1953 paper on "The Meaning of Relativity," which included his controversial unified-field theory.

The bottom line is that the brain, like other organs of the body, has considerable reserve. Neuroscience research findings offer conclusive evidence that it is possible to have reduced brain size without reduced mental or bodily function.

We need to put to rest the idea that normal shrinkage of the brain over time causes either aging or inevitable problems with how our brain performs in later life. Intellectual capacity is not necessarily compromised by the loss of some brain cells. If cell numbers were all that counted, it would be important to note that by the time we are born—certainly by age two—we have nearly all the brain cells that we will ever have for higher intellectual capacity. While we have more brain cells at two than we have at twenty-two, you would not want your two-year-old to do your taxes. While it is true that we lose cells with age, we gain in the number of essential connections between cells, and research suggests that if we mentally challenge ourselves through work or play, the number of these connections increases, independent of age. The latest research even points to some regeneration of neurons.

The Brain and Creativity

Alexander Romanovich Luria (1902–1977), the Russian psychologist considered one of the founders of the field of neuropsychology, wrote The Working *Brain in 1973, when he was seventy-one.*

Too many people view the aging brain as an organ that, on the one hand, no longer responds to challenge and, on the other hand, only loses cells. Neither view is accurate, as reflected in extraordinary new findings from neuroscience research. These recent studies in neurobiology and neuropsychology have revealed capacities of the brain that once would have been viewed as science fiction and have turned contemporary thinking in the brain sciences upside down.

Landmark experiments show not only the brain's plasticity—its ability to change with use—but also its remarkable capacity for responding to environmental challenge. In effect, these new findings confirm the folklore advice to "use it or lose it." They illustrate the profound effect our behavior can have on our biology, including the biology of the aging brain. The diagram below helps to illustrate these points: In this simple drawing we see a 100,000-fold magnification of

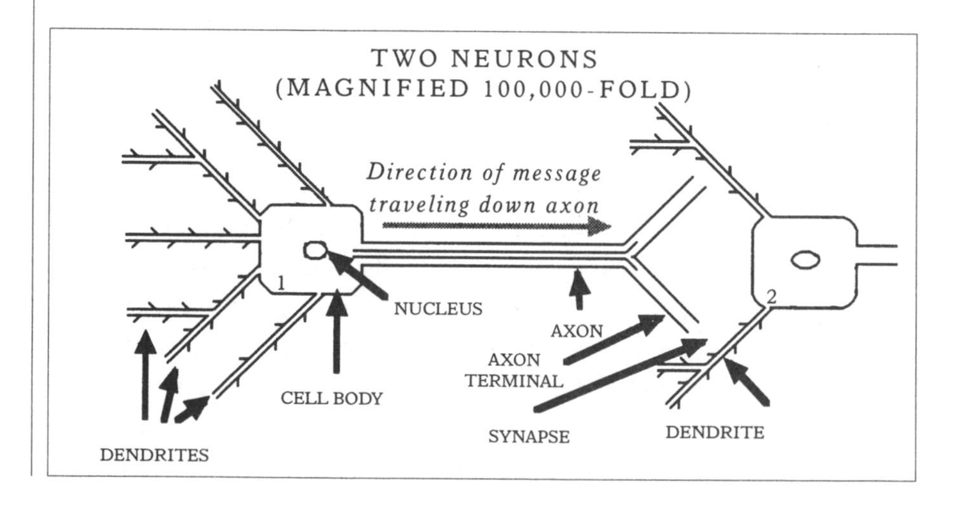

two neurons in the gray matter part of our brain—the brain cells responsible for higher intellectual functioning.

We see on the left one entire neuron, with its different component parts—the *cell body* with its nucleus, which houses the genetic information and command information for the neuron. The long, thick offshoot to the right, projecting from the cell body, is the *axon,* which contains inner filaments that act like telephone wires sending messages down the length of the neuron. The smaller, branchlike extensions off the cell body and axon are *dendrites,* which are involved in making communication connections among different neurons.

Andrew Ellicott Douglas (1867–1962) was an American astronomer and father of "dendrochronology," a term he coined meaning tree dating, in his three-volume work Climatic Cycles and Tree Growth. *He completed the third volume at age sixty-nine (1936). Douglass noted variations in the widths of the annual growth rings of trees that corresponded to sunspot and climatic phenomena.*

Humans have over 15 billion of these neurons. Neurons communicate with one another in two ways: through the release of chemicals known as *neurotransmitters,* and through the dendrites. Neurotransmitters are released and exchanged between the dendrites of neighboring neurons much like squirrels jumping from the branches of one tree to another. The more dendrites that exist, the easier the communication. Researchers have discovered that when laboratory animals are exposed to a more challenging or enriched environment, their brain cells sprout additional dendrites. For example, laboratory rats challenged in a more complicated maze developed more dendrites than rats in a less complicated maze.* Moreover, additional dendritic spines—even more smaller branches that help with communication among brain cells—also sprouted.

Other changes—both anatomical and chemical—also resulted from increased brain challenge. While the number of neurons did not increase, the cell bodies and nuclei—or control center—of existing neurons increased in size. An enzyme that contributes to memory and thinking became more active. The number of supportive cells in the brain that help nourish the neurons grew. Finally, the *cerebral cortex* as a whole—the thinking part of the brain—was found to have thickened.

"Minds, like bodies, will often fall into a pimpled, ill-conditioned state from mere excess of comfort."

—CHARLES DICKENS

Contrary to the image of the brain dimming with age, *all of these changes in response to environmental and/or behavioral challenge continued with aging.* In effect, the aging brain was found to respond

*These experiments were conducted by Marian Diamond and her colleagues and reported in Marian C. Diamond, "An Optimistic View of the Aging Brain," in *Mental Health and Aging,* ed. M. A. Smyer (New York: Springer Publishing Co., 1993), 59–63.

The great German dramatic composer Richard Wagner, in his autobiography, My Life, *wrote about a dream image he had in that borderline state between waking and sleeping: "I sank into a kind of somnambulistic state, in which I suddenly had the feeling of being immersed in rapidly flowing water. Its rushing soon resolved itself for me into the musical sound of the chord of E flat major, resounding in persistent broken chords; these in turn transformed themselves into melodic figurations of increasing motion, yet the E flat major triad never changed, and seemed by its continuance to impart infinite significance to the element in which I was sinking." What Wagner heard in his dreamlike state would become the major motif of his monumental opera* The Ring of the Nibelung. *Wagner continued composing until his death,*

to mental exercise in much the same way that muscle responds to physical exercise. This dramatic influence of behavior on biology has profound ramifications for creativity in the context of everyday life as we age.

Sleep: Rejuvenation and Stimulation Enhance Creative Brain Activity

When I first entered college, one of my professors told my class that the best way to learn something was to read the material, "sleep on it," and then read the material over again the next day. Sleep was part of the learning process. Similarly, when students taking standardized tests are stumped on a question, test advisers recommend skipping the question and returning to it later. They contend that the mind will unconsciously work on that question even though the test taker has moved on to the next problem. This advice has long been a part of folk wisdom. There are also many examples of individuals dreaming of answers or having an answer come to them in a moment of creative inspiration. While there are no formal studies showing a direct link between creativity and sleeping or dreaming, there is enough respectable information to suggest that such a connection exists.

One of the most common pieces of historic dream lore is the story of the renowned German chemist Friedrich August Kekulé, who had been desperately trying to determine the atomic structure of the chemical benzene, which was becoming increasing valued in the creation of synthetic dyes. Knowing its structure could significantly accelerate progress in its usage. Then one day in 1865, while riding on a streetcar, Professor Kekulé dozed off and began to dream. He dreamed about atoms whirling in a dance, taking the form of "a snake eating its tail," resembling a spinning ring. Upon awakening, he was startled to realize that the dream had provided him the insight that the fundamental structure of benzene was that of a ring—which became known as "the benzene ring."

It was Elias Howe's dream in 1844 that led to his invention of the modern lockstitch sewing machine. He had been attempting to develop such a machine for years, but his most recent needle design, with a hole in the middle of the shank, did not work. His frustration mounted. As the tale goes, one night he dreamed of being captured by a tribe of savages. The king of the tribe bellowed, "Elias Howe, I command you on pain of death to finish this machine tonight." But in the dream, too, he could not come up with a successful needle design. His patience exhausted, the tribal king ordered his followers to execute Howe. With his eyes focused on the end of the approaching spears, Howe noticed an eye-shaped hole. As the terrifying spears came yet closer, he suddenly awoke. Shaking off the frightened feeling, he could still see this vision of the spears, each with a hole at the tip. Things clicked. Howe then designed a needle with an eye-shaped hole near the point, and it worked.

In my own struggle over a period of months with how to portray creativity in a different and dynamic manner, it was a dream that ultimately helped me envision my theory clearly in waking hours with the $C = me^2$ equation.

Research is expanding in the field of sleep, but as yet the function and benefits of it are not clear. Theories about sleep suggest that it enforces conservation of energy; provides our bodies with an opportunity to recuperate; allows the brain time to process the overwhelming amount of information it receives; and enables the brain to process and consolidate experience and information into meaningful memories.

We know that at a cellular level in the brain, when neurons sprout new branches of dendrites, the communication among neurons is enhanced, and with that the potential for higher-level thought processes increases as well. We also know from sleep studies that sleep influences the levels of different brain hormones and neurotransmitters. We may speculate that during sleep this rich chemical bath of hormones and neurotransmitters enhances brain cell activity and dendrite growth. Perhaps in sleep, neurons forge new communication pathways across dendrites, enabling a greater exchange of information in patterns that differ from those used during conscious, waking thought.

I theorize further that as these connections among neurons are made, images occur in our minds, during the dream phase of sleep. If the information activated in the sending neuron fits with the informa-

creating Parsifal, *which many consider his greatest opera, at the age of sixty-nine.*

Kath Walker (1920–1993), the Australian poet and activist for Aboriginal rights, became the first Aboriginal poet to be published in English in 1964 (at age forty-four) with her work We Are Going. *In 1972, she wrote a book of stories,* Stradbroke Dreamtime, *in traditional Aboriginal form. Winner of many awards, including the Mary Gilmore Award and a Fullbright Scholarship, she wrote* Quandamooka, the Art of Kath Walker *in 1985, when she was sixty-five. She adopted the tribal name of Oodgeroo Noonuccal and directed a Center for Aboriginal Culture, for children of all races, on Stradbroke Island. She wrote* The Rainbow Serpent *in 1988, when she was sixty-eight.*

tion activated in the receiving neuron, then a comprehensible dream image emerges and the connection between the neurons endures. If the information from the sending neuron is incompatible with that of the receiving neuron, then a nonsensical or bizarre dream image arises, and the connection between the two neurons fades away. Since a neuron can communicate with numerous other neurons simultaneously, it is possible that both kinds of information—that which fits and that which doesn't—could be communicated at the same time.

When this occurs, I suggest that meaningful and nonsensical dream images are superimposed upon one another—the latter camouflaging the former. The camouflage may at times serve to protect against emotionally charged or painful thought connections; at other times, it may operate merely as background noise. This could explain why various dreams require interpretation to make sense; the interpretation is, in effect, filtering out the camouflage.

My theory of dream activity is largely speculative, but it is based on established theories and objective findings about the brain and may help explain the nature of dreams and why we think more clearly about an issue when we've had a chance to "sleep on it." We have literally billions of brain cells involved in higher intellectual functioning, and since each cell can have literally thousands of dendrites, we have trillions of opportunities for novel connections among dendrites, producing novel connections for ideas. We're not talking small numbers or limited possibilities here. And this process knows no endpoint with aging. This biological uncertainty of connections—which neuron will interact with another and how—carries with it remarkable possibilities for each of us, every minute of every day.*

As sleep relates to aging, again we find mistaken negative assumptions. Many people mistakenly believe that sleep disruption is a natural part of aging and an unavoidable contributor to mental decline. In truth, major changes in sleep with age do not appear to be caused by aging but more often are the result of changes in lifestyle or the effects of illness, such as arthritis, prostate problems, bladder problems,

"People who don't have nightmares don't have dreams."

—ROBERT PAUL SMITH

*An overview of sleep is presented in T. C. Neylan, C. F. Reynolds, and D. Kupfer, "Neuropsychiatric Aspects of Sleep and Sleep Disorders," in *Textbook of Neuropsychiatry*, 3rd ed., ed. S. C. Yudofsky and R. E. Hales (Washington, D.C.: American Psychiatric Press, 1997), 583–60.

depression, or other health problems. Studies following healthy older persons into their eighties find sleep patterns similar to healthy young persons, or slightly different in ways that do not appear to detract from the quality of the sleep. In fact, contrary to the notion that sleep problems are part of an inevitable decline in brain function, research suggests that some sleep and mood disorders can be reversed by challenging the brain and developing a sense of mastery in a given area. This only confirms the power of creative endeavor in the promotion of health for any of us at any age. *

The real story of the aging brain is one of what *can be* with aging, and what for many has been achieved while growing old. It is a story not only of the positive developments that can accompany aging, but what can be added late in life even in the midst of loss.

Mr. Brown's Story: No Miracles Needed, Just Nature Nurtured

When I was a third-year medical student in 1968, I had an unexpected experience that profoundly influenced how I approached very sick patients, especially those with a poor prognosis. One of the first group of patients I was assigned to follow included Larry Brown, a sixty-seven-year-old government worker who had suffered a very serious stroke the day before we met. When I saw him, he was awake, but could not express any words or move any parts of his body except his eyes, which most of the time simply stared forward. I was working under the supervision of a third-year internal medicine resident, a doctor in specialty training to become an internist, and four years ahead of me in education. The resident said he was sorry for Mr. Brown and for me, because the severity of Mr. Brown's stroke meant his future was bleak and I would see very little, if any, change in him.

***George Friederic Handel (1685–1759) suffered a stroke when he was fifty-two, but went on to create* Messiah *five years later. At age sixty-five he composed* Jephthah.**

*Sleep in relation to aging is examined in C. F. Reynolds, M. A. Dew, T. H. Monk, and C. C. Hoch, "Sleep Disorder in Late Life: A Biopsychosocial Model for Understanding Pathogenesis and Intervention," in *Textbook of Geriatric Neuropsychiatry*, ed. C. E. Coffey and J. L. Cummings (Washington, D.C.: American Psychiatric Press, 1994), 323–31.

I asked the resident why no improvement was expected, but he could offer no specific physiological reason, except to say there was too much brain damage and his experience with stroke patients like this was that there was little hope for improvement. I was dismayed by this presumption of hopelessness and couldn't accept it. I thought, Well, that isn't *my* experience—of course, I had no experience with stroke victims at all—and I decided to approach Mr. Brown as a man who could benefit from a determined rehabilitation program. The resident was reluctant at first to approve the rehabilitation treatment plan, but finally gave me the go-ahead.

As I requested, nurses diligently exercised Mr. Brown's limbs for him so they would not begin to stiffen abnormally because of lack of movement, and I coached the family to do the same on their visits. Three days later there was essentially no change, and some of my colleagues voiced renewed skepticism. I felt it was still too soon for conclusions about Mr. Brown's potential for recovery. The rehabilitation treatment continued and after a week had passed, Mr. Brown started to show some movement on his right side and express a few unintelligible words. After the second week, he began to regain movement on his left side, and he could utter more words. By the end of the third week, his movements were more robust and we could begin to understand his words. After four weeks had passed, his muscle strength had improved significantly and he could speak in short intelligible sentences.

Étienne-Maurice Falconet (1716–1791), the French sculptor known for his figures of Venus that epitomize the Rococo style, suffered a stroke in 1783, at age sixty-seven. Following his stroke he gave up sculpture but turned to writing art history, publishing nine volumes by the time he was seventy-one, in 1787.

The resident was quite surprised and rationalized that Mr. Brown was a rare exception to the rule. But for me and my experience, he *was* the rule. The family looked at me as if I were a miracle man, but I said what I believed: It was nature taking its course, helped by all of us, and that we needed to continue our efforts to support this healing process.

The other fortuitous part in this experience for me was that the attending physician in charge of the unit who had assigned patients to the students also wanted us to follow two of our patients over a longer time—a full year—to get a better sense of the course of different diseases. I chose Mr. Brown as one of my patients.

After a month had passed, Mr. Brown had improved enough to return home, where his family wanted to care for him. In addition to getting the advice of the attending physician and the medical resident, they asked me what I thought they should do. My advice was influenced by my growing preference for specializing in psychiatry, and I knew it was as important to pay attention to the mind as the body. I recommended that in addition to continuing physical rehabilitation activities at home to exercise his body, they should also help him exercise his mind though conversation, reading to him, asking him to read to them, and any other ways they could find to keep him mentally active.

During the next several months, Mr. Brown's family and friends were enthusiastic partners in this mind-body rehabilitation effort. His minister visited him and, upon learning of the rehabilitation treatment plan, suggested that the family get Mr. Brown involved in the community center that the church had set up for its older members. The family was at first skeptical, because Mr. Brown had never been very social outside his family. But the minister was very persuasive about the potential for this activity to contribute to Mr. Brown's progress by providing physical and intellectual activity.

Mr. Brown listened. He began to attend the community center, at first in a wheelchair, and then, as he improved, assisted only by a walker. Continuing improvement allowed him to trade the walker for a cane. He got involved in card games and in a newly created wood shop, where he started to make practical objects, from doorstops to small storage chests that he would paint decoratively. All of this was new for Mr. Brown and gave him great satisfaction, and his family was delighted beyond description.

Mr. Brown was not able to return to the job he'd held before the stroke because of the long hours and complex paperwork that were part of that position. But he had been launched on a new course of productive, satisfying, creative activity that enhanced the quality of his life.

As my experience with brain-diseased patients grew, I saw more and more people like Mr. Brown, who, in the absence of continuing strokes, showed unexpected improvement and the capacity to experiment with new, personal "small c" creative activities that were part of their rehabilitative program. A number of these patients showed subtle but specific improvements in motor and intellectual functioning over two, three, or even more years.

> ***"Keep your face to the sunshine and you cannot see the shadow."***
>
> —HELEN KELLER

Initial improvement in a patient like Mr. Brown is typically viewed as stabilization following a major medical emergency such as stroke, or bleeding from or blockage of a blood vessel in the brain. Ongoing, long-term improvement is less well understood. But based on what we know about dendritic sprouting in response to a stimulating environment, it would seem that appropriate ongoing challenges for persons who suffer a stroke should be part of a continuing rehabilitation effort.

These challenges may encourage dendrite growth that functions like bridges, allowing new communication among brain cells previously cut off from one another owing to gaps created by lost cells destroyed by the stroke. If impairments are the result of severed communication between certain cell groups, then perhaps the bridging of new dendritic sprouting may restore those connections, improving function. Lost cells are generally not being replaced, but the gaps between remaining cells may possibly be reduced by these dendrite branches.

Biological Complexity Promises Continuing Potential for Creativity

"If you've broken the eggs, you should make the omelet."
—ANTHONY EDEN

All this said, there remains considerable mystery about how the brain functions and positively responds to disease and injury. In fact, there remains far more mystery than understanding. Recent research, for example, has identified various patients with a form of dementia that affects a particular portion of the brain—the frontotemporal lobe—who suffer significant intellectual impairment while at the same time, remarkably, show newly acquired or enhanced artistic skills.* It appears that the damage done by the unwanted deterioration also destroys something that has caused blockage of activity in the artistic arena.

This research hints at the profound potential in identifying new biological dimensions that influence creative expression or result in its

*Research among various patients with dementia in the frontotemporal lobe resulting in newly emergent or enhanced artistic skills was reported in B. L. Miller, J. Cummings, F. Mishkin, K. Boone, et al., "Emergence of Artistic Talent in Frontotemporal Dementia," *Neurology* 51, no. 4 (1998): 978–82.

awakening. Surely there are other avenues for change within the brain, opportunities for us to use specific stimulating activities that could physically alter the obstacles to various creative processes, just as the disease process does in these patients with frontotemporal dementia. The challenge is that we have not yet clearly identified these biological blocks to creative expression, nor do we fully understand how a stimulating environment and activities actually cause physical improvements in the brain.

The challenge of this complexity requires that we open our thinking about what we do know, and see it differently, if we are to find new pathways of understanding. Here, as in many instances in nature, we must believe that complexity is in the service of stability. It is the brain's complexity that acts as a protective labyrinth, buffering the effects of any single disturbing event or influence. We can look for different interpretations of the changes we commonly consider negative attributes of aging, and in those qualities traditionally viewed as more positive qualities of aging, we can find new potential for growth.

For example, as our brains age, information typically does not get processed as quickly. This can affect how we receive or understand new information or how we respond to new situations. If we suppose that this slowing down serves a purpose in nature, and look for it, we might acknowledge that most of life does not—or does not have to—operate in a beat-the-clock mode.

We might explore the possible benefits of this slower process. In most situations, taking a little more time to adjust helps us digest the information and respond thoughtfully, rather than simply react under pressure. Older pianists, for example, whose playing is affected by not being able to move their fingers as fast across the keys, may creatively rearrange a composition, ever so subtly altering its tempo and rest periods between chords so that the music, though technically different, remains just as appealing and creative. Harmony, melody, and beauty, after all, are not dependent on velocity.

***American pianist Arthur Rubinstein (1887–1982), who made more than two hundred recordings during his life, was still performing at eighty-eight, and at ninety-two (1980) he wrote his autobiography,* My Many Years.**

It is also important to note that changes in reaction time are subtle with aging, hardly dramatic in most people. Recent research on persons age sixty-five and older who use computers found that with practice both the *speed* of their response and the *accuracy* of their selec-

Noah Webster (1758–1843), American lexicographer, published in two volumes the great **American Dictionary of the English Language**—*now called* **Webster's New International Dictionary of the English Language**—*in 1828, at the age of seventy.*

Oliver Wendell Holmes Jr., known as "The Great Dissenter," was appointed associate justice of the U.S. Supreme Court at the age of sixty-one (1902). He sat on that court for the next thirty years, retiring just before his ninety-first birthday. The newly inaugurated President Franklin Roosevelt called upon the retired justice and found him reading Plato. The President inquired, "Why do you read Plato, Mr. Justice?" The ninety-two-year-old scholar replied, "To improve my mind, Mr. President."

tions increased. Learning and training can have significant and long-lasting effects, independent of age, and they commonly compensate for normal age-associated changes of this kind.

In other instances, we see changes with aging that would seem to contradict one another. On the one hand, many people in later life experience increased difficulty in word finding—coming up with the word one wants to say, with it often stuck on the tip of their tongues. On the other hand, vocabulary has been found to increase into the eighties among older persons who continue to challenge themselves intellectually with reading, writing, crossword puzzles, word games, and the like. With aging we can experience a simultaneous growth and decline in a particular kind of brain work.

Meanwhile, there are a host of positive changes that come with age that present vast opportunities for creative expression. For instance, it may be easier to define problems and come up with problem-solving strategies over time. Just as our vocabulary builds, so do general knowledge, career experience, and life experience.

We typically use the phrase "older and wiser" to refer to the more experienced insights that come with age. But what is wisdom? What might be the biological basis for wisdom and what other potential might that hold for us? In addition to wisdom making us better judges, might the same biological process also potentially make us better learners?

The dictionary definition of wisdom includes "sagacity"; a sage according to Webster is "very wise"; especially an elderly person, widely respected for "wisdom, experience, and judgment." Typically we think of wisdom in terms of *knowledge*. Certainly knowledge is a critical component. But there are two other key ingredients—*emotional understanding* (emotional intelligence) and *life experience*. All three of these elements accrue with time. They can't be bought and they can't be rushed, so it is not surprising that wisdom, though not unique to later life, is associated more often with aging.

Emotional understanding is a particularly complex component of wisdom. It builds with time and our ability to learn from past experiences with people or situations, and uses that experience to heighten our understanding of people and situations new to us. Such emotional awareness is a great asset to a judge and a diplomat, and again helps explain why so many high-level judges—those on the U.S. Supreme Court, for instance—and diplomats are quite advanced in age.

Just as we have begun to identify certain biochemical links in conditions such as Attention Deficit Disorder, depression, and other mood disorders, enabling us to provide more effective medical interventions, it is reasonable to expect that there are intricate biological and biochemical processes that bring about wisdom as we see it in everyday life.

Just as folk wisdom advises us to "use it or lose it," science now tells us the same thing. Modern basic neurobiological research has finally caught up, showing the soundness of this advice through discoveries of the remarkable anatomical and physiological responses of brain cells to stimulating interaction with our environment and one another. Today we have scientific evidence that confirms the importance of creative stimulation to maintaining brain health, and that a healthy brain in turn maximizes our capacity to deal successfully with our environment and the health challenges there for us.

Creativity as Preventive, Healing "Medicine"

We know from studies of stress, particularly in older persons, that prolonged stress has adverse effects on the immune system; findings reveal that chronic stress lowers the levels of protective immune system cells moving throughout the body. In this situation, our resistance to infection and perhaps other illness is lowered, our health becomes more vulnerable and our healing ability is compromised as well. Research that combines the study of psychological, neurological, and immunological influences again suggests that the negative psychological effects of chronic stress block or disrupt normal function of the brain cells that send messages to the immune system. Remember that the brain is the body's command center or control tower, and when it is adversely affected, it gives out bad information to other parts of the body.

Experimental studies indicate that creative activities and their consequent positive effect on mood and morale can lead to an increased production of protective immune cells. We don't know why this is so.

Black Elk (1863–1950), was an Oglala Lakota holy man and traditional healer. He had lived through the last of the U.S. and Sioux wars and the start of government policies that he felt threatened his culture. Many in the Lakota Nation feared the dissolution of their culture and strove to find ways to preserve their sacred knowledge and information. Black Elk committed himself to this undertaking, and at the age of sixty-seven (1930), he dictated his life story to John Niehardt in the book **Black Elk Speaks.** ***This book contributed enormously to preserving Lakota culture and was reprinted many times, read not only by Lakota Indians but by the general public. Black Elk continued to serve as a guest speaker at various gatherings until his death at age eighty-seven.***

Perhaps, in the same way that sustained stress appears to lead to insidious, then serious problems with overall health, the sustained experience of the positive, health-affirming nature of the creative process delivers a heightened, satisfying, positive health effect.

When we look at the way creativity may influence the course of illness, preliminary scientific findings suggest that sustained creativity can promote recovery from acute health problems, such as infections and injuries, as well as improve the course of chronic or even terminal illnesses. This is not to suggest that creativity can cure a terminal illness, but rather that it enhances relief through better coping abilities.

Hanya Holm (1893–1992), the dancer and choreographer, choreographed more than a dozen Broadway musicals, including **Kiss Me, Kate**, *at fifty-five (1948),* **My Fair Lady**, *at sixty-three (1956), and* **Camelot**, *when she was sixty-seven (1960).*

The popularity of expressive arts therapies—art therapy, dance and movement therapy, and music therapy, for instance—among patients with serious illness testifies to this enhancement, as do research findings that reflect the positive impact of these creative interventions. Research confirms what I have seen in so much of my work with individuals and families whose lives are touched by the most devastating of disorders, but find their lives improved by creative activity and expression.

Recent findings from research on Alzheimer's disease—perhaps the most dreaded of all age-associated brain disorders—also suggest a positive contribution from sustained creative challenge to mental functioning. There is some scientific evidence suggesting that individuals at risk for Alzheimer's disease, who have over the years continued to challenge themselves mentally, on the whole may have a delayed onset of the disorder.

These preliminary findings suggest that perhaps through ongoing, prolonged challenges for our minds, a reserve in brain function is developed that forestalls onset of Alzheimer's in those at risk for it. This theory also suggests that these individuals may have built up a richer, more dense network of dendrites that preserve over a longer time the important connections between remaining brain cells not damaged or destroyed in the insidious progression of Alzheimer's. These studies point to the role of creativity in preserving brain function alongside the more apparent role in promoting positive function.

Imagery: Creativity as a Therapeutic Tool for Healing

Jeanne Achterberg, a pioneering researcher, has been instrumental in helping us explore the healing power of creativity through systematic mental imagery. In her book, *Imagery in Healing,* she quotes Thomas Largewhiskers, a hundred-year-old Navajo medicine man and sage: "I don't know what you learned from books, but the most important thing I learned from my grandfathers was that there is a part of the mind that we don't really know about and that it is that part that is most important in whether we become sick or remain well."

Rachel Naomi Remen, medical director of the Commonweal Cancer Help Program, spoke well in talking about the therapeutic use of imagery when she described the connection between our creative powers and our health: "Health is the movement towards wholeness. Imagery is the movement towards wholeness made visible."

My colleague and wife, Wendy Miller, an expressive arts therapist who uses imagery as both a creative and therapeutic tool in her work with medically ill clients, described to me the case of Kathy, a lawyer in her fifties, who struggled with breast cancer.

While receiving medical treatment for her cancer, Kathy described to her treatment team a recurring image she experienced of a dinosaur eating raspberries. At that time, efforts were underway to help her elevate her white blood cells. Although she did not describe the image of the dinosaur eating raspberries as disquieting, she was advised to work on altering her imagery because of the likelihood that the dinosaur represented the cancer devouring fragile protective cells represented by the raspberries. She was told that since dinosaurs are so much stronger than raspberries, her immune system didn't have a chance. It was then suggested to her that she develop an image in which the dinosaur would be killed off, or be distracted from eating the raspberries or simply not be interested in eating fruit. The hungry dinosaur image continued to recur periodically, but the hostile interpretation of it did not feel right to her. Meanwhile, the cancer was found to have metastasized and aggressive medical treatment was applied.

Cancer researching physician Elise Strang during her sixties and early seventies (from the late 1930s to 1950) pioneered in organizing clinics attempting to prevent cancer (especially cervical) by early diagnosis. At the age of seventy-three, she was awarded the prestigious Albert Lasker Award of the American Public Health Association for her "application of preventive medicine to cancer control."

At the same time, Kathy was referred to Wendy for expressive arts therapy. Wendy used exploratory conversation, art making, and art-as-meditation to better understand the meaning of Kathy's recurring dinosaur imagery. What emerged was something different from the earlier interpretation.

To Kathy, the dinosaur appeared to reflect her old way of being in the world, an outdated, aggressive, and controlling style. She experienced the raspberries as fresh and sweet, and thought they might reflect a fragile but newly growing sense of self. This "self" was characterized by a more receptive nature, a more "feminine approach," as she described it, to being in the world. Kathy realized that each time the dinosaur ate a raspberry, she felt calmer and more at peace with the possibility that she had a chance to heal.

Kathy now felt that it was important for her not to resist the image of the dinosaur eating the raspberries but to foster it—allow the dinosaur to enjoy the raspberries—and allow her old ways of experiencing things to give way to the newly emerging sense of being comfortable with a new lifestyle and circumstances that offered her a greater feeling of peacefulness, even in the midst of her terrifying cancer.

Kathy is no longer called a cancer patient, but a cancer survivor. She attributes the positive turn in her clinical course to the combination of new state-of-the-art medicine in cancer treatment and to the longstanding state-of-the-art healing imagery in treating one's soul. In Chapter 6 we will look in more depth at behavioral and biological explanations to see why treating the mind through creative interventions helps the body—especially the aging body—in the face of adversity.

Conclusion: Biology Offers Promise, Mystery, and Incentive

Raymond Chandler, author of "private eye" novels, continued to create new adventure for his Philip Marlowe character in* Playback*, written in 1958 at age seventy.

I love a good mystery—scientific or fictional—and one of my personal favorites on the fiction front is Agatha Christie's *Murder on the Orient Express*. In it, her renowned detective Hercule Poirot was enmeshed in an exceedingly complicated maze involving twelve major suspects all coincidentally riding on the same train—in my view, something akin to the line-up of major theories attempting to identify the key to aging. Poirot struggled through extraordinary efforts to identify the guilty party. He pondered the evidence, came to a startling conclusion, and explained:

> I was particularly struck by the extraordinary difficulty of proving a case against any one person on the train, and by the rather curious coincidence that in each case the testimony giving an alibi came from what I might describe as an 'unlikely' person . . . I said to myself: This is extraordinary—they cannot all be in it! And then, Messieurs, I saw the light. They were all in it. For so many people connected with the . . . case to be traveling by the same train through coincidence was not only unlikely; it was impossible. It must be not chance, but design. . . . I saw it as a perfect mosaic, each person playing his or her allotted part. . . . The whole thing was a very cleverly planned jigsaw puzzle, so arranged that every fresh piece of knowledge that came to light made the solution of the whole more difficult . . . the case seemed fantastically impossible!

At the age of eighty-four, Dame Agatha Christie (1890–1976) oversaw the 1974 revision of the movie **Murder on the Orient Express,** *based on her novel of the same name. She wrote up until she died at age eighty-six. Her books have sold more than 100 million copies.*

Alas, the biology of aging, too, remains a mystery. Perhaps the perfect complexity of it, like Poirot's challenge on the Orient Express, is the mystery and the explanation all in one. But whether we believe, as some scientists do, that the aging process is caused by a number of mechanisms, or we believe as other scientists do, that there is an ultimate biological culprit lurking, we must not allow the mystery to fuel misunderstanding, negative stereotypes, or negative expectations of aging.

There are many illnesses for which we don't know the causes, but we do know the treatment. We don't always understand life, yet we move forward. We don't understand all there is to know about aging, but we know there continues to be tremendous potential for intellectual growth and creative expression.

Mary Roberts Rinehart, best-selling author of mystery books, was preeminent in the genre of fusing humor with the detective story. Writer of novels and plays, her highly successful play **The Bat** *was revived, with her collaboration, when she was seventy-seven, for television, and starred Zasu Pitts.*

We know that the brain remains active—our "wiring" remains flexible—and that it responds positively to challenge, creating new connections that strengthen our capacity to respond to new ideas and generate them. We know that creative stimulation enhances our health, both biologically and emotionally, and that some mental functions actually improve with age and experience. We know that even in the face of illness or disability, creative expression has the power to transform our lives with new opportunities and experiences of healing.

"For age is opportunity
no less
Than youth itself, though
in another dress,
And as the evening
twilight fades away
The sky is filled with stars,
invisible by day.

—HENRY WADSWORTH LONGFELLOW, "MORITURI SALUTAMUS"

Sen. Claude Pepper, who held court in Congress into his nineties, once said, "Life is like riding a bicycle. You don't fall off unless you stop pedaling." In the presence of an aging healthy brain there is no reason for mental activity to stop in later life. With creativity, like learning, or like life, for that matter, the trick is to keep going at it.

Clearly, aging presents a great scientific opportunity for exploration, but more important, aging and creativity present an unparalleled opportunity for us as individuals, to *grow* as we grow older, in ways that in younger years we could not even have dreamed.

3

Transition and Transformation: Creativity Across Our Changing Inner Landscape

And the day came when the risk to remain tight in a bud
was more painful than the risk it took to blossom.

—ANAÏS NIN

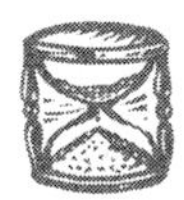

NANCY, A FORTY-THREE-YEAR-OLD MOTHER of three, confided that she looked forward to reaching her fifties, because she hoped by then to have a calmer, richer kind of wisdom than her frantic life as a middle-aged mother seemed to offer. Ted, fifty-two, had achieved significant success as a management consultant, but blamed his divorce from his wife of many years, and the subsequent emotional estrangement from his children, on years of self-defeating decisions about work, money, life, and relationships. "I just wish I could start thinking like a grown-up—see things more clearly, develop some perspective, and make better choices," he said.

"Nothing can bring you peace but yourself."
—RALPH WALDO EMERSON

Despite our culture's preoccupation with youth and staying young, at a deeper level there remains in each of us a desire to be "a grown-up"—to be competent and confident out in the world. With our first breath of life, we begin a developmental journey that, step by step, enables us to grow into our world through progressively more complex use of movement and language, and physical and emotional expression. The young child "learns" to crawl, walk, and talk with nature as her first and most powerful resource. Encouragement plays a strong role in that forward progress, but at the heart of it is a developmental drive dictated by nature.

The dramatic physical, intellectual, and emotional changes we see in adolescence are, again, a matter of nature's urge to grow, shaped by a combination of genes and life experience—nature *and* nurture. In the course of a lifetime, a sequence of psychological stages shape the patterns of thought, emotion, and behavior with which we approach life. Although each stage has some common identifying characteristics, the way they unfold in any one of our lives is unique, shaped by our particular mix of psychological and social influences—our experience of family, friends, and community, and our inner life. Unlike the physical changes we see so clearly as our height, weight, and general appearance reflect our years, our psychological growth and development moves in less obvious steps toward a future wide open with creative potential.

"Even if you're on the right track you'll get run over if you just sit there."
—WILL ROGERS

About fifty years ago, American psychoanalyst Erik Erikson offered the most comprehensive and enduring blueprint of human emotional development throughout life, which he summarized in fairly simple terms as the "Eight Ages of Man." Erikson's theory, which remains widely accepted as a basis for understanding emotional development, suggests that life unfolds in eight stages of emotional growth, each one featuring a key emotional issue or developmental task that builds on the one before and establishes the foundation for continued emotional growth.

Regardless of our age, the degree of success we have learning the lessons of each age shapes our emotional health—or distress—in the years to come. Beginning with trust, and working through autonomy, industry, identity, and intimacy, Erikson mapped out the psychological issues for infancy, early childhood, school age, adolescence, and young adulthood, respectively.

Adulthood and old age were the remaining two age stages, with the key psychological issues being, first, generativity, or an interest in guiding the next generation through personal action or a legacy of work; and later, integrity, which means coming to terms with our successes and disappointments in life and our relationships. This final step allows us to look squarely at life, feel at peace with it, and believe our lives have had meaning.

This pattern of psychological transitions over time not only shapes our emotions, thinking, behavior, and overall identity, or self-view, but also influences our creative potential—that ability to think about things in new ways. Just as a small, hard seed transforms day by day into a vibrant flowering plant, we change as we grow, and every transition provides the context for the next phase of growth and expression.

Creativity itself also follows some developmental steps that are influenced by our inner resources, experience, and life situation, producing different results at different ages and under different circumstances. Joseph Wallas, in his 1926 classic book, *The Art of Thought,* described the creative process in four steps—preparation, incubation, illumination, and verification—which can occur at any age and for any length of time.

Preparation is the stage in which we lay the groundwork for new thinking, perhaps by mastering a body of knowledge, immersing ourselves in a problem or perceived area of opportunity, and engaging in speculative thinking, limbering up the mind for action. This could take years—even a decade—or just days, depending on the subject and how much we already know.

During the incubation stage we let ideas "simmer," cultivated, sometimes even unconsciously, by the mind. Here, too, the process might take anywhere from a few hours to years.

In the illumination phase of creativity, we transform our insight into action. When Thomas Edison, the prolific American inventor, made his provocative statement that genius is 2 percent inspiration and 98 percent perspiration, he described this transformation of idea into action.

The last stage—verification—is the time it takes for a new idea to gain acceptance, both by ourselves and by others. This becomes significant when we look for the reasons why, for instance, in certain fields of endeavor such as math and science, innovators and achievers tend to be

"Discovery consists of looking at the same thing as everyone else and thinking something different."

—ALBERT SZENT-GYÖRGYI

recognized early in their careers, while in psychology and philosophy that recognition tends to come much later in life. Is it really that whole fields of bright, critical thinkers lose their spark with age, or is there something about the evaluation stage? This is something we will explore in greater detail in Chapter 4.

Innovative thinking can take place at any or all stages of human development—including stages in the second half of life that we'll explore shortly. But the stages of the creative process don't just happen. The social and emotional influences that shape our experience also influence our readiness to launch a creative process.

Our inherent capacity to step outside the lines, to explore foreign territory, is demonstrated in our dreams. The noted French writer and film director Jean Cocteau reflected on such: "One of the characteristics of the dream is that nothing surprises us in it. With no regret, we agree to live with strangers, completely cut off from our habits and friends." Cocteau continued to direct films into his early seventies. He directed* Orphée *in 1960 at age seventy-one.

For example, many people first experience the awakening of their creativity only when their children leave home or they retire from the workplace, when they finally feel they have time to devote to their own interests. Research also shows that older adults are more in touch with their unconscious feelings, through dreams and daytime reflection, so they experience less psychological resistance to difficult emotional issues; as a result, they are able to draw upon this rich material more creatively than they did at a younger age. This accessible inner realm is an exciting source of imagery and understanding and explains why a number of artists first emerge or fully realize their potential only in later life.

The psychoanalyst R. Maduro, who conducted cross-cultural research into the psychology of aging in the early 1970s, noted: "With increasing years artists say they are 'more open' to the nuances of internal chaos and pure intuition, to 'conceiving,' and to the 'unfolding of the self' . . ." rather than imposing order on that creative energy. Whether we express our creativity through art, or through travel, cooking, gardening, friendship, community action, business, science, or technology, age can enhance our intuitive powers for self-expression.

It is the combination of your experience, your interests, and your readiness—different at different ages—that can launch you in new directions of your choosing. Your creative potential at any age is built upon your life experience, but not limited to it. Another early researcher in aging, psychoanalyst, Martin Grotjahn, observing the unpredictable creative chemistry of age, development, and experience, said it well: "Insight occurs just because it is high time."

Where Understanding Stops Short: Aging and Creativity as Unexplored Territory

You can see that even in Erikson's thoughtful outline, five of the eight ages occur by adolescence; six of the eight developmental stages are in the first half of life. Daniel Levinson, whose original research into middle age is credited with identifying the "midlife crisis" as a developmental transition, expanded our understanding of that life predicament, but, like Erikson, stopped short of dealing in depth with life after middle age, or with the exciting potential of middle age itself. In scholarly papers and textbook discussions of human development generally, most of the emphasis has been placed on the first half of life, especially the earliest stages of infancy through adolescence.

This emphasis on developmental issues in the first half of life is echoed in the multitude of parenting books, TV and radio shows, and conversation among parents, teachers, and others who live or work with children. Children themselves are encouraged today to see their lives in developmental terms, with school assignments such as drawing time lines of their lives, marking highlights along the way.

Far less attention has been paid to developmental stages of midlife and beyond—what we commonly call the second half of life—even though these are the decades of adult life that actually offer the greatest potential for us to take the initiative and act not just on the dreams of our youth, but on new visions of our life desires and potential.

This lack of attention to the fuller developmental dimensions of adult life is no small oversight. It represents a troubling gap in scientific study, in public policy, and in popular perception that leaves us with a very limited view of adulthood, as if our intellectual and emotional growth reaches some level we call "mature" and simply stops there, or erupts in crisis, before declining with advancing age.

Nobel Laureate Anatole France published* The Bloom of Life *as he continued to bloom at the age of seventy-eight (1922).

With scant meaningful information or discussion about the full range of development in later adult life, naturally there has tended to be a much stronger focus on social and emotional crisis and conflict resolution in adulthood rather than on the emotional growth and creative

William Golding (1911–1993), the English novelist and author of **Lord of the Flies** *at the age of forty-three, wrote five highly regarded novels after he was sixty-five, including* **Rites of Passage** *at age sixty-nine, which won the Booker Prize and* **The Fire Down Below** *at age seventy-eight.*

The great Russian writer Leo Tolstoy (1828–1910) recorded in his diary, "I remembered very vividly that I am conscious of myself in exactly the same way now, at eighty-one, as I was conscious of myself, my 'I' at five or six years of age. Consciousness is immovable."

opportunity possible with aging. Any recognition that as adults we continue to experience significant developmental transitions is generally reduced to the stereotypical midlife crisis.

Gender stereotypes further reduce our understanding of that particular midlife passage to its most narrow terms: A man presumably trades in his family car and wife for flashier models; a woman presumably struggles with menopausal hot flashes, empty-nest blues, and an urge for cosmetic surgery. Sex and money are subjects of continuing consternation. Some contemporary commentators label each decade of age with catchy slogans—"The Serene Sixties," for instance, to quote from one—which suggest that we progress through our lives much as we might a theme park, moving together with our age peers from one developmental realm to the next.

The reality of adult life is a much richer and more complex tapestry of struggle, growth, and creative potential. Our developmental growth progresses in fits and starts and sometimes waves that take us forward, and sometimes backward for a spell, as we grow. We are, at forty, fifty, sixty and older, not so very different from children of four, five, six, or older, who struggle through developmental transitions and life changes. We progress at our own pace, each of us. If we struggle or hesitate at times, it is not because we're older and less capable, but because we are in the process of developmental transition, which often goes unrecognized and therefore unsupported by friends, family, or our culture. As a result, we often misunderstand the nature of our struggle and overlook the tremendous opportunities for growth.

It would be absurd to suggest that a child who throws a temper tantrum at age two is experiencing a developmental crisis, or that a child who can't read at age three will never be a reader. And yet, we judge ourselves just that harshly when we limit our expectations of life at age fifty, or any age, to what we are or what we know or what we can do at that age, instead of seeing ourselves as works in progress, capable of lifelong learning, growth, and change. These developmental steps require the same leaps of faith, risk taking, and emotional vulnerability as they did when we were five and learning to tie our shoes or say goodbye to our parents at school each day. They also offer a similar potential for discovery and delight as we age. Just as we celebrate the toddler's struggle to walk as the first step of many to come, we need to recognize the steps of adult development as a building process, not a crisis or a dead end, and celebrate the creative potential possible for each of us on our separate journeys.

ROBERT HENRY'S STORY: THE POWER OF THE PAST SHAPES THE FUTURE

"We have need of history in its entirety, not to fall back into it, but to see if we can escape from it," wrote Spanish essayist and philosopher José Ortega y Gasset. In our own lives, just as in the lives of nations, we must recognize the power of the past as well as the fresh potential that awaits us, and find a way to use them as catalysts for creative growth. Among the forces that influence our psychological development and related patterns of behavior in adult life are past experiences in the developmental stages of our youth. All the developmental stages play major roles in shaping our identity; those who go through a stage with significant unresolved emotional conflict often face an ongoing struggle to establish a healthy sense of themselves. Similarly, the effects of major experiences at different stages remain powerful influences on the way we think and act for the rest of our lives.

Robert Henry, the eighty-eight-year-old man I mentioned in Chapter 1, who became a documentary photographer in his later years, came to me first in a study I carried out on people in good mental health after age sixty-five. Robert arrived for the first time in my office carrying two stuffed briefcases. He sat down, pointed to the briefcases and explained that he had a long and unusual story, and he assumed that I, as a scientist, would want validation of what he said. I thanked him and invited him to tell me something about himself. He began by saying that he was finally back to normal after an ordeal that had started a year earlier. I asked him to explain.

At that time, he said, he had been engaged in his new late-life interest, documentary photography, with a sense of adventure. On one self-assigned photography mission, he was in the mountains of Colombia, filming a small cathedral, when he and his guide were attacked by a small band of robbers. He was stabbed and brutally beaten, suffering a

Alfred Eisenstaedt, the American photojournalist (1898–1995), started freelancing as a photojournalist in his twenties, and in 1936, at age thirty-eight, became one of the original photographers working for Life *magazine, where he continued to publish photographs over the next thirty-six years until he was seventy-four. His publications include* Witness to Our Time, *published at age sixty-eight;* The Eye of Eisenstaedt, *published at age seventy-one;* Photojournalism, *published at age eighty-three;* Eisenstaedt on Eisenstaedt, *published at age eighty-seven.*

Nathan Dane (1752–1835), a nineteenth-century American lawyer, published his nine-volume General Abridgement and Digest of American Law *from 1823 to 1829 when he was seventy-one to seventy-seven. It was the first comprehensive work on American law. He was also a delegate to the Continental Congress.*

collapsed lung and two displaced vertebrae. But he survived, completed rehabilitation, and now was ready for his next photo adventure.

Until his first retirement at age seventy-three, Robert had worked as a lawyer for the government. Upon retirement he drew upon his experience as a lawyer, as well as his schooling and experience that included accounting, and went into business for himself, dealing with estates and trusts. He continued this until age seventy-eight, when he retired again and became more active in camera work. He had always had an interest but never enough time for it. Over the next decade he became a highly skilled documentary photographer.

When Robert was eighty-one, following the death of his wife after fifty-five years of a very close marriage, his photography took a turn to the more adventuresome. Two remarkable series that had become very popular in presentations he made at his retirement community were a documentary on Alaska developed from an extensive set of pictures taken from a helicopter, at times under unexpectedly challenging wind conditions in uninhabited places. Another was a documentary of Tahiti that followed two years of research preparation and extensive negotiation with the French government about aerial filming near militarily strategic off-limits locations.

"You seem to gravitate to challenge, adventure, and, at times, risky situations," I commented.

He nodded and acknowledged that things had pretty much always been this way. When I asked him to talk about his early life, Robert explained that he had grown up in the Midwest, one of six kids, in a family with roots back to pioneer days. He was proud of his family, and described his relationship with his grandfather as particularly close, as was his relationship with his mother.

"What about your father?" I asked.

Robert described a tumultuous relationship with his father, who was very strict. For instance, when Robert was approaching his teenage years he was not allowed out after 5 P.M., because he was required to devote himself to homework and be in bed by 8 P.M. He became increasingly rebellious in reaction to his father's strictness, especially as he entered adolescence, and his father became increasingly disapproving of him and beat him on occasion as a form of discipline. Robert recalled getting into a lot of fights at school, defending his older brother, who was frequently the victim of name calling because of his big ears. Hearing about these fights, his father would beat him again.

The abuse brought their relationship to a crisis point when Robert was fourteen. As he recalled it, one day he was walking down the road after school with his younger brother, when a trouble-making boy shot the brother in the eye with a BB gun. Robert rushed his brother to the emergency room, where everything turned out okay, and the hospital staff praised him for his quick response. Then Robert called the town mayor about the neighborhood menace with the BB gun. The mayor called the boy's father, who was very embarrassed and punished his son.

John Taliaferro Thompson (1860–1940), an American soldier and inventor, patented the "Tommy Gun," the Thompson submachine gun, a .45-calibre gun weighing ten pounds, in 1920, when he was sixty.

Robert's father heard about this from the boy's father, who was a friend. That day, when Robert arrived home, his father was furious at him for calling the mayor and embarrassing his friend, and he started to take a swing at Robert. In that instant, Robert recalled, "I thought, 'No more of this!' and I swung at him." Robert ducked his father's blow and landed a punch of his own on his father's chin, knocking him out. His father never attempted to beat him after that.

When World War I broke out, Robert enlisted in the army. At twenty-one he became the victim of chlorine gas poisoning that caused blindness and serious chronic nosebleeds. Distraught about the blindness, he wished to die, and his condition began to decline abruptly. A perceptive nurse and hospital administrator searched for someone there who could rekindle the young soldier's desire to live. Coincidentally, visiting the hospital was a young new entertainer by the name of Arthur Godfrey, and he was asked to talk with Robert. He told Robert that it obviously took guts to soldier as he did, and that Robert should turn that courage toward a desire to live.

Godfrey's sickbed visit was a moving experience. Robert's fighting spirit, honed sharp by the years of abuse at his father's hands, revived and he grew determined to live, after all. He agreed to some new experimental treatments for chlorine gas blindness, and his vision eventually returned.

Upon leaving the army, he went on to college and became a lawyer, eventually landing a job with the Department of the Treasury, where he became one of the chief investigators in the federal government's effort

Sir Michael Foster (1689–1763), the English judge, had a great influence on the development of modern criminal law, publishing **Crown Cases and Discourses upon a Few Branches of the Crown Law** *in 1762, when he was seventy-three.*

to snare Al Capone on tax evasion. As his case against Capone grew stronger, so did gang threats on Robert's life, resulting in a number of harrowing escapes for him. At one point, I told Robert his story sounded like a movie, and he replied that it had been the subject of one later, receiving President Roosevelt's approval. He then proceeded to take out of his briefcase newspaper clippings verifying his story. Then he showed me his Department of the Treasury ID card, which he had borrowed from the National Archives.

Clearly, after Robert's boyhood with an abusive father and the follow-up bout with chlorine gas in World War I, Capone was a few steps back in the line of things that intimidated him. The severely challenging life events that had shaped the early and late parts of his adolescent development created in Robert a "resistance fighter" response, a capacity to brave danger in pursuit of his objectives, which was ideal preparation for taking on Al Capone.

Just as his difficult adolescent developmental period had shaped Robert's career choices as an adult, his retirement shaped a new phase of his adult development, allowing him the freedom to take a very different road, though one that still reflected his ease with challenge, adventure, and risk taking that took shape during his adolescence. Instead of dealing with the risk of gunshots—from boyhood BBs to bullets on the job—he engaged in "shoots" of a different kind, creative photo shoots, reflecting a new developmental influence that shaped his activities into his nineties.

A New Perspective on Adult Development: The Stages of Human Potential

Developmental growth can't be forced; you can't really teach a child to read until his brain, body, and emotions are ready for the task. When he is ready, learning looks less like hard labor and more like a blossom growing toward the light. By the same token, certain qualities of mind and action in adulthood that are developmental in nature unfold in their own good time and offer unique and exciting potential for us as we grow older.

Wisdom comes to us this way, largely a developmental product of age, smarts, and emotional and practical life experience. Jean Piaget, the Swiss psychologist noted for his landmark work on the stages of intellectual development, described "postformal thought" as a thought process that helps integrate the subjective and the objective, feeling and thinking, the heart and the mind, and emerges with aging. It plays a role in allowing us to understand and express emotions—an asset for any of us pedestrians along the walk of life. Postformal reasoning also fosters the ability to respond to complex situations with more than one right answer. Postformal thought transforms our life experience into what we commonly call "wisdom."

Jean Piaget (1896–1980) published **The Early Growth of Logic in the Child** *at age sixty-two. At the age of sixty-nine he created the International Center for Genetic Epistemology, which he directed until he died at age eighty-four. He continued publishing nearly up until his death.*

There are a host of other positive changes that open up new opportunities for creative expression as we age. It may be easier to define problems and come up with strategies over time, for instance. Our increasing knowledge, our emotional history and our social, career, and life experience all add to the inner resources we tap during the creative process. However, in order for us to take advantage of this developmental impetus, we have to recognize it in our lives.

In my thirty years of work as a doctor, a therapist, and a scientist, my formal training has been greatly enhanced by my practical education in the company of my patients, my family, my colleagues, and the many others with whom I have been fortunate to work and live. Scientific literature may be thin on the second half of life, but the older adult experience has been my "office" for all these years, and I have developed my own working theory of adult developmental stages in order to help others understand the significant obstacles and opportunities those years present.

This is significant, because today, as in no other time in history, there is more freedom of choice exercised by individuals in regard to when they have children or add new constellations of family to their lives through remarriage; layoffs and downsizing create "new opportunities" where in previous generations long careers followed by retirement were the norm. It is a new world, in many ways, but we are creatures of historic habit. We need a new frame of reference in which to picture ourselves growing, and recognize how the confluence of inner resources and life circumstances can present us with opportunities to revive our lives in meaningful, satisfying ways.

Betty Friedan (born in 1921), the American feminist author, published **The Feminine Mystique** *at age forty-two, which explored the identity and causes of the frustrations of modern women in traditional roles. At age seventy-two she published* **The Fountain of Age,** *where she explodes misconceptions about aging; and at age seventy-six she published* **Beyond Gender: The New Politics of Work and Family,** *where she contends that the time has come for women and men to move beyond identity politics and gender-based, single-issue political activism.*

Nearly all of us experience emotions in common as we get older, whether it is distress or desire that occupies our thoughts. If we recognize these feelings as natural developmental markers in our lives, we can tap the underlying developmental energy to boost our efforts to make desired changes.

Four developmental phases shape the way our creative energy grows and the way we express it. Each phase itself is shaped by our chronological age, our history, and our circumstances. And each phase is characterized by changes in how we view and experience life in a combined psychological, emotional, and intellectual sense. I call these *human potential phases*, and they are as follows:

1. *Midlife Reevaluation Phase*. During this time creative expression is shaped by a sense of crisis or quest. Although "midlife crisis" is the phrase we hear so often, most adults in this Phase actually are motivated by quest energy to make their life or work more gratifying. Midlife is a powerful time for the expression of human potential because it combines the capacity for insightful reflection with a powerful desire to create meaning in life. This Phase typically occurs in those between their forties and early sixties.

2. *Liberation Phase*. In this Phase, typically occurring in those approaching their sixties to early seventies, creative endeavors are shaped with the added energy of a new degree of personal freedom that comes both psychologically from within us and externally through retirement. Creative expression in this Phase often includes translating a feeling of "If not now, when?" into action. People tend to feel comfortable about themselves by this time, knowing that if they make a mistake it won't undo the image others have of them, and more importantly, it won't undo the image they have of themselves. This psychological and emotional understanding provides a new context for experimentation, and retirement often provides a new feeling of finally having free time to try something new. Both these inner and outer elements are liberating and additive.

3. *Summing-Up Phase*. This Phase sees creative expression shaped by the desire to find larger meaning in the story of our lives, and to give

in a larger way of the wisdom we have accrued. In the role of "keepers of the culture," the lessons and fortunes of a lifetime are shared through autobiography and personal storytelling, philanthropy, community activism, and volunteerism. This Phase typically occurs among those in their seventies or older.

4. *Encore Phase*. This is the time of advancing age, in which creative expression is shaped by the desire to make strong, lasting contributions on a personal or community level, to affirm life, take care of unfinished business, and celebrate one's own contribution. This Phase typically occurs among those around their eighties or older.

John Harvey Kellogg (1852–1943) and Will Keith Kellogg (1860–1951) were American inventors who formed W. K. Kellogg Corp. in 1906. In 1930, with both brothers in their seventies, The W. K. Kellogg Foundation took its place as one of the leading philanthropic institutions in America.

In Chapter 2 we discussed the neurobiological response of the brain to a stimulating environment. I also explained the phenomenon of dendritic sprouting by which brain cells sprouted new branches (dendrites) in response to behavioral challenge. Other findings from the biological study of the brain reveal that between one's early fifties and late seventies there is actually an increase in both the *number* and *length* of branches from individual brain cells in different parts of the brain involved with higher intellectual functioning.* Gerontologist George M. Martin has referred to these changes with aging as reflecting "sagging." These branching changes compensate for brain cell loss that can occur over time and further reflect the "plasticity" or modifiablilty of the brain as it ages. *Even more interesting about these neurobiological findings is that they directly correspond timewise to the unfolding of the above human potential phases,* pointing to a possible biological connection to the change in human development in the second half of life.

These human potential phases combine elements of age-based developmental stages as described by Erikson, with the greater fluidity of life transitions that we experience today. Sometimes we might experience a phase in synch with others our age, but not always; the age of occurrence varies. Sometimes they coexist, intersect, even synergize or combine in a way that adds even greater energy to the mix.

*This research was conducted by Stephen Buell and Paul Coleman and reported in Dorothy Flood and Paul Coleman, "Hippocampal Plasticity in Normal Aging and Decreased Plasticity in Alzheimer's Disease" in *Progress in Brain Research* 83 (1990):435-443.

Thomas Hardy (1840–1928), the great English writer, after writing novels, turned to poetry at age fifty-eight with the publication of **Wessex Poems**, *continuing his poetry until the age of sixty-eight, the year he died, when he published* **Winter Words**.

The significance of these human potential phases is that they set the stage for a new creative thrust at different points in our lives. Our awareness of these phases can help close the gap between recognizing our potential and actually harnessing it. Knowing that the natural course of our inner development in the second half of life brings us closer at different times to tapping our creative potential can provide a much needed measure of confidence or faith we need to begin, change, or energize our creative efforts.

Voices of Experience Tell Us There Is More to Come

A series of personal reflections by a diverse group of men and women over fifty reflect these adult life phases and the underlying common experience of continued growth in different ways at different times. Sometimes the comments offer a clear reflection of a single phase, other times they reflect transition or overlapping of the phases. For instance, Gwen, an eighty-seven-year-old homemaker, says, "I have grown as a person in ways I never imagined in my younger years. There is a freedom to be who you are and speak your mind that is such a relief. I can't even describe it, but it's wonderful." Her comments show a strong Summing-Up Phase influence, but they also reflect the influence of the Liberation Phase, where her new sense of freedom is apparent.

As you read their comments, listen for the different influences that combine to create this fresh, new outlook for each person.

MIDLIFE REEVALUATION PHASE

The kids are finally on their own. Now it's my turn. I'm raring to go.
—Joan (fifty), homemaker, college graduate.

After twenty-five years of working in pediatric clinics, I am looking forward to changing my focus from direct care to teaching and writing a book on raising a healthy and happy child.
—Nancy (fifty-one), pediatrician

I figured it was time to leave big bureaucracy, where I worked in environmental health, and change course to be on my own, in my own small business. I've discovered I'm a really good consultant on safety in the workplace. My early education was in both fields.

—Jacob (fifty-two), left mid-level management to consult

Four years ago, I divorced. It was a bad and sad marriage. She wasn't the only one to blame. With me, everything came first before my family life. I paid a steep price and learned my lesson the hard way. Now that I'm engaged again, I'm determined to reverse my priorities between work and home.

—Chad (fifty-five), business executive

LIBERATION PHASE

I've never been much of a risk taker, but I feel now that if something came up where I had to do something, I know I would do what needed to be done.

—James (sixty-five), retired insurance agent

I find that I stand up for myself more now, and that applies to many other older women I know. I'm on the board of directors of our retirement community, speaking my mind.

—Emily (sixty-eight), retired secretary

My dreams are fanciful stories with adventure in them. I enjoy them. I feel I now have the time and have developed the ease for learning and trying something different—with both my family life and new activities. For the first time in my life I've become politically active.

—Juan (seventy-one), retired accountant

Since sometime in my sixties, I've been more accepting of myself. That's a big change for someone of my generation, because when we were younger adults, women especially had such limited opportunities and we expected to conform to everyone else's expectations of us. If you didn't conform you were punished. That's something it felt good to outgrow. There's a kind of lessening of the struggle to be what everybody else expects you to be. It feels more like a liberation.

—Marijoy (seventy-four), retired high school teacher

Mahatma Gandhi (1869–1948), the great Indian leader and peacemaker, successfully completed negotiations in 1947 (age seventy-seven) for Britain to grant India its independence. The next year he was assassinated.

SUMMING-UP PHASE

Katherine Porter (Anne Maria Veronica Callista Russell), the American writer (1890–1980) and author of* Ship of Fools *(1962, age seventy-two), published her* Collected Short Stories *in 1965 (age seventy-five), which was awarded a Pulitzer Prize.

What are my goals? I want to write memoirs for my children and grandchildren—filled with interesting anecdotes. I just learned how to use the computer to start the process. My wife, who is also approaching eighty, said I wasn't going to leave her out, and she did the same.

—Daniel (seventy-nine), retired economist and his wife Grace (seventy-eight), retired grade school teacher

I see more clearly now the importance of volunteerism and paying back, the importance of people who know things and know how to do things sharing that with the rest. Our communities really do need us.

—Celia (eighty-one), retired librarian

My husband and I worked hard and faced many challenges. But we ended up doing well. He died and left me a modest inheritance. I want to honor him by giving to charity and those in need.

—Deborah (eighty-five), homemaker

I understand life's issues better now, and it helps me when I work on canvas.

—Will (eighty-seven), artist

ENCORE PHASE

Frank Lloyd Wright (1867–1959), internationally recognized American architect, designed the famous* Fallingwater*—a house projecting out over a waterfall—at age sixty-nine (1936). He later designed the Guggenheim Museum in New York in 1959 at age ninety-one, the year he died.

I enjoy these projects [in documentary photography] and hope to do them as long as I can; I don't ever want to get them out of my system.

—Robert (eighty-eight), retired attorney

I was always good at golf, and I like going out on the course, getting a par here and there at different holes. I can still do it. There are other things, too, that I came to do well—and am still good at—like helping people solve problems.

—Nate (ninety-two), retired career military person

In my nineties, there's the wonderment that you have survived this long, and then you begin to think of the positive side, which is, I can do pretty much what I want and no one cares.

—Catherine (ninety-three), retired legal secretary

I've come to feel at peace with my life; it wasn't easy. I would like to live long enough to see the world at peace. I don't know if I have enough time.
—Christine (one hundred one), retired social worker

Midlife Reevaluation/Quest Phase

The fourteenth-century middle-age Italian poet Dante Alighieri, in the opening lines of his great work *The Divine Comedy*, wrote:

> *Midway life's journey I was made aware*
> *That I had strayed into a dark forest,*
> *And the right path appeared not anywhere.*

So saying, Dante confronted the dark unknown, and began his search for a "right path" toward a meaningful life.

Six centuries later, despite the changes in the way we live, we continue to travel the same inner paths through the unsettling landscape of midlife. What is it that turns our sense of life's journey from a simple walk in the woods to a frightening experience of being stranded in a "dark forest" with no promising path in sight?

"It is not easy to find happiness in ourselves, and it is not possible to find it elsewhere."
—AGNES REPPLIER

Some would suggest it is the disheartening physical changes that are presumed to accompany middle age, undesirable changes so familiar that they represent a whole category of jokes about hair loss, weight gain, and limping libido. Change in our fitness and appearance can certainly have a sobering effect. However, the most disturbing aspect of middle age, the thing about middle age that so profoundly challenges our sense of self, is a dramatic, though often overlooked, change in the way we think about death.

"Far away there in the sunshine are my highest aspirations. I may not reach them, but I can look up and see their beauty, believe in them and try to follow where they lead."
—LOUISA MAY ALCOTT

At some point in life, typically in our forties or fifties, our thoughts of death change from abstract to concrete, from something that *happens* to something that *will happen*. From the time we are young, we look forward to each birthday, eagerly counting off the years that distance us from the labels of childhood. Middle age, for most of us, is the first time that we pause a bit uneasily as we contemplate the passing years, with a thought to how many we may have left. It is at this point in our lives, for the first time with depth of consciousness, that we confront our mortality. We look to the horizon and see the sunset rather than the sunrise. If the uncertainty of life leaves us daunted, the certainty of death fills us with sudden dread.

Not surprising, research on aging has found that this shift in our perspective, along with other physical and emotional transitions of middle age, have a dramatic effect on our emotional stability. The resulting angst, or profound anxiety often accompanied by depression, is a familiar hallmark of middle age. We see it in anxious or turbulent expressions of art, music, and literature. And we see it in the everyday medical symptoms of middle-age: restlessness, edginess, apprehension, worry, or irritability; muscle tension, fatigue, sleep problems, and anxious dreams; trouble concentrating or the mind going blank; the spoken and unspoken fear of death, which is, according to research, greater at middle age than in old age, when it realistically grows closer.

"Between my head and my hand, there is always the face of death," wrote Francis Picabia, French painter and poet, when he was forty-four.

John, a forty-six-year-old patient of mine, said in therapy: "Something new is happening to me. I try to look into the future in an effort to plan, but it is as if a heavy screen blocks my view and makes me feel very uneasy inside."

Barbara, forty-three, explained that she had recently grown uncomfortable about flying, a problem, since travel continued to be necessary for her work. "I was never afraid of flying before, but now I feel anxious about it," she said.

Diane, a forty-six-year-old patient, described a new, unpleasant turn in her dream life: "I was daydreaming about a beautiful butterfly flapping its wings above some flowers; then all of a sudden it was eaten by a crow. I'm having more and more daydreams like this, where something ominous occurs."

At the age of sixty-five, Aldous Huxley (1894–1963), author of **Brave New World**, *wrote his essay "Brave New World Revisited" (1959).*

Ronald, forty-four, in middle age began to experience a number of dreams in which he found himself in places from his past that were familiar—college, for instance—but in the dream he found himself having to make decisions in situations that offered no clear right choice. In one dream segment, he struggled to decide whether to get involved with a woman he had known only briefly in the past, or in taking an exam, and he was uncertain of the answers. In effect, he was going back in time, second-guessing himself at paths taken long ago, and what had seemed like familiar territory now seemed threatening, with a sense of the unknown and uncertainty about making correct choices. He was also having dreams about unfamiliar environments: buildings with complicated corridor systems and feeling lost in them; a train station where he was not sure which train to take or even what direction he was supposed to travel—east or west.

This angst is a natural defensive response to the dramatic shift in our life view at middle age, when we lose the youth-based frame of reference that has provided us a sense of order and personal control, before we have an "older, wiser" view of life to put in its place. With the emotional structures that have stabilized us through youth altered or displaced by our recognition of our mortality, our first response is fear. We remain trapped by anxiety until we regain our emotional balance and are able to devise a viewpoint that accommodates aging and life's end. This is often reflected in anxiety dreams in which we experience free falling; things seem out of our control in our universe when our perception of our lifetime changes so abruptly.

Interestingly, angst can lead either to the "midlife crisis" we recognize in desperate or impulsive attempts to reclaim the youthful body or vision, or it can be transformed into energy that drives a quest to reevaluate our life and unleash new creative energy that affirms it. Just as every crisis offers an opportunity for action that can bring about good, the angst of middle age need not be labeled "bad" just because it's painful or uncomfortable. It is emotional energy, and what matters is what we do with it.

"Anxiety is the handmaiden of creativity."

—CHUCK JONES, WARNER BROTHERS ANIMATOR

JOHN WENTWORTH: MIDLIFE QUEST MAN

John Wentworth was an assistant district attorney with a formidable passion for winning convictions against defendants in criminal cases. He got a job in the state district attorney's office right out of law school in his mid-twenties and immediately got people's attention with his aggressive and highly effective trial skills. He had always been aggres-

Studs Terkel, America's popular oral historian, had planned to practice law, but after failing his first bar exam, he decided not to pursue a career as an attorney. He subsequently embarked on a career as a radio actor, and this was followed by work as a radio disk jockey, commentator, sportscaster, and television host. Through his interviews and commentaries he emerged as an enormously engaging oral historian. At the age of seventy-two (1984), his work **The Good War: An Oral History of World War Two** *was awarded a Pulitzer Prize.*

sive and effective, a personality style already noticeable when he was in the ninth grade and a member of his school's debating team, steamrolling over opponents. At every age, his personality was part of his reputation: no one wanted to get on his wrong side. Over the next twenty years, he built up an extraordinary record of successes, and people naturally began to talk about his promising future should he seek the leadership position of state's district attorney.

However, upon turning forty, John started to become introspective and questioned what he was doing with his life, particularly after experiencing a series of related and disturbing dreams where a growing number of notches were appearing on his gun handles. He began to ponder his invincibility, his mortality. He began to ask himself, "Is this what I want to do for the rest of my life, putting away all these people?"

Four years later, opportunity triggered his decision to leave the district attorney's staff and criminal law altogether, enabling him to pursue a new quest. A college friend had successfully recruited a group of investors to fund a new biotechnology company focused on experimental genetic engineering approaches to conquering cancer. The company wanted a highly competent and aggressive chief executive officer with a background as an attorney.

John chose this new career path, recasting his crime-fighting instincts to fighting cancer instead. For John, this was more satisfying than his previous work and made him feel very much alive, making him more comfortable in dealing with his anxiety about his own mortality.

EVELYN'S STORY: NEW LIFE BORN OF MIDLIFE STRUGGLE

Evelyn was forty-two years old when her husband Jack divorced her. They had been married for eight years, but three years into their marriage, strain had developed, which she had attributed to a combination of her husband's frustration with his job and their difficulty in having a baby. She had been struggling to establish herself as a freelance journalist, writing articles for different magazines. But with the mounting stress in her marriage and her concern that she was quickly growing past the age for pregnancy, she had begun to feel increasingly fatigued and on edge to the point that her writing suffered. At forty she had been told, following extensive fertility workups, that she would not be able to conceive and was advised to consider adoption. Her husband had always said he was not interested in adopting and became even more distanced. Shortly afterward he had an affair and moved out. A year later Evelyn and Jack were divorced.

Initially, Evelyn was devastated and felt her future to be bleak. She described the low point occurring during that Easter, when she had a dream about carrying a basket of eggs, then stumbling and dropping them, with all the eggs breaking; she awoke in an extreme anxious sweat. Fortunately, she had very supportive friends who were a great comfort and pointed out the painful truth that Jack was bad for her, that things in her marriage would only have gotten worse, and that now she had a second chance. She also entered into psychotherapy.

Two years had passed since her divorce, and Evelyn met Stephan, a forty-eight-year-old philosophy professor at a community college, also divorced and with no children. They were strongly attracted to each other right from the start, and a year later got engaged and married. Stephan's first wife had not wanted children, although he did, and pushing fifty he was feeling the pressure of time, just like Evelyn. Stephan was very supportive about adopting, and together they initiated the formal process.

Remarkably, ten months after their marriage the opportunity to have a baby through adoption occurred. Four months later they were parents. They moved into a new home in the town near the campus where Stephan was teaching. When the baby was about a year old, Evelyn pursued a part-time job at the small local newspaper in the town where they lived. The editors were very impressed with her writing samples and offered Evelyn her own column, which finally gave her the chance to develop her creative writing skills fully. After a period of great pain and turbulence, Evelyn's crisis passed; now in her late forties, she has put her life on the path that for so long had eluded her.

Ida Tarbell (1857–1944) was an American journalist and chronicler of U.S. industry. Her* History of the Standard Oil Company *(1904), which she wrote at age forty-seven, focused on the unfair competitive practices John D. Rockefeller used against small petroleum producers. The book made visible the new role of women as muckraking journalists. She later wrote the history of* The Nationalizing of Business *in 1936 at age seventy-nine; this work became a standard reference on American economic growth after the Civil War. Her last book was her autobiography,* All in the Day's Work, *written when she was eighty-two.

Mary Baker Eddy (1821–1910), founder of the Christian Science Church, founded* The Christian Science Monitor *at the age of eighty-seven.

Elizabeth Cady Stanton (1815–1902) was one of the leaders of the women's rights movement in the United States. In 1840, when she got married at age twenty-five, she insisted that the word obey *be deleted from her marriage vows. In 1848, at thirty-three, she and fifty-five-year-old Lucretia Mott (1793–1880) organized the first women's rights convention in the United States at Seneca Falls, New York, launching the women's suffrage movement. Mott remained active in the movement until her death at age eighty-seven. In her seventies, Stanton teamed up with Susan B. Anthony (1820–1906) and Matilda Gage (1826–1898) to write the monumental* History of Woman Suffrage, *completed in 1887 (Stanton was seventy-two; Anthony was sixty-seven; Gage was sixty-one). Elizabeth Stanton subsequently wrote her autobiography,* Eighty Years and More, *in 1898 at the age of eighty-three.*

Coming to Terms with Middle Age

Gradually, as middle age progresses, a healthy level of emotional denial helps us overcome fear of death. By that I mean, we regain a sense of emotional balance that allows us to meet fear with the right flow of courage and inspiration to take on change and the process of engaging in exploration, innovation, and creativity. This is the "healthy denial" that characterizes our species, enabling us to explore the great reaches of space, tackle great social problems, or paint great canvases. Once the temporary distortion of fear and anxiety is becalmed, the positive pull of new development stages—human potential phases—kicks in. It is this dynamic combination of healthy defenses and development that drives our creativity forward.

Someone who has not adequately negotiated earlier stages of development and enters midlife with a sense of not being fulfilled—with career, family, or self-image—or worse, a sense of failure in life, may be moved to despair or panic resulting from this double blow of feeling profoundly unfulfilled and confronting mortality. These are individuals at risk for depression and/or midlife "crisis." Fortunately, at this stage, as well as all the others, most crises can be resolved. Sometimes sage guidance and support from significant others point toward a brighter path; sometimes a tumultuous period of trial-and-error experimentation and self-absorption with new endeavors and relationships and uncertain outcomes follows; sometimes therapy provides new insights.

One of the great things about the human body is that it moves toward equilibrium once things are disrupted; this is built in. If we get an infection, our immune system responds, releasing white cells to combat the infection; our temperature increases to speed up the reaction of the white cells; and so on. Initially, the white cells are overwhelmed by the challenge, but then they catch up. Our psychological defense system works in a similar way. A disturbance or disorder—anxiety or depression, for example—triggers our psychological mechanisms of defense, such as denial and rationalization. While we initially may feel overwhelmed, given the proper support and time we begin to adjust and restore our emotional equilibrium. Again, it's how our minds work. When an infection is too great, we go for antibiotics, rest, and chicken soup. When anxiety is too great, we may need extra external help to regain our balance: support from others and perhaps therapy and medication.

However the challenge of this phase is experienced, it offers exciting opportunities for creative growth and new forms of expression. This finding is consistent with those of the MacArthur Foundation study on midlife that reported uncovering less midlife crisis than expected among those age forty to sixty who comprise more than sixty million Americans. Of course, even if only 5 to 10 percent in this age group experience turmoil of crisis proportions, it still amounts to several million people. Also, many who do experience turmoil short of a full-blown crisis eventually experience restored equilibrium and find that the rough waters stirred them to chart a more creative course. And many who go through a crisis do the same.

While the MacArthur Foundation study highlighted finding less *crisis* than anticipated in the middle years, what it did not articulate was the magnitude of *quest* that occurs during this stage of one's life, quest catalyzed by the psychological dynamics of the midlife reevaluation phase of human development. This stage infuses us with new energy to fire up our inner life experience in the "e^2" component of the $C = me^2$ creativity equation, fostering new potential for creative growth during midlife.

"The man who views the world at fifty the same as he did at twenty has wasted thirty years of his life."

—MUHAMMAD ALI

BRAD AND BETSY'S STORY
WORK-LIFE ISSUES IN TRANSITION

Brad was a forty-one-year-old workaholic attorney on Capitol Hill. Since age twenty-nine he had worked for a Congressman who was always worried about being reelected, and this obsession played out in his placing great demands on those who worked for him—something Brad, already too much a captive of his work, didn't need. Brad had been in several relationships with women since working on the Hill, but he exhausted the patience of each of them with all the dates he would break at the last minute because of the latest crisis with the Congressman.

Turning forty did catch Brad's attention and he began to get increasingly impatient over little annoyances at work. He also started to develop some resentment toward the Congressman, whom he came to view as controlling his life. Then Brad met Betsy.

Betsy, thirty-seven, also a lawyer, worked on the Hill, too. But she had reached her limits and was starting to contemplate a lifestyle change and the idea of starting a family. They had actually known each other superficially for several years, but became close while working together intensely for several months on legislation that their Congressmen employers were going to cosponsor.

Jeannette Rankin (1880–1973) was the first female member of the U.S. Congress, serving two terms—1917–1919 (ages thirty-seven to thirty-nine) and 1941–1943 (ages sixty-one to sixty-three). In 1968, at the age of eighty-seven, she led 5,000 women, calling themselves the "Jeannette Rankin Brigade," to the foot of Capitol Hill in Washington, D.C., to protest the war in Vietnam.

They fell in love and discussed getting married. But Betsy also recognized Brad's workaholic nature, and she knew that his working on Capitol Hill could place a great deal of strain on a marriage.

She began to push him to think about a job change, pointing out to him how his job appeared to be getting to him, describing his increased irritation with it. Betsy also informed him that she was resigning from her job in six months even if she didn't have another job in place; she had already given notice.

Brad was incredulous. He could not conceive of someone leaving a job without another job already lined up. Brad was also in a rut. He couldn't take the next step and seriously think about change. He was becoming increasingly anxious. The three colleagues he had grown closest to on the Hill had all left. Each had gotten married. All were starting families. Brad was wondering what was happening to him, or more accurately, what *wasn't* happening to him?

As he became increasingly anxious, he started to wonder, should he get married, could he handle it with everything else? Then he began asking those questions one often asks at his stage of life. Who am I? Where am I going? Why and for what? All of this questioning only made him more anxious.

Then circumstances lent a hand. His Congressman lost reelection. Come January Brad would be out of a job. At first, it really made him anxious, but Betsy suggested that this was the break he needed—the chance for a fresh start that he'd been unable to initiate himself. It was now or never, she said.

When I later saw the two of them in counseling, they recounted Brad's hesitation about coming. Brad had obsessed endlessly about his predicament, asking over and over again, "What am I going to do?"

When Betsy suggested he seek counseling, he refused. "Not me," Brad said, "I don't believe in it; I'm not going to join the ranks of the worried well in endless psychoanalysis." Betsy had countered that he was indeed worried and didn't look at all well.

Brad reluctantly agreed to give couples counseling a try for at least four visits. In counseling he was asked if he felt he was in control of his life. He answered honestly, "No." He was then asked what would give him control. "A job," he said. Betsy added, jokingly, "A seventy-hour-a-week job." Brad laughed, too, and saw the truth in her comment. The way he usually worked, the job took control of him rather than vice versa. He was asked what his ideal job might be. Betsy again piped in: "One that locked the employees out before nine A.M. and after five P.M. and all day on weekends!" Brad agreed it would be great if the job set those limits. He simply felt he couldn't.

"It's easy to come up with new ideas; the hard part is letting go of what worked for you two years ago, but will soon be out of date."

—ROGER VON OECH

They tried to identify jobs that could set limits to allow a normal lifestyle. Betsy had begun to think about teaching law with built-in summers off. The thought of teaching was intriguing to Brad, as well, in part because in his former job he had given several lectures a year at the local universities, drawing upon his Hill experience; these had been some of his most satisfying diversions. Why not try making the appealing diversion the mainstay?

Betsy was encouraging, and Brad gave it further thought but wondered whether it would pay enough. Betsy pointed out that the pay wasn't much different from that of his previous job, and further, she pointed out, with the two of them pooling their earnings they could pick and choose work that would give them more of a life together. They stayed in counseling twelve weeks, during which time Brad actually did pursue teaching possibilities and got a job as an assistant professor at one of the local law schools. Betsy did not find a teaching job, but found a very flexible part-time position with a public interest group that promised her lengthy periods off during the summer. They then got married, committed to each other and committed to a future that promised new adventures in work *and* free time together.

Hardinge Stanley Giffard (1823–1921), an English lawyer, supervised the development of the digest **The Laws of England** *(1905–1916), from the age of eighty-two until he was ninety-three.*

When you look at the midlife stories of Brad and Betsy, Evelyn, John Wentworth, and many others, these aren't stereotypic stories in which midlifers in crisis turn everything upside down and throw away the past to start something completely new. They are instead stories of the developmental struggle—especially challenging in middle age—to harness the emotional energy of the age and use it to move through sometimes difficult life experiences and on to the next level of creative potential.

Benedetto Croce (1866–1952), considered the foremost Italian philosopher of the first half of the twentieth century, with great courage protested the rise of Fascism, writing in opposition to Mussolini with such works as **History as the Story of Liberty** *(at age seventy-two). He survived considerable censure as he acted upon his conscience. With the fall of Mussolini in 1943, Croce, at age seventy-seven, played a leading role in helping to resurrect liberal institutions in Italy. At age eighty-five he published* **Philosophy, Poetry, History.**

Liberation Phase: Risk Taking and Courage

There was a time when the number sixty-five meant one thing: retirement. For anyone with a paying job, this was the year you left it behind; the day you retired was, in many important ways, the first day of the rest of your life. Your income, your schedule, your responsibilities, and your circle of human contact changed instantly to retirement mode, a long-awaited liberation for some, a dreaded period of loss for others unprepared for the freedom of time and movement. For homemakers, a similar liberation and shift in relationships came on the heels of children departing "the nest" to start lives on their own.

Today, the liberation we once associated with the sixth and seventh decades of life now occurs across a wider range of ages. Corporate downsizing, layoffs, and early retirement turn younger adults out to pursue new paths. Some studies that have looked at career paths of managers and workers found that the average worker changes jobs six to eight times before settling into a stable employment relationship, while managers often change jobs even more frequently. Divorce, remarriage, delayed childbearing, and the return of adult children to their parents' homes has scattered in the wind any age-based concept of the empty nest.

If we look beyond age markers alone and search instead for the underlying developmental phase of adult life, we find that it is defined by a kind of personal liberation combined with life experience that lifts inhibitions and gives the courage to ignore social conventions that restrict our creative expression.

Mark Twain (1835–1910) published **"The Man That Corrupted Hadleyburg" and Other Stories and Sketches** *at age sixty-five.*

"The seventieth birthday!" wrote Mark Twain upon reaching his. "It is the time of life when you arrive at a new and awful dignity; when you may throw aside the decent reserves which have oppressed you for a generation and stand unafraid and unabashed upon your seven-terraced summit and look down and teach—unrebuked."

This new sense of available time and personal liberty in later life, combined with significant life experience, produces new feelings of freedom, courage, and confidence commonly described by men and women of advanced age. Here, too, contrary to negative stereotypes, the feeling of being more free allows older individuals to experiment, to take a risk, to try something new. Most of us, as we head into our sixties, at least have become comfortable with who we are; if we make a mistake while trying something new, it doesn't threaten our identity or shatter our image among friends. So, while someone in his twenties may not take an art class for fear of looking incompetent, the same person in his forties, fifties, or sixties will be much less concerned about appearances and much more interested in experimenting with new ways to learn. In this frame of mind, we're more likely to take a chance on a class or a cruise or some other novel experience than we would have been at a younger age.

Retirement is like a patron, providing time and resources for many to explore new interests rather than having to focus just on making ends meet.

Research underscores the adventurous nature of adults in this liberated phase of development. Studies show that older adults who are not handicapped by extenuating circumstances—those resulting in significant physical limitations or financial constraints—are just as venturesome as their younger counterparts. This greater freedom and courage that many older adults exhibit help explain why throughout history so many older adults about or beyond age seventy have assumed the role of shapers or shakers of society. Socrates, Copernicus, Galileo, Mahatma Gandhi, Golda Meir, and Nelson Mandela are but a few among myriad individuals who have risen to greatness in these later years.

Golda Meir (1898–1978) was Prime Minister of Israel from 1969 to 1974 (between age seventy and seventy-six).

It is evidence of the resilience of the human spirit that this self-liberation of the creative spirit can bloom even after longstanding adversity and despite extraordinary psychological traumas that challenge our ability to develop normally, both emotionally and behaviorally. It is never too late for that liberation to occur, never too late to surmount trauma, and in many, many lives, this liberation takes place only in later life.

FRIEDA LASKA: SURVIVAL AND THE LATE BLOOMER

Frieda Laska, sixty-seven, struggled simply to survive the first six decades of her life, suffering abuse and neglect throughout her childhood and through middle age, which left her emotionally scarred and isolated, with feelings of low self-worth, shame, and self-doubt. I met her when she reached her sixties, and both her changing social circumstances and the new developmental phase she was entering—the liberation phase—uncovered new paths for her.

Frieda was born into a family with six brothers and two sisters; she was the third oldest, with two older brothers. She described her father as an alcoholic who treated her in a fun-loving way but abused his wife, Frieda's mother. Her mother, in turn, was a harsh disciplinarian who whipped Frieda for disobedience, frequently sent her to bed without supper, and kept her home from school to maintain strict control. Her father would not intervene to stop her mother's abuse. Steeped in despair as a child, she said, she often contemplated suicide and made one unsuccessful attempt.

Her mother managed the money in the family but never bought Frieda a doll or a new dress, only used ones. She received her first new clothes and her first doll from the nuns in parochial school when she was in the fifth grade.

Charles Perrault (1628–1703), a French writer, studied law, then at the age of sixty-nine (1697), by retelling half-forgotten folk tales, created the versions of "Cinderella," "Sleeping Beauty," "Little Red Riding Hood," and others that were to establish the classical form and standard of modern literary fairy tales.

When she was about twelve, Frieda was raped by her two older brothers, and suffered continuing sexual abuse by them for several months until her mother, without explanation, took her out of school and sent her to a nearby farm to live and work. Her pay was sent home. A woman at the farm took a liking to Frieda and bought her a beautiful new green dress; Frieda said she felt like Cinderella. The woman would also talk to Frieda, counsel her, and make sure she was well fed. This woman became a caring mother figure in Frieda's life, and other adults in the rural community responded to Frieda with similar positive attention or genuine affection. Her godfather treated her kindly, as did the town baker, who treated her to rides in his delivery buggy. Frieda also returned to school and found comfort in the friendships she made there and at her church.

Though she felt she had incorporated in her own life some of her father's positive side—his fun-loving qualities—she also had incorporated his legacy of abuse in her first marriage, as is often the case in the lives of adults who have been abused as children.

Frieda married when she was twenty-one, remaining so until her husband died when she was sixty. She described him as autocratic, not allowing her to buy anything, never complimenting her, and often criticizing her. She described him on one occasion giving her a list of thirteen things about her that he didn't like. She wanted to dance, but he wouldn't let her. She was also discouraged from driving—"You'll scratch my car," he would complain. If she raised her voice at him, she'd get the silent treatment for as long as two to three weeks. She often longed to die, though never tried to commit suicide.

"No one can make you feel inferior without your consent."

—ELEANOR ROOSEVELT

She felt, in retrospect, that her first husband reflected the abusiveness of her father toward her mother and her mother's coldness toward her. Three years after his death, she married again, and saw things go from bad to worse. Husband number two wanted only her money. Now in her mid-sixties, she felt a new courage and listened to her friends who said she should get into therapy and divorce him. She did both. Her second marriage ended after six months.

Her greatest new insight was that she should move to a place that would offer a supportive, not a stressful or abusive, environment. She realized that she should never again get married. She had always been good at making friends, so she thought a retirement community with a strong social program would be good, and without an autocrat over her—as her mother and husband had been—she might finally have a chance to emerge into the world. And emerge she did.

This was truly a liberation period for Frieda. Avoiding strongly negative interpersonal relationships for the first time in her life, she was fully able to tap into the liberating dynamics of her retirement. She had retired, or more accurately, resigned from her past as a daughter, then housewife, under siege.

She was a Cinderella set free. Over the next several years as she entered her seventies, she gradually grew comfortable with the idea of using her money to buy new dresses, go to good restaurants, venture on trips to see new places, and in general to treat herself well. She took swimming lessons to overcome a lifelong fear of water. From her ther-

Margaret Rudkin (1897–1967) started the Pepperidge Farm bakeries in 1937 with a few loaves of home-baked whole wheat bread. In 1963, at sixty-six years of age, she wrote* The Margaret Rudkin Pepperidge Farm Cookbook, *which went on to become a bestseller.

apy she learned that if negative memories began to color her current thoughts and behavior, she could reverse this downhill emotional slide by focusing on positive life experiences—her kind godfather, the friendly baker and his buggy, the farm woman who bought her the beautiful green dress and took her under her wing—people who had valued her and tried to help.

It was an extraordinary revelation for her that she could dare to give a second thought to a longing and then act on it. Her newfound ability to listen to her own thoughts and her own desires reflected emotional growth for Frieda; she had entered a new developmental phase of her life and was learning to deal differently with both the inner and outer obstacles to self-expression in her life.

She was launched on a new creative path. She now viewed her future as "a time when my dreams will come true." She described a list of new ventures she wanted to get involved with, indicating her goal was to come up with thirteen different things she could feel good about. I commented that her first husband would have appreciated that number; we both laughed. She had already begun to move up that list.

The liberation phase may foster creativity with a big *C*—creative achievement that could change the course of one's community or culture—or it may inspire creativity with a little *c*—creative accomplishment that could change the course for oneself or one's family. No matter what the scope of the action, at the heart of it is the inner freedom that moved Jenny Joseph to write in her 1969 poem *miss rosie*: "When I am an old woman I shall wear purple."

Late-Life Summing-Up

With increasing age, across all fields of human endeavor, there is an increased desire, and even urgency, to sum up our life's work, ideas, and discoveries and to share them with our family or society. The desire to sum up late in life becomes profound and inspired in many, driven by varied feelings—wanting to complete one's life work, needing to give after receiving much in life, sensing there may not be much time left. The result is that we discover or create important opportunities for sharing and expression.

Autobiography, for example, becomes one of the most dynamic and enduring ways of transmitting multiple dimensions of knowledge about an area to the next generation. From philosophy to physics, from politics to prose, leaders in virtually all fields have displayed a tendency to write or convey their autobiographies in later years. Autobiography becomes a significant source of social creativity in the second half of life. It also builds upon natural tendencies with aging to reminisce and elaborate stories, either in oral, written, or visual form. This summing up process in general also comprises a key dynamic underlying the role of older persons as keepers of the culture. We'll explore autobiography as therapy and legacy in Chapter 8, but for now it's important to recognize that this "urge to tell" is innate and, I believe, part of nature's plan to pass the wisdom of human experience on from one generation to another.

This desire to "give back," to leave a legacy, written or otherwise, also shows itself in interesting patterns of philanthropy and volunteerism in later life.

Annie King Phillips, whose first career of twenty-seven years was as a teacher in the public schools of the District of Columbia, embarked on a second career in public health administration upon obtaining her master's degree in public health at the age of fifty-five. She "retired" at age sixty-six only to embark on a vigorous new career as a volunteer, creatively incorporating all that she had learned in both education and health to help the disadvantaged in her city. At age seventy-five, she began writing autobiographical poetry that draws upon her combined rich African-American and Native American heritages, adding another dimension to her role as a keeper of the culture. At seventy-nine, she made this mission a major part of her life.

When we share our life stories, the telling has distinct therapeutic effect. You might be surprised at the significant number of people past eighty who explore psychotherapy for precisely this reason. More and more, we are a "psychological society," a culture increasingly at ease with the idea of introspection, and more older people today are well aware of the potential benefits of therapy, even if they haven't tried it before; as they confront the issues of advancing age they are more comfortable accessing counseling services.

Geronimo (1829–1908) was an Apache chief born in Arizona. His Indian name was Goyathlay ("one who yawns"). For generations the Apache had resisted white colonization by both Spaniards and Americans from the East Coast. For decades, Geronimo heroically and effectively continued that tradition, achieving fame, before finally being captured. At the age of seventy-seven he dictated his autobiography, titled **Geronimo: His Own Story.**

Ella Deloria (1889–1971), a Yankton Sioux Native American linguist and author was a true keeper of her culture. She translated thousands of pages of ethnographic texts written in the Sioux language and compiled a Lakota (a dialect of the Sioux) grammar and dictionary. At the age of seventy-three, in conjunction with the University of South Dakota's Institute for Indian Studies, she received a large National Science Foundation grant to compile a Sioux dictionary. She continued working on her dictionary, publishing articles and lecturing, until shortly before her death at age eighty-two. Her activities played a significant role in ensuring the survival and continued strength of the Sioux language.

During the twenty-five-year longitudinal study I conducted in a high-rise apartment building for older persons living independently, every two to three months a person over 80 or one of their family members would contact me. The oldest person I was asked to see was 104, and she concluded that even the one visit was "very worthwhile." These are people of an age who are generally unafraid of what they'll find out about themselves and instead are curious to find it out.

I first saw Mrs. Elizabeth Broyer when she was eighty-nine; I was twenty-eight. She was suffering from anxiety then, heard there was a psychiatrist—*shrink* was her actual word—in the building and thought she would give it a try. She had never seen a shrink before. In the past year she had first lost an older sister, and then, six weeks prior to our meeting, her younger brother. Even though she had been fairly close with her family, she was not sure that all that she had wanted to say had been said and shared with her lost siblings.

We reviewed her relationships with them, and she came to realize that nothing major had been left unresolved. There had been a few things she would have liked to discuss with them, but she eventually felt all right about it. Over a period of several months she also discussed unresolved concerns about her life in general and came to feel that here, too, there was much to feel good about; she had done well by others and by herself. The relatively minor background doubts she had had were brought to the forefront and exaggerated by the grief that she experienced around the loss of her two siblings. The grief passed and the doubts cleared, and we terminated therapy.

Seven years later, now ninety-six, she called me again, saying she had a recurrence of her anxiety, and asking if we could meet again. She walked into my office, sat down, stared at me, and commented: "The last time we met, you were young and your face was clean." With this statement, she passed the preliminary mental status test, because the last time we met I hadn't had my current beard. While this time, too, she had anxiety, it was of a different quality and upon further evaluation it turned out to be a symptom associated with a cardiac arrhythmia for which she started treatment. She spent the next six months re-reviewing her long, interesting life in our sessions, this time with pride instead of doubts—a creative summing-up that I was able to persuade her to share with her daughter. As a result, she was enriched by a new appreciation for her own life and by how others appreciated it, and she was better able to enjoy the time she spent with her family.

The Encore Phase: No "Swan Songs" for Creativity

This latest-blooming human potential phase is often referred to as the "Swan Song" stage, named in ancient fable for the sweet song supposedly sung by a dying swan and connoting the last act or final creative work of a person before death. I don't see it that way for a number of reasons. First, it suggests a single event—a kind of grand exit—rather than a whole phase of human potential. Then, there is a sadness about the term, a feeling of ending rather than a feeling of celebration more appropriate to this creative encore. And the notion of a final event implies that there can be no more. This is most untrue and is another negative stereotype of aging that denies the fresh contributions of thought and activity that the eldest in our society routinely and repeatedly share.

Lionel Hampton, American jazz musician (b. 1909), introduced the vibraphone into jazz and became the first musician to record on the vibraphone. He recorded with Louis Armstrong in 1930 (at age twenty-one), played in Benny Goodman's band, formed his own big band in 1940, continuing as a bandleader into his seventies and continuing to perform past age eighty.

There can be more than one or even many encores. In the advancing years of late life, there is a desire—a developmental urgency—to affirm life in any number of ways. It might be in a creative work, the resolution of a longstanding problem, a statement waiting to be said, or the right thing to do that had been on hold for years. The powerful quality of that love of life is conveyed in the last two lines of Shakespeare's Sonnet 73:

> *This thou perceiv'st, which makes thy love more strong,*
> *To love that well which thou must leave ere long.*

The encore phenomenon taps the inner pressure that many feel to do or say something before it's too late. Not to overlook the obvious, the phrase applies strongly to the field of music, reminding us of how many noted musical achievements have come late or at the end of a musician's or composer's career or life cycle—like the late works of Verdi, Liszt, and Stravinsky.

The great Italian composer Giuseppe Verdi (1813–1901) composed his operatic masterpiece Otello *at age seventy-four.*

Manuel Patricio Rodriguez García (1805–1906), the Spanish singing teacher and inventor of the laryngoscope, taught singing at the Royal Academy of Music in London until the age of ninety.

Falstaff was Verdi's final opera, composed in 1893, when he was eighty. *Falstaff,* a great comic libretto, was produced at La Scala and vindicated Verdi in the realm of comedy in that his prior attempt fifty-five years earlier in the same theater had been a sad failure; it was an area of his work that he felt, until then, was incomplete. Nineteenth-century composer Franz Liszt's vocal and piano works in his last years, when he was in his seventies, though viewed as strange at the time, were markedly experimental and considered prophetic of twentieth-century developments. Igor Stravinsky, born in 1882, throughout his career personified innovation in rhythm and harmony in twentieth-century music, still working at it until he was eighty-eight, shortly before his death in 1971. In his late seventies, Stravinsky, in one of several bursts of innovation in his career, integrated diverse twentieth-century schools of music in his compositions *Canticum Sacrum, Agon, Threni,* and *Movements for Piano and Orchestra.*

Artists, Encores, and Us: "Late" Style or Fresh Perspective?

Because artists express in some visible, audible, tangible way the universe of human emotions, we can look at artists' lives and works, and the way they have been interpreted, to see how the encore phase offers us new creative energy and expression as long as we live.

Some art historians and observers suggest that certain qualities characterize the "late style" work of artists, writers, and composers. For instance, they say older artists and musicians tend to emphasize unity and harmony. Painters and other visual artists express unity and harmony through decreased tension in the content, muted colors, and calmer tones. In musical composition, these qualities result in greater simplicity to the melody. The late-life work of poets, too, has been described as having elements of harmony through a calm, meditative tone. Other common characteristics of "late style" in creative work point to a conciseness in art, music, and writing alike. Artists are said to have more economy in their brush strokes; composers are said to have shorter works; writers are said to be more sparing with their words. Late works are also depicted as being more subjective than objective in content, and often more introspective, focusing more on inner emotions and experiences than on outer world scenes and events. This is especially true with writers. And some observers note a greater attention to themes of aging and issues of death in late-life works.

These views are not restricted to the arts. In many fields, there seems to be a process of paring down or an integration of ideas, as reflected in the many writings of histories of fields, textbooks, memoirs, observations, and philosophy accrued over a lifetime.

While a number of patterns are justified and do exist among numerous artists, they by no means occur universally in the creative works of older persons. For example, while the work of late-life writers has been described as being more concise and sparing of words than their earlier works, the noted literary scholar Leon Edel found American novelist Henry James's writing style to have become more complex with age. James, who wrote into his seventies in the early twentieth-century, used longer and more complex sentences in his late-life writings. Also, while there are those portraying late-life poetry as calm and meditative, others point out late-life writings that reflect anger and cynicism.

Liberace (1919–1987) played piano by ear at four. At fourteen he appeared as a soloist with the Chicago Symphony Orchestra. At age sixty-six (1985), he broke all box-office records at the massive Radio City Music Hall in New York with his flamboyant performances.

In music, many examples contradict the typical patterns of late style creativity. Johann Sebastian Bach, for example, composed right up until his death at age sixty-five, working on a masterly piano series titled *The Art of Fugue*. Rather than moving toward simplicity, though, these fugues were arranged in a general order of increasing complexity, where Bach used ever more difficult and abstruse contrapuntal devices, though always handled with masterful ease.

The late work of Richard Wagner also departs from these patterns. Wagner is viewed as having reformed the whole structure of opera. *Parsifal*, staged when Wagner was sixty-nine, is considered perhaps his greatest opera. Rather than based on inner life, it was inspired by a great piece of literature—one of the King Arthur stories. Parsifal, one of the heroes from King Arthur's Round Table, eventually became the guardian of the Holy Grail.

In art, too, it is not difficult to find examples that go against this late style stereotype. The late-life work of American painter Georgia

The noted twentieth-century sculptor Louise Nevelson, who continued to sculpt until she was well into her eighties, changed the materials used in her sculpture in 1966, when she was sixty-seven, as she began to use Plexiglas and aluminum.

O'Keeffe, her *Sky Above Clouds* series, contained some of her most expansive, as opposed to most concise, works. *Sky Above Clouds IV*, done when she was 78, is 8 by 24 feet. Moreover, the clouds do not represent death or the afterlife. On the contrary, there are feelings of life and optimism with her blue sky above these clouds—reminiscent of Grandma Moses' painting *Rainbow* when she was 101. As for harmony in late style work, the very talented twentieth-century sculptor Louise Bourgeois created her formidable painted wood, latex, and fabric environmental sculpture titled *Confrontation* at age sixty-seven—an unsettling, complex work that is 37 feet long by 20 feet wide—hardly concise.

Statements or actions from politicians in their later years that appear to be departures from earlier stances are a form of the encore phase and social creativity. So too, with philanthropists, many of whom become prominent in their later years. After many decades of acquiring wealth, these individuals have a desire to make a different—if not final—statement by giving. At a personal level, reconciling difficult relationships, doing imaginative volunteer work, and creating memoirs to hand down resonate as encores that represent creativity with a little c. Clearly, the encore phase is neither a swan song nor a winding down of creative energy. As it applies to all of us and in everyday life, regardless of our field of endeavor we are reminded that it is never too late for creative expression.

ELEANOR AVERY: A SECRET SONG

I visited Eleanor Avery in the nursing home. She was an eighty-eight-year-old widow, dying from lung cancer. I had just started conducting my study on life in the nursing home. Eleanor saw me walking down the corridor several times and asked the nurse who I was. When she learned what I was doing, she asked the nurse if she could participate in the study.

"Sometimes you just gotta trust that your secret's been kept long enough."
—ANNE CAMERON

On my third visit with her she told me, "I'm eighty-eight and have said many things to many people, but I realized I've told you things I've never told anyone before." I told her I was both very flattered and very appreciative, and that such depth of sharing would help make my study important to others. She then said, "I have a deep secret that I have kept for seventy years; I have never told anybody about it, not even my parents back then, but I have always wanted to talk about it." I told her she had my rapt attention.

She said that when she was eighteen she was married for the first time, meaning that she had been married twice. Nobody ever knew about her first marriage. She had never told anyone, concerned about the impact this would have in her small town. In this small town, as she was growing up, James, the boy down the street, was the one her family always thought she would marry, and James courted her from the day she turned sixteen; James was eighteen. And she always thought she would marry James, even as a little girl, when she had first developed a crush on him.

When she was seventeen she had her first opportunity ever to leave home during the summer break before entering her senior year in high school. That summer while visiting relatives she met Tommy, and by their second date they were passionately in love. Tommy was also visiting relatives and lived across the country. They were heartbroken at the end of the summer to have to go back home, far from each other, but vowed that when they came back the next summer, which they were each determined to do, if they were still in love they'd get married. Eleanor told me that when you're seventeen and haven't seen the world, things like that can happen to you.

The next summer each did return and the romance burned just as strong. They again talked about marriage, but Tommy agonized that his family expected him to go to college in order to prepare to take a role in the family business. He said they would be furious if they thought he wanted to get married, but he told Evelyn he loved her very deeply. Evelyn, surprising herself, asked him if they could get married secretly, and when the time was right tell their families. They were both just eighteen. Tommy agreed and they were secretly married, again each going to their separate homes at the end of the summer, planning to write and wait for the right moment to break the news.

Upon returning home, James proposed to Eleanor, and Eleanor's parents were quite pleased. They were very fond of James and were closest of friends with James's family. Eleanor felt in a terrible bind, but things got even more complicated. Shortly after Tommy arrived home,

Claudine-Alexandrine Guérin de Tencin (1681–1749), a French writer and courtesan, was the author of various romances, including* Les Malheurs de l'amour, *written in 1747, when she was sixty-six.

he learned that he had developed leukemia. Not knowing then how rare and aggressive it was, by letters they planned a visit, but six months later, before the visit materialized, Tommy developed pneumonia and died.

Eleanor was devastated and in even greater stress, because she felt that if she revealed that they had gotten married, her parents might never forgive her and that her friendship with James would be over. She also felt that if Tommy's parents knew, it would tarnish their last views of him. So she kept the secret, a terrible burden for a eighteen-year-old young woman already in deep grief.

Eleanor grieved her loss deeply and delayed any plans of marriage with James, though she never explained why. Three years later she married him. It was a long and good marriage, and James had been a wonderful husband. Eleanor had now been a widow for seven years. All through the years, though, Eleanor had felt she couldn't tell her secret to anyone. She didn't want to hurt James's feelings, and even after he died she didn't want to alter her children's image that their parents' marriage had always been very special. Of course, it had been very special, but Eleanor felt divulging her secret would only complicate her loved ones' feelings about her and their family life, which had been rich and full. But you could tell from the expression on her face and the sweet sadness of her tone that something had been left unfinished.

She said, "Last night I dreamed about Tommy; it was a very beautiful dream. I think I dreamed about him because this is the month when Tommy and I got married. I also knew I would be seeing you today, and I always wanted to tell somebody, and I knew," she said with a smile, "that a psychiatrist is trained to keep secrets." We met several more times and she talked about more special thoughts and feelings that had been locked in the secret diary in her mind. She died five months later. That was twenty-five years ago, and this is the first time I have written about her story.

Berthold Goldschmidt (1903-1996), the German composer, helped to complete Mahler's unfinished Tenth Symphony and conducted its first performance in 1988. Goldschmidt was eighty-five.

It might seem odd to include Eleanor's story here, in the company of Johann Sebastian Bach and Grandma Moses and such renowned examples of creative spirit in late life, but in essential matters of the heart, they shared a similar quality of the encore phase expression.

Eleanor's life was like a CD full of rich, wonderful tunes from a life fully lived, but her secret was the song that had never been sung.

Her story of tragic love was something beautiful, while bittersweet, that had always been a part of her inner life, a part silenced all those years. In her act of sharing the story with me, she was, at last, presenting herself fully and freely, without caution, without concern for consequences. It was something she was able to do because life presented her with the opportunity at the right time and in the right place, with the right person. She was pleased to be able to contribute her life story to something larger—my research study—and at this point in her life, she wanted her story to express who she really was; she wanted to be whole.

G. Stanley Hall (1844–1927), the noted psychologist, educator, and founder of the **American Journal of Psychology,** *at age seventy-nine published* **Life and Confessions of a Psychologist.**

The Career Curve: Why the First Isn't Necessarily the Best

The idea that we *grow* as we grow older—that our potential for creativity continues to develop—goes against what is widely considered popular wisdom or "common sense." Whenever I speak at professional conferences or community meetings about the unrecognized potential of creativity with aging, I hear challenges to the idea. I call them "gotcha" questions, because they are usually raised by people who sincerely believe they have evidence that contradicts my optimism.

By age sixteen Mozart had composed twenty-five symphonies. Of course, since he only lived to be thirty-five, we never had a chance to see what he could do in his late years.

One of the gotcha challenges I hear most often has to do with career achievement and the observation that the greatest accomplishments of humankind's best and brightest minds typically occur early in their careers. At first glance, it might seem to be true: mathematicians and poets, in particular, are typically viewed as reaching the height of their creativity as younger adults.

If we look more closely, however, we see that the evidence tells a much more intriguing story that only underscores the power of creativity, as well as the power of negative stereotypes to obscure the truth. Misconceptions and negative stereotypes about aging are so ingrained in our culture that even experts in a given field fail to see an accurate picture of the potential for aging members of their own field.

Poets and mathematicians, for instance, are typically described as reaching their creative peak early in life, producing at relatively young

Arthur Glyn Prys-Jones edited the first anthology of Welsh poetry and later published several verses of his own, including "Valedictory Verses" in 1978 at age ninety. He was president of the Welsh Academy from age eighty-two (1970) until his death at age ninety-nine.

Christine de Pisan (1363–1431), a prolific French poet who composed several works championing women, wrote at age sixty-six in celebration of Joan of Arc's early successes.

ages their exceptional works of literature or theory that redefine the realm. Keats, Shelley, Byron, and Dylan Thomas, for example, were all writing accomplished verse in their early twenties. But like Mozart they all died young, not providing an opportunity to show what later life might have brought. Thomas died at age thirty-nine; Byron at thirty-six; Shelley at twenty-nine; and Keats at twenty-five.

When poet Stanley Kunitz won a National Book Award in 1995 at age ninety, for his book *Passing Through,* another noted poet offered the following praise: "One of America's great poets. Most poets dry up at fifty. For him to be writing poems at ninety is just incredible."

I was particularly struck by the comment "Most poets dry up at fifty." This certainly was not my impression in reviewing poetry across a span of nearly three thousand years—from the Greek epic poet Homer (eighth century B.C.) to the Irish poet William Butler Yeats (1865–1939), to the American poet Maya Angelou, born in 1928, the poet at President Clinton's 1993 inauguration.

One of the ways I evaluated creativity with aging among contemporary poets was to review the book *The Best American Poetry of 1997.* Of the seventy-four included, 46 percent of those whose ages were provided were fifty or older. There were 14.5 percent age sixty-five and older—a percentage greater than the number of people age sixty-five and older in the population as a whole. In effect, the older poets were *overrepresented* from a statistical standpoint. From this group, it would be impossible to conclude that most poets dry up after fifty. Incidentally, the poet who made that comment—Mark Strand—was himself included in this "best American poets of 1997" group; he was sixty-three.

What about mathematics, the field in which aging stereotypes may be greatest? They reveal several patterns that also apply to most if not all fields. First, there are those, despite the stereotype, who remain creatively active in elaborating mathematical theory and discovery throughout their lives. Three of the greatest mathematicians of all time, Archimedes, Sir Isaac Newton, and Carl Friedrich Gauss (Einstein was more a theoretical physicist, using mathematics in the service of physics), were very active up to or close to their deaths, Archimedes and Gauss in their late seventies, Newton in his mid-eighties.

Despite the celebrated nature of their earlier work, many mathematicians make significant and original contributions in later life. The great eighteenth-century Swiss mathematician Leonhard Euler made his greatest discovery the year he died, at age seventy-six, in 1783, and that work became an essential part of modern number theory. Over the course of his life, right up to the end, he published over eight hundred different papers and books on every aspect of pure and applied mathematics, physics, and astronomy known at that time. Similarly, the French mathematician and astronomer Pierre-Simon de Laplace in 1825, at age seventy-six, completed the fifth volume of his monumental work *Celestial Mechanics (Traité de mecanique céleste)*, considered the greatest work on celestial mechanics since Newton's *Principia Mathematica*.

In many fields—mathematics in particular—a scientist's first and most original theory is viewed as his or her most creative expression. But their most creative contribution may not be the theories per se, but how, in general, they have influenced their field.

Consider the noted Russian mathematician Andrey Nikolayevich Kolmogorov (1903–1987), whose work influenced several branches of modern mathematics, with new theories flourishing throughout his fifties. In later life, though, he paid great attention to problems of mathematical education of schoolchildren. He was appointed chairman of the Commission for Mathematical Education under the Presidium of the Academy of Sciences of the USSR. Under Kolmogorov's leadership a new state program of training in mathematics in the Soviet school system was developed. This program helped the Soviets keep pace as a global superpower in science.

When we consider the significance of these lifetime contributions, using Kolmogorov as an example, do we conclude that his greatest impact was on mathematical theory in his early adulthood and middle age, or on education that advanced the growth of mathematics for his entire society in his later life?

Many mathematicians remain creative in highly novel ways in later life, though not necessarily in the area of mathematics. The German mathematician and philosopher Gottfried Wilhelm Leibniz, a contemporary of Newton, also invented calculus, independent of Newton; many consider Leibniz's the more complete method. But Leibniz's best-known works are the highly influential philosophical treatises he wrote when he

Archimedes (287–212 B.C.) was the most famous mathematician and inventor of ancient Greece. He was reported to have been killed at the siege of Syracuse, in the year 212 B.C., by a Roman soldier whose threat he ignored while immersed in a mathematical problem. He was seventy-nine. The capture of Syracuse was reportedly delayed owing to the deployment of war machines designed by Archimedes. In general, his work influenced mathematics over the next two thousand years.

Sir Isaac Newton (1642–1727), in addition to inventing calculus, published his masterpiece **Philosophiae Naturatis Principia Mathematica** ***around 1687 (at age forty-five). It contained his three laws of motion and is considered the fundamental work for the whole of modern science. He published his second edition of*** **Principia**, ***with***

extensive alterations, at age seventy-one, and his third edition with yet further changes at age eighty-four.

Carl Friedrich Gauss (1777–1855) had a long career, advancing the application of mathematics to physics, astronomy, and geodesy (the mathematical determination of the shape and size of the earth's surface). He developed the "intrinsic-surface" theory—by which characteristics of a curved surface could be found solely by measuring the lengths of the curves that lie on the surface. This theory in turn inspired one of his students, Bernhard Riemann, whose ideas provided the mathematical basis for Einstein's general theory of relativity. Over his career, Gauss made numerous mathematical discoveries, including pioneering contributions to expanding the domain of algebra. At age seventy-one he prepared a new updated edition of his earlier proofs

was in his late sixties, works that laid the foundation of eighteenth-century Rationalism and had a major influence on modern symbolic logic and the thinking of such twentieth-century giants as Bertrand Russell. Such works included *Systema Theologicum* and *Monadologia.*

Bertrand Russell, the well-known English mathematician and philosopher, published his noted *Principles of Mathematics* in 1903 (when he was thirty-one) and *Principia Mathematica* with Alfred North Whitehead between 1910 and 1913. But he also published his very important work *An Enquiry into Meaning and Truth* at age sixty-eight, his best-selling *History of Western Philosophy* at age seventy-three, his *Human Knowledge: Its Scope and Limits* at age seventy-six, and his highly informative *Autobiography*, written between 1967 and 1969 when he was ninety-five to ninety-seven. He was awarded the Nobel Prize for Literature when he was seventy-eight (in 1950).

In his late eighties, Russell became a public world figure in his protests for nuclear disarmament, having been imprisoned for such during a provocative demonstration at the age of eighty-nine. Albert Einstein similarly became socially creative in later life through his protests against nuclear weapons.

Career Curve Versus Age Curve

There is an explanation for the way these exceptional careers would appear to peak earlier in certain fields than in others. It comes from Dean Keith Simonton, a leading researcher on creativity and aging in the Department of Psychology at the University of California, Davis. Simonton emphasizes the influence of a "career curve" as opposed to an "age curve" in explaining whether or when one peaks in a given field.

In other words, creative output is influenced more by experience in a field—"career age"—than by chronological age. Different careers in different fields of study require different amounts of time to master.

Philosophy, for example, is a field in which some of the most profound works have been produced by thinkers in their later years. It is almost inconceivable to imagine Immanuel Kant or Aristotle fully formulating their ideas and receiving broad acceptance of them at, say, age twenty. Similarly, in psychology, a theory that is introduced when one is young may take years or even decades to be accepted, and even then acceptance occurs only after a large number of people agree that it's sound.

In contrast, with math or theoretical physics it may take only one or two or at most a few highly respected authorities to say a theory is sound. The net result is that peaking will appear to occur earlier in math because the nature of the field allows an idea to gain recognition and acceptance earlier; again this is not an age effect but a field or career curve effect.

Also important is the comparative length of time it takes for an idea to gel, to fully take shape and be recognized, in one field compared with another. Here, too, we find field or career curve differences more significant than an age factor. I'll again use the fields of math and psychology to illustrate the point about this time factor for recognition and acceptance: math has a circumscribed and objective knowledge base that can be mastered more quickly than some other fields of study, and when one comes up with something new, emphasized above, it is easier to determine whether that something new is valid and important than the same kind of evaluation in some other fields.

By contrast, in psychology, Dr. Benjamin Spock's *Baby and Child Care* is still subject to debate on various issues, for instance, whether it is ever appropriate to spank a child. This hardly seems as significant as Einstein's $E = mc^2$, but unlike $E = mc^2$ it doesn't elicit universal agreement.

Once an idea is established and accepted, conditions for career peaking exist. While the career curve discussion above helps us understand why in some areas one may peak earlier than in other fields, it does not fully explain why one doesn't keep peaking with comparably original work. Why didn't Einstein later discover several other equivalents of $E = mc^2$? After an artist creates a seminal piece, why doesn't he or she create several other seminal pieces?

It's not that such never occurs. Highly infrequently will a scientist win a second Nobel Prize (e.g., Frederick Sanger in 1958 in chemistry for his determination of the structure of the insulin molecule, and in 1980 in chemistry for his development of chemical and biological analyses of DNA structure). Or, rarely will an artist be viewed as having more than one pivotal piece. For example, Picasso's *Les Demoiselles d'Avignon,* painted in

of the fundamental theory of algebra. He continued to work on mathematical theory until he died at age seventy-eight.

Maria Gaetana Agnesi (1718–1799) was an Italian mathematician and scholar. A child prodigy who spoke six languages by age eleven, she later published books on philosophy and mathematics. Her mathematical textbook* Instituzioni analitiche, *which became famous in Italy, was published when she was sixty-six, in 1784. She is particularly remembered for a cubic curve known as the Witch of Agnesi.

Frigyes Riesz (1880–1956), the Hungarian mathematician, at age seventy-two wrote a classic textbook with Bela Szökefalvi-Nagy in 1952, **Lessons on Functional Analysis.** *He did pioneer work in functional analysis, which led to important applications in mathematical physics.*

1907, influenced the beginning of Cubism, and his *Guernica,* created in 1937, contained the first reference in his work to political events.

Yet, most often individuals are said to have peaked once they have created their ultimate work. This isn't a reflection of the value of their work; it reflects the value judgment placed on an initial work expressing a new idea, in contrast to later ones that fully develop and go far beyond the initial idea. Typically the initial idea is viewed as seminal, while the later, further advanced ones are diminished by being viewed as derivative.

This is thin thinking. The sustained creativity and intellectual energy required to explore an idea fully is at least equal to—and often greater than—that required to launch it. It is senseless to declare that a creative individual in any field has peaked, when in fact the initial idea so highly regarded continues to be expanded and, quite often, made even better. An original idea deserves recognition as such, but our expectation of the contributor need not be forever fixed on that single moment.

When we look at career peaking from a different perspective, using the $C = me^2$ formula, it clearly represents the ultimate synergy of the multiple facets of our creativity equation: the mass of material that you have accrued in a given body of knowledge and of your "*e*" outer world experience and inner "e" world experience. That's not easy to achieve repeatedly, but as we grow older and explore new areas of interest and new forms of expression, our creative potential increases.

Recognizing Obstacles and Opportunities

While age-related changes do influence how we can express ourselves, most of those obstacles can be overcome with support and a strong desire for change. Karl Abraham, one of the giants in the early field of psychoanalysis, wrote a classic paper on psychoanalysis of patients at an advanced age in which he said that he found these patients to be among his most successful.

The "big three" categories of obstacles that hold people back are fixed psychological patterns, fixed ideas, and social situations. Fixed psychological patterns are those responses we have used for years and continue to use, even when they work against us. Fixed ideas are simply biases we may have about doing new things or doing things differently. And social situations refer to the external context of family, friends, and others, and life circumstances, that shape our lives.

Sometimes two of these or even all three intersect and combine to create a formidable obstacle to change. To liberate ourselves at any age, we need to ask ourselves if we, or those around us, are holding us back with rigid thinking or oppressive traditions. If so, we need to post a mental sign that says "Reconstruction Underway" and begin to reexamine these limiting factors to find or build a way around them.

ETHEL'S STORY: AN INNER SELF HIDDEN TOO LONG

Ethel was the oldest child in a family of nine children. She was like a second mother to her youngest siblings, playing a major role in bringing them up. She never had anything approaching teenage years relatively carefree of major household responsibilities that so many kids in small nuclear families experience. This sense of magnified responsibility toward others carried over into her adulthood, where, without skipping a beat, she deferred to the needs of her husband, her husband's business—a small consulting business where she assisted with administrative matters—her children, and then her grandchildren. She did all this with grace and dignity, but never gave equal opportunity to her own talents.

"The life of every man is a diary in which he means to write one story and writes another; and his humblest hour is when he compares the volume as it is with what he vowed to make it."

—JAMES M. BARRIE

When she was in grade school one of her teachers had said she had a real talent for drawing. Her family was quite poor, though, and her heightened sense of responsibility kept her from asking them for drawing materials. When she married, she again felt her time belonged to her family. This pattern continued for the next fifty years until her husband retired and closed his business.

Struggling to deal with her free time, she started volunteering at a local community center, working with children in arts and crafts. While so doing, she created a few sketches of her own, which came to the attention of the admiring community center coordinator. The coordinator asked her if she had ever showed her work, and Ethel explained she had none—no "work" to show. The coordinator was stunned and asked her how that could be—her drawings were so moving. Ethel explained that she had never really had time to pursue art and had always had many other responsibilities. The coordinator, who later told me about Ethel, asked her, "What about now?"

"If you have got a living force and you're not using it, nature kicks you back. The blood boils just like you put it in a pot."
—LOUISE NEVELSON

Ethel was taken aback and just shook her head, saying, "I can't." The coordinator, a thoughtful counselor as well as administrator, asked Ethel if perhaps her desire to help with the children's art class reflected, in part, her own inner self knocking at a locked inner door, wanting very much to come out and pick up an artist's brush, something she likely had always wanted to do but which she had denied herself for the sake of others. Ethel said maybe that was so, but she couldn't take the next step; she was still locked in a seventy-year pattern, not owing to her advancing age but to psychological forces that had been established at a young age.

The community center wasn't just for children, and, coincidentally, it was starting a new art group for older participants. The coordinator nudged Ethel to attend, cleverly saying it would improve her ability to help the children, secretly hoping it would finally escort her onto a new path for herself. The nudge worked. Ethel attended the adult art group, and when they saw her potential they were so supportive that they were able to liberate her from her psychological imprisonment. A year later Ethel's work was in a group show—her first ever. She was radiant with her newfound self and the emergence of the talent that had been stilled for so long—for *decades*.

Ethel's story reminds us that no matter how circumstances may have conspired in our younger days to shape our psychological development away from creative growth and self-expression, it is never too late to get out of a rut, even if that rut is a deeply ingrained psychological one. It's important to remember that the creative process is a process—not a simple solution—and to recognize the power and the potential of all the factors: psychological, social, and economic. Ethel wasn't simply an undiscovered artist who needed to sign up for night classes; her story was much more complex, as are all our lives, and each facet of her life played a part in the quality of her earlier constrained years as well as in her self-discovery and explorations at an older age. Her personality and psychological pattern of chronic self-sacrifice, her social role as the oldest in her large, poor family when growing up, and as a wife in a marriage relationship that included family business responsibilities imposed a kind of self-denial on her. To free Ethel from her self-imposed artistic exile, it was necessary to recognize her social and emotional needs, and help her find ways to honor them, too.

I have a favorite story about a man who accomplished a great feat in his older age through combining fortitude of body with creativity of mind. Described in his autobiography *The Gypsy Moth Circles the World,* Francis Chichester sailed around the world alone when he was sixty-five.

Chichester's voyage in his 54-foot boat, *The Gypsy Moth,* began in August 1966. He celebrated his sixty-fifth birthday at sea on September 17, 1966, and completed his circumnavigation in May 1967. In the process, he established seven world records, including the fastest voyage circling the earth by any sailing vessel—almost twice as fast as any other—and the longest passage that had been made by such a vessel before making a port call. When he arrived back in England, a crowd awaited him with much fanfare and public spectacle. One of his friends wrote of the event:

"Chichester could not see himself as the crowd of cheering Londoners saw him. I did. Slight (until you caught a glimpse of the muscle in wrist and forearm), weather-beaten . . . Chichester gave himself no airs, and when he acknowledged the Lord Mayor's address of welcome, the crowd's cheers, he spoke more of Sheila his wife and Giles his son than of himself. He was the nation's hero, but to me he seemed to epitomize not scarlet and lace, but that incredible endurance of men who sailed with Drake, Anson, Cook, and Nelson, for England. And that, I think, is what everybody felt. And that is why we cheered."

After his return, Chichester was knighted by the Queen of England with the very sword given by Queen Elizabeth I to Sir Francis Drake nearly four centuries earlier.

What always strikes me about the story of Chichester and his accomplishment isn't so much that he sailed around the world by himself at age sixty-five, but the attitude he had in completing his goal. Chichester shows us a glimpse of this attitude while writing in a log he kept while at sea:

> People keep at me about my age. I suppose they think I can beat age. I'm not that foolish. Nobody can be more aware than I am that my time is limited. I don't think I can escape aging, but why

British-born Colin Fletcher, an old-fashioned adventurer, became the guru of the serious hiker with books like* The Thousand-Mile Summer *(1964), describing his hike from Mexico to Oregon. But for years what he coveted was to become the first to run the length of the Colorado River, from source to sea, on a raft—all 1,700 miles to the Gulf of California. He did it in his late sixties (1989), and wrote about it in his 1997 book,* One Man's Journey Down the Colorado, Source to Sea. *He strove for a "genuine journey," wanting to "pare the fat off my soul . . . to make me grateful again for being alive."

beef about it? Our only purpose in life, if we are able to say such a thing, is to put up the best performances we can—in anything, and only in so doing lies satisfaction in living.

Chichester recognized that the infirmities associated with old age are unavoidable for many, but we should not let these challenging effects cut short our goals in life or our fulfillment in later years. One colleague described Chichester as "at last releasing the dream." We should find our own dreams and not let misconceptions about old age, self-doubt, or even initial failure bring us down.

Former U.S. President Jimmy Carter climbed Mount Fuji at age seventy.

Ours is a species whose spirit inspires us ever to seek challenge and discovery—to climb mountains, sail around the globe, fly to the moon. Now that spirit has transcended the age barrier, where society both sees and celebrates the possibility for such quests, recognizing no endpoint for them in the life cycle. That an astronaut in his late seventies, Sen. John Glenn, could, with a sense of societal exhilaration, be approved for a space flight, reflects such social change. He embodies the changing view of aging—that having "the right stuff" knows no age limit.

The great nineteenth-century American poet Walt Whitman, who published until he died in his seventies, wrote in *Leaves of Grass,*

Youth, large lusty loving—
youth, full of grace, force, fascination,
Do you know that Old Age may come after you,
with equal grace, force, fascination?

"The biggest temptation is . . . to settle for too little."
—THOMAS MERTON

This grace, force, and fascination of which Whitman writes is there for all of us as we age, if we embrace our creativity in whatever form it takes. It may be creativity with a "big *C*" or creativity with a "little *c*." It may be creativity in the expressive arts, or it may be creativity in a social context. It may be public or personal. It may be creativity involving you alone, or it may be a collaborative creativity with others.

The possibilities are infinite, and the developmental energy for them is built in. Creativity is a natural, vibrant force throughout our adult lives and a catalyst for growth, excitement, and a meaningful legacy in each of our lives.

4

The "When" of Creativity: Opportunities That Change with Age

When I was young I was amazed to learn that the elder Cato (a Roman statesman)
began at the age of eighty to learn Greek. I am amazed no longer.
Old age is ready to undertake tasks that youth shirked
because they would take too long.

—SOMERSET MAUGHAM, *THE SUMMING UP*

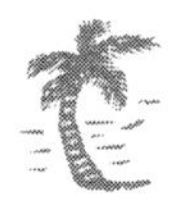

WILLIAM SOMERSET MAUGHAM BEGAN his distinguished career as an author after completing an education to become a doctor, and his trenchant insights about human behavior reflected his medical understanding as well as his thoughtful observations of the human condition. When Maugham noted in his mid-sixties that advancing age brings with it a distinct power of focus and enterprise, he touched on the two fundamental aspects of aging that drive the extraordinary potential for creative expression in the second half of life. The first is the *capacity to experiment.* The second is the *significance of time.*

In earlier chapters we have explored the powerful capacity of the

In Rome during the height of the glorious Roman Empire life expectancy from birth was only twenty-two years; people reached old age, but average longevity was low because of disease, complications of childbirth, famine, and war. In contemporary

America, life expectancy after age 65 is approaching twenty years.

brain to continue to make new connections and to process and manage information differently as we age. We learned, too, that as adults our psychological development progresses through growth phases—human potential phases—that create rich opportunities for creative thought and expression at even the most advanced ages. We examined some negative expectations of aging and other obstacles to creativity that need not be, and we confronted the power of middle-age angst to obscure our vision of our creative potential—of what *could be* in our lives. High on the list of those obstacles, at least in midlife, is the fear of time slipping away, the dread of time spent trapped in the "dark woods" of aging, or simply a sense of time as the enemy, a force that works against us. In the throes of angst at any age it is impossible to think of time in a neutral way.

Traditionally, in Judaism, the bar mitzvah was an orthodox religious celebration marking the adulthood of a boy at age thirteen. My mother, Lillian Cohen, always regretted not having the opportunity to have such a ceremony for herself. By the time my mother reached adulthood, numerous Conservative and Reform Congregations had instituted a separate ceremony to mark, also at age thirteen, the adulthood of girls, called bat mitzvah. Approaching age seventy, my mother decided she wanted to get her bat

There is no question that our capacity to experiment remains strong not just despite our age, but often *because* of it. "Live and learn," we say wryly on the heels of an unexpected lesson. But it is true in the longest sense of time: as we live, we learn, and in so doing we expand our capacity to learn more, and differently, from life. Also true is this: No matter how strongly we believe in our ability to grow and change, it is our perception of time that dictates our hope and enthusiasm for the task. If we want to act on what we know—which is that we can reinvigorate our lives at every age—then we need to embrace the passage of time as an asset, an opportunity, a framework for accomplishments and dreams as we age.

The human potential phases we explored in Chapter 3 *require the passage of time*. Midlife reevaluation isn't something you can work ahead on at age twenty-six. The liberation phase of adult life comes only after you have spent some considerable years in the harness of commitments and priorities of an earlier age. It is useful for us at any age to reflect on the purpose and meaning of our lives, but the summing-up phase of later adult life is uniquely empowering, because it embraces the complexity of decades of life experience. And the encore experience is so named precisely because it comes as a spontaneous gift of creativity that follows the main event.

This enriching quality of time was brought home to me again during the longitudinal study of mentally healthy older adults that I initiated around 1980. My goal was to discover what contributed to ongoing sound mental health apart from having good genes. During the course of the study I interviewed Mrs. Malloy, an eighty-one-year-old woman, who had spent most of her life raising a large family. In her sixties, when her children reached adulthood, two of them developed serious marital problems, while a third suffered a major medical illness. Mrs. Malloy wanted to help them in any way she could; the responsibility she felt toward her family consumed her every moment.

At last, in her eighties, her life had settled down and she experienced a new freedom of time that allowed her finally to pursue her passion: reading biographical and historical novels. During the eight months prior to our interview, she had devoured eighteen of these lengthy books. I was red-faced when she asked me how many I had read during that time. Her formal schooling had gone no farther than high school, but as an octogenarian she launched her own form of continuing education and creative enrichment.

mitzvah. She creatively pursued her goal by taking conversational Hebrew for two years, brushing up on what she had learned in her youth, then taking a formal training program for the bat mitzvah. She completed the ceremony at age seventy-four, the oldest having done so in her synagogue. Not only were she and her family extremely proud, but she provided a model for her community that it was never too late to pursue your dreams.

Categories of Creativity with Aging

Once we clear away the fear and other emotional fog that darkens our view of time passing, we can see the more exciting relationship between time and creativity across our life span. This is the reality that so many "seniors" are living as they book continuing education cruises to Alaska or the Galapagos Islands, fill their schedules with special-interest classes at the local community center or library, or enjoy quieter pleasures alone or with special friends or family members. As they find new ways to enrich their experience of time, they are stoking the coals of creativity. This is also the source of the equanimity, the centering of the spirit, that enables some men and women to seek and find joy in their lives despite complications of health or finances. Aging and creativity intersect in distinctly different ways at different times to produce new opportunities for personal growth and discovery:

When you are completely absorbed or caught up in something, you become oblivious of things around you, or of the passage of time. It is this absorption in what you are doing that frees your unconscious and releases your creative imagination.

—DR. ROLLO MAY

- Creativity that *commences* with aging, or first becomes apparent in later life.

- Creativity that *continues, sometimes changing* with aging, evident in those who continue to be creative in a particular field of focus throughout their life, and those whose creativity takes a new turn.
- Creativity that *connects with loss,* which develops in response to loss or adversity.

Henri Matisse (1869–1954), the great French painter, at ages eighty to eighty-two, designed the stained glass for the Dominican Chapel at Vence, near Nice.

Our creative potential is expanded still further, because, just as people are intelligent in different ways, they may be creative in different ways. There are multiple domains—different forms—of creativity: musical, linguistic, logical-mathematical, spatial, bodily kinesthetic (movement), and social, for instance, as Howard Gardner has discussed. Creative expression is not limited to one particular domain. You might be creative in a social situation as was Grandma Higginson in her ability to solve problems in my kindergarten classroom, or you might be creative in an artistic way like the French painter Henri Matisse, considered one of the greatest artists of the twentieth century.

As discussed earlier, too, there is creativity with a "big *C*" (creativity on a public scale) and creativity with a "little *c*" (creativity on a personal level), as well as collaborative creativity that can emerge in activity with others wherever we go. Any of these forms of creativity can occur at any point along that time line, *commencing, continuing, or changing,* and *connecting through adversity* with age.

Individual factors that can support creative growth at these times include retirement that allows new use of time and financial resources to engage in self-discovery activities, the courage to try new things, and the maturity to better understand yourself and your potential. Despite extensive research to identify isolated features of personality or thought processes that produce creativity, the most significant conclusion to be made from it all is that no one type of person has a corner on creativity. Each of us has the potential to think, learn, and act anew. What changes with time and age is the way we go about doing these things.

Why is time such a positive and significant factor in our creative growth? Remember our $C = me^2$ equation, illustrating the idea that creative expression C occurs when the special knowledge we have accumulated in a given area (*m*ass of material) interacts with the combined experience (e^2) of both our outer and inner worlds. All the ingredients in this brew are in a constant state of mixing and changing. Doing something new or creative changes our base of information and our life experience of the outer world and the feelings that alter the inner world of our emotions. Aging, by itself, is not the determining factor here, but rather time and the natural psychological development over time that affects what we do and how we feel about it.

You may have the *m*—the mass of material—necessary for a creative act, but your outer world experience may not yet be right, or your inner world experience may not yet be ready. You may have been working at a job or under life circumstances that didn't add much to your knowledge base, or the *m*. Your experience of your inner and outer worlds may improve only after changing fields, perhaps with the courage and freedom of later life. Or you may experience a synchrony, or optimal balance, in later life, and then decide to immerse yourself in a new area out of which creative growth and new expressions of it are bound to emerge. There is no one right age for $C = me^2$ to produce the best results, but time and experience tend to enhance each of the pieces. For many people that optimal combination of knowledge, experience, and emotional readiness occurs most dramatically in later life.

All three categories of creativity offer exciting potential, especially if you recognize them as natural launching points for new creative growth and you put some focused energy behind that launch.

Thomas Hobbes (1588–1679), the great English political philosopher, wrote his masterpiece Leviathan *at age sixty-three (1651); it presented a synthesis of metaphysics, psychology, and political philosophy. He wrote with renewed vigor in his eighties, writing an autobiography in Latin verse at age eighty-four and verse translations of the* Iliad *and the* Odyssey *from their original Greek—the former at age eighty-seven, the latter at age eighty-eight.*

Katharine Graham, retired publisher of the Washington Post, *wrote her first book at seventy-nine, her autobiography,* Personal History, *which won a 1998 Pulitzer Prize.*

Creativity That Commences with Age

In 1980 at the Corcoran Museum of Art in Washington, D.C, I saw an exhibit that was the culmination of a formal study of folk art in the United States, covering the period from 1930 to 1980. Almost half of the best work during this fifty-year period was done by minorities, especially African-Americans, and particularly from along the Mississippi–Alabama corridor. Many of these people were deceased.

I went to the show not only as someone who appreciates art, but also as a gerontologist, always searching for new insights into aging and the lives of older adults. Reading the artists' brief biographies posted by

Silas Claw and Bertha Claw were husband and wife and Navajo potters. In 1968, at age fifty-five, Silas Claw, in beginning to work with clay, broke his first taboo—men do not pot among the Navajo. His transition was clever and represented an artful gray zone regarding tradition in that he did the pottery with his wife; Silas made most of the pots and appliquéd figures on them, while Bertha handled the sanding and the painting. Their Wedding Vase, *created when Silas was seventy-six, is a good example of innovative work. The Claws produced approximately fifty pots a year, along with assorted other art objects. Their work is shown and sold in galleries in the Southwest.*

their work, I discovered that of the twenty exhibitors in the show, sixteen of them—eighty percent—had started their art or reached a recognizable mature phase as artists after the age of sixty-five. Thirty percent of these were eighty or older.

After this show I carried out a more formal study of folk art in the United States and found that across the ethnic and racial diversity of our society, folk art has been dominated by older adults. Many of these individuals were free to pursue their personal interests only after other responsibilities were out of the way.

In the Corcoran show, I was particularly drawn by artists such as Bill Traylor, whose work was on the cover of the museum's catalog. Traylor was born a slave in 1854 outside Montgomery, Alabama. Following Emancipation he remained as a farmhand on the plantation where he had worked all his life. At the age of eighty-four, his wife having died and his approximately twenty children having gone their own ways, Traylor moved to Montgomery. He worked for a while in a shoe factory until "rheumatism" made it too difficult for him to continue. He started to receive some meager financial assistance, but he would still sleep nights in the storage room of a funeral parlor and spend his days on a sidewalk seat in front of the pool hall or by one of the fruit stands in the downtown street market area.

Approaching the age of eighty-five, in 1939, Traylor began to draw despite his arthritis. It just came to him, he once told a newspaper reporter. He then began to hang his drawings on a fence behind him and occasionally sell them to passersby. His work was eventually discovered, and his first show took place at the art center in Montgomery in 1940, when Traylor was eighty-six. National recognition soon followed.

Another artist in that Corcoran show was William Edmonson, one of my heroes because of the impact his life had on future generations. Edmonson was an African-American whose career had been a mixture primarily of cooking and janitorial jobs. In his early sixties, during the Great Depression of the 1930s, he was working as a janitor in a Nashville hospital. The economic crisis of the times caused the hospital to fail financially. Edmonson lost his job. As he later described, in an attempt to cope with this crisis, he had the inspiration to carve. In his mid-sixties, Edmonson emerged as a gifted sculptor. A photographer captivated by his work sent a portfolio of pictures of Edmonson's sculptures to New York's Museum of Modern Art (MOMA). In 1937, at the age of sixty-seven, Edmonson became the first black artist in the history of MOMA to have his work exhibited in a one-man show. In so doing, he and MOMA opened the doors to diversity for the generations that followed.

In the more formal study of American folk art, I found that older people continued to dominate, regardless of racial or ethnic background. For example, in another well-known folk art exhibit—the Hemphill Collection at the National Museum of American Art—the cover of the catalog showed a sculpture by Irving Dominick, an American artist of European ancestry in his late sixties. Dominick's sculpture, *Marla,* is shown to the right.

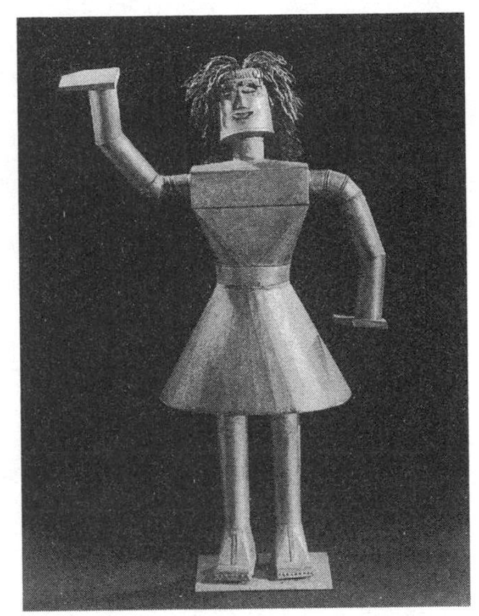

Marla, Irving Dominick, 1982 (age sixty-six)
NATIONAL MUSEUM OF AMERICAN ART, WASHINGTON DC/ ART RESOURCE, NY

Looking closely at the image, especially the head, neck, and shoulders, you can see that it looks very metallic and cylindrical. Interestingly, up until he retired in his mid-sixties, Dominick worked in a heating and air-conditioning company making ductwork. After retirement he turned his duct-making skills to sculpture and achieved national recognition as an artist.

So, what is it that brings previously unexpressed creativity forward in later life? Sometimes it's a change of situation, or a psychological shift in perspective. Often it is both, reflecting the combined energy, or synergy, of chronological time, emotion, and developmental readiness reflected in the phases of human potential we explored in Chapter 3.

For instance, creativity that commences with aging for the midlife adult can arise from greater attention to the inner life (Midlife Reevaluation Phase) and a refocusing of emotional energy. If not at midlife, then it may be the greater allowance of time, financial resources, or emotional freedom of the Liberation Phase that stirs creative energy into action. Still later, it may be the emotional process of the Summing-Up Phase that first motivates us to want to add new chapters to our life stories. In unusual circumstances of emotional deprivation, creative expression may have been stifled for nearly a lifetime and yet still be responsive to Encore energy and desire for creative self-expression. You

Eddie Arning, an American folk artist from Texas, whose work has been represented in many of the foremost museum collections as well as in numerous private collections, did not start drawing until he entered a nursing home at the age of sixty-six (1964). Prior to that he had been committed to a state mental hospital for thirty years. He is known for his bold interpretive drawings, often reflecting a narrative style.

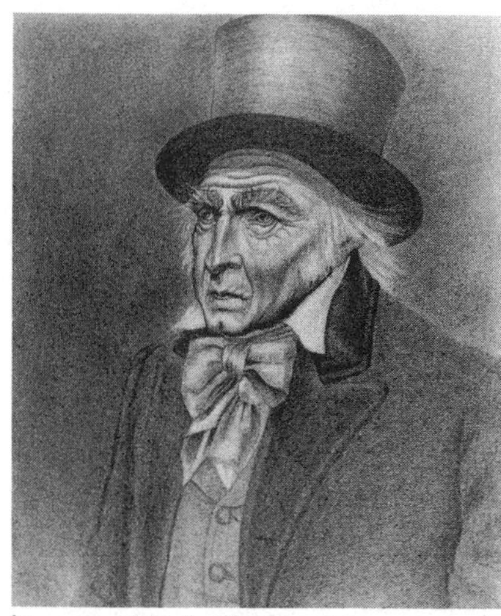

A mean-spirited old man
DRAWING BY MILDRED BALDWIN

are never too old and it is never too late to experience creative growth and find new, satisfying forms of expression.

One of my favorite case studies of creativity commencing with age was originally reported 150 years ago, but I shared it anew in 1987 when I was called to testify before the U.S. Congress regarding funding for mental health programs for older adults. Some Congressional leaders wondered whether it made fiscal sense to support treatment for late-life depression; they questioned whether psychotherapy could do any good for patients of advanced age. The skeptics' sentiment was that if, as the saying goes, "You can't teach an old dog new tricks," then there's no point in paying for the lessons.

I went on to present a famous case from the mid-1800s concerning a well-known figure from London, who at that time was reported to have been a melancholic, mean-spirited, misanthropic old man, someone who took pleasure in making the lives of all around him miserable. It was said at the time that "the cold within him froze his old features, nipped his pointed nose, shriveled his cheek, stiffened his gait, made his eyes red, his thin lips blue, and spoke out shrewdly in his grating voice." These qualities had evolved over a period of decades, culminating in his later years. By historical accounts, he then received a home visit by a multidisciplinary team, although this was more than one hundred years before the health and mental health outreach movement became popular. This team used psychodynamic, dream-oriented psychotherapy to help this man, more than fifty years before Freud's *The Interpretation of Dreams*. The effectiveness of this intervention was complete and since renowned. The old man, awakened to his potential for creative living, staged a dramatic turnaround, transforming his depressive energy into vitality that enhanced his experience of life and the lives of those all around him.

The "patient" here was none other than Ebenezer Scrooge (above, left), the celebrated grouch of Charles Dickens's great story *A Christmas Carol*, written in 1843. This enduring tale from the nineteenth century reflects the truth about old age and fresh starts even as we start the new millennium, and that is this: No matter how late in life, no matter how

Jean-Étienne-Dominique Esquirol (1772–1840), the French physician who was a pioneer in treating and teaching about mental disorders, wrote Des maladies mentales *at age sixty-six.*

The catalog of Elizabeth Layton's (1909–1993) one-person show, which toured the country and eventually made it to the National Museum of American Art, sums up her experience: "The twentieth-century folk artist Elizabeth Layton launched a twenty-year

severe the circumstances, when our knowledge, experience, and emotional readiness are in synch, creative change can transform our lives.

I see the essence of Scrooge's life story in countless other lives.

Alan Hendel described himself as the son of an abusive alcoholic father. Alan saw himself carrying on the grim tradition of alcohol abuse, and recalled how in college, it had interfered with his relationships as well as his studies. Whenever a relationship grew closer, his drinking intensified and inevitably destroyed the bonds of friendship or intimacy.

Following college he obtained a middle management job in a large insurance company. He was very good at what he did, but he felt his career advancement was limited by his alcohol-related behavior. Increased stress at work would trigger heavier drinking, even during lunch breaks; the alcohol would alter his behavior, lowering his inhibitions to emotional expression, which took the form of sarcastic comments or loud, verbally hostile interactions with coworkers. His supervisors warned him that the drinking and verbally abusive behavior had to stop, and Alan occasionally sought counseling or attended meetings of Alcoholics Anonymous (AA), but then drifted away from sources of help. Gradually, he was assigned solitary work without responsibility for supervising others.

Problems with relationships continued, and he retired early at age sixty, a loner. Without the structure of work, his drinking problem temporarily worsened. Then came the turning point. One day after lunch, at which he downed three drinks, he was driving home through his neighborhood when suddenly a neighbor's six-year-old child rode his bicycle into the street in front of the car. Alan's reflexes were blunted from the drinking. He hit his brakes and turned the steering wheel very late, but miraculously just scraped the back wheel of the boy's bike. The boy was knocked to the ground, but fortunately received only minor bruises. Alan was severely frightened and deeply humiliated by the event, especially since it had occurred in his own neighborhood. Tragedy dreams filled with accidents and people weeping tormented him for the next few weeks, and he developed new resolve to overcome his drinking problem. He was further motivated when a medical checkup showed that the alcohol was beginning to take a noticeable toll on his liver and stomach.

painting career in her late sixties . . . In the fall of 1977, a sixty-eight-year-old woman from Wellsville, Kansas, stared into her looking glass and drew herself. These self-portraits, besides reflecting the hopes and fears of the world, allowed her to win a thirty-year struggle with depression. In the few years since, almost without trying, the artist gained armloads of friends and national recognition. Certainly without intending to, she wrote an unexpected but inspiring chapter in the history of art and human achievement."

The protagonist in what is generally considered one of the first American short stories was a man who essentially slept away his youth with a drinking problem only to finally overcome it upon entering later life and become a model citizen of his community—Rip Van Winkle from Washington Irving's 1819 classic.

He enrolled in a combination counseling and AA program, and this time they worked. I saw him in my Well Aging study seven years later, and he had not had a drink since that day of the collision. He also described a change in his feelings about himself and his life, and for the first time about being a partner in enduring, satisfying relationships. He also had assumed a leadership role in self-help alcohol groups, and to his great satisfaction found himself in growing demand as an inspirational speaker.

Long held captive by alcoholism, and then released by his sobering turnaround, Alan's creativity blossomed and was accompanied by new emotional growth and a greater feeling of self-worth. Stories like Alan's show that it is possible to "turn over a new leaf" and begin to tap our creative energy even in the face of chronic mental health problems. It does not require a stretch to realize what is possible in the face of sound mental health.

Creativity That Continues with Age

John Boyd Orr, Scottish biologist, at age sixty-five (1945) was the first director of the United Nations Food and Agriculture Organization. His outstanding work in improving the world's food situation brought him the Nobel Peace Price in 1949 (age sixty-nine). His book **As I Recall** *was published when he was eighty-six.*

My Uncle Sumner (Bud) Strashun was a very talented and dedicated food technologist, whose work involved important research into the development, processing, and preservation of foods. He was also a food plant consultant, helping companies develop plants to process different types of food. Uncle Bud always wanted to make a difference in the quality of life for people, and this goal translated into a very intense and innovative approach to his work that never stopped. He vigorously continued to make contributions to his field right up to his death in his early eighties.

Though he never retired, when he entered retirement age in his mid to late sixties he was able to reduce the time he spent at his occupation to liberate time for volunteer work. These efforts took him to a whole new level—international consultation to developing nations in Africa, Asia, and Eastern Europe. He provided technical assistance on the development of feasibility studies to establish food plants in many nations all over the world, completing his last trip not long before he died at eighty-two. He enjoyed the challenges that pushed his creativity to a new level in planning for countries dealing with economic limitations and special food needs. While he volunteered his time, his expenses as well as those of his wife, Claire, who accompanied him, were covered by a private nonprofit agency supporting such efforts. In addition to this program providing a creative infusion into his life's work, it also provided a new creative infusion into his marital and family life with the rich experiences that he and his wife participated in together in their travels and in the wonderful sharing of those experiences with the extended family.

Uncle Bud and other older adults like him are at work all around us every day. I see them in their roles as mentors in the worlds of business, industry, and scholarship, as volunteer tutors for young people in the schools, helpers at homeless shelters, and community activists or consultants where they see a need. Despite this evidence, however, the stereotype of creativity dimming with age is a stubborn one. Even Freud started as a doubter of flexibility and creative potential in later life. In 1905 he wrote that patients near or above the age of fifty lacked the "elasticity of the mental processes, on which treatment depends." He also doubted if people in this age group were still "educable" or could handle heavy amounts of information.

It is ironic that Freud wrote this as he was nearing his fiftieth birthday, a period in his own life demonstrating considerable elasticity and educability. Ironic, too, is that Freud's regard of "the greatest masterpiece of all time," *Oedipus Rex,* was written when Sophocles was seventy-one.

Certain cultural views have reinforced the bleak stereotype. The once steadfast tradition of retirement at age sixty-five supported that image of being "burned out" or "turned out to field." Some people still mistakenly believe that age automatically compromises our ability to continue our work with the same momentum or capacity of younger years. More often, in truth, it is external factors, and not the internal influences of age itself, that compromise our performance or outlook in everyday life.

The art world offers us an easy view of continuing creativity as well as age discrimination so prevalent in many cultures. The Renaissance painter Titian was considered the greatest portrait painter of

Harvey Washington Wiley (1844–1930) was an American food chemist who became chief of the chemical division of the U.S. Department of Agriculture in his thirties. In that position he carried out major analyses of foods with the purpose of improving their purity and reducing risks of harmful effects. Overcoming many obstacles and opponents with vested interests, his efforts led to the establishment of the Pure Food and Drug Act of 1906 when he was sixty-two. He continued his crusade for food purity until his death at age eighty-six, along the way writing* Not by Bread Alone *in 1915 at age seventy-one.

T. S. Eliot (1888–1965), the American-born British poet and winner of the Nobel Prize in Literature, published* The Confidential Clerk *at sixty-six and* The Elder Statesman *at seventy.

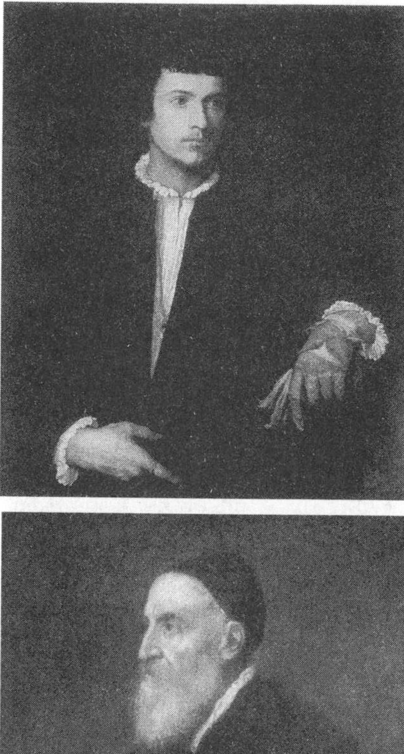

(Top) **Titian:** ***Man with a Glove*****, age 39**
COURTESY MUSÉE DE LOUVRE
(Above) **Titian** ***Self-Portrait,*** **age 78**
COURTESY MUSEO DEL PRADO

that period and an artist who continued to be productive over the course of his lifetime. His story also shows that when an older person changes his work, however subtle the change, there is too often a rush to judgment that the difference represents decrement. This is true even when the individual is at the top of his or her field.

Let's look at Titian's work in the context of three stereotypes about aging: (1) creative vision invariably diminishes with age; (2) physical dexterity deteriorates with advancing years; (3) the willingness to try new things—to take risks—fades out.

Consider first Titian's portrait *Man with a Glove* (top, left), which the artist painted when he was thirty-nine. Much can be said about the painting in terms of its poignancy and beauty, but for the purposes of my discussion, one feature in particular should be noted: how well defined the figure is in the portrait. Now look at the self-portrait he did when he was seventy-eight, exactly double this age. It's regarded by art historians as being as comparably poignant and beautiful as *Man with a Glove.* Some feel it is even more powerful. But others have wondered if there was any change in Titian's skills, since on reexamination of the painting the outline looks less well defined.

Next, let's look at Titian's work five years later—when he was eighty-three. His portrait (facing page, top) of *Tarquin and Lucretia*—the rape of Lucretia—is regarded as a very engaging painting, but has been quite controversial because of its decidedly more vaguely defined appearance. Critics believed it was a sign of Titian's failing power as an artist. But then, we discover that Titian did a second painting of *Tarquin and Lucretia*—also at the age of eighty-three—and, remarkably, it looks as if it had been done at the same time as *Man with a Glove,* forty-four years earlier in terms of how well defined the outlines of the figures are (facing page, bottom).

What is the explanation for this more amorphous, or loosely defined, image, if not as a reflection of failing hand or vision? I suggest that this highly successful portrait painter felt extraordinary pressure from his Renaissance public to continue to paint in his "trademark" style. This commercial pressure is one that many successful artists experience and that they must defy when they seek to express their creativity in new styles or forms. I look at Titian's "shapeless" style and I see this old master scoffing at the critics, asserting his creative independence at age eighty-three, as if to say: "I want to do something different. I want to explore. I want to innovate."

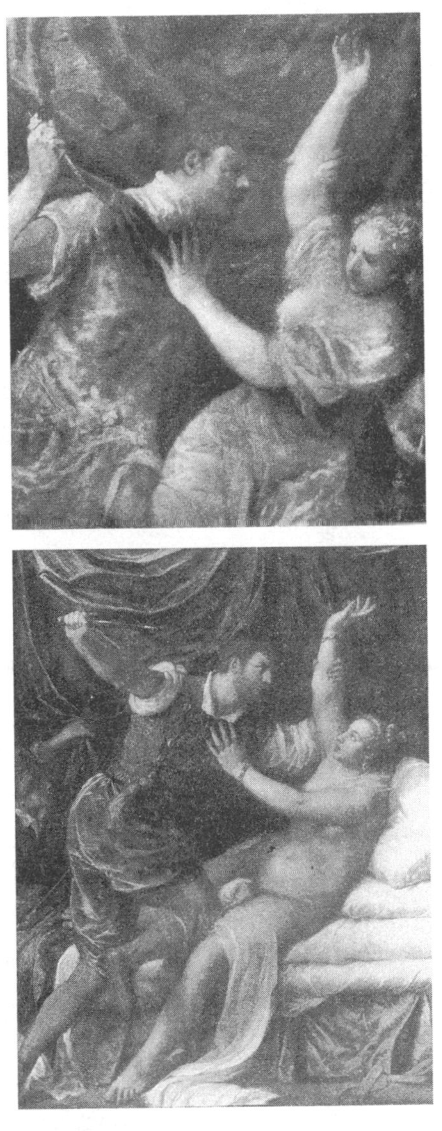

(Top) *Tarquin and Lucretia* (painted at age eighty-three)
COURTESY GEMÄLDEGALERIE
(Above) *Tarquin and Lucretia* (painted at age eighty-three)
COURTESY FITZWILLIAM MUSEUM, CAMBRIDGE

By comparing all four paintings it becomes clear that Titian's creative vision did not decline with aging. The second *Tarquin and Lucretia* painting illustrates that there is not an inevitable marked progressive deterioration of physical dexterity with aging. I suggest that the first *Tarquin and Lucretia,* rather than indicating Titian's decline as an artist, reflects instead risk taking and innovation, and that rather than being seen as having become more amorphous, or shapeless, perhaps it is more *impressionistic,* anticipating the Impressionist movement by three centuries. Dismissive attitudes toward Titian's later work underscore the popular assumption that when an older person does something different and unexpected, it is a sign of some ill effect of old age. Creative experimentation is assumed to be the realm of young artists and young people. Adults who seek to be innovative or novel in their thinking face age prejudice and general skepticism.

Not only can creativity continue with aging, the outcomes of its expression can grow, often building upon one another and becoming an expanding knowledge base and a series of discoveries that add to one another. As a young woman in late nineteenth century America, Annie Jump Cannon became deaf through contracting scarlet fever. She later entered Radcliffe College and took up the study of astronomy. Over the years she discovered numerous stars and novae. At the age of seventy-five she was named William Cranch Bond astronomer at Harvard and continued her course of discovery and contribution. Annie Jump Cannon's accomplishments not

Mary Cassatt (1844–1926), the Impressionist painter renowned for her studies of domestic scenes, painted her noted work **Fillette au Grand Chapeau** *at the age of sixty-four.*

Francisco de Goya (1746–1828) the great Spanish painter, following an illness, became permanently deaf at age forty-six. Afterward, his art took on new character, freer in expression and rich in imagination. He continued to paint outstanding works until his death at age eighty-two. Some among the many of his great late-life works included **The Duke of Wellington** *(at age sixty-six);* **Ferdinand VII in an Encampment** *(at age sixty-eight);* **Self-Portrait with Doctor Arrieta** *(at age seventy-four);* **The Milkmaid of Bordeaux** *(completed at age eighty-one); and* **Don José Pio de Molina** *(at age eighty-two).*

only illustrate creativity against a backdrop of loss—her loss of hearing—but even more dramatically both *continuing* creativity and an *ongoing growth* as she aged.

Reflecting an inner drive contributing to a continuing creativity is the unfulfilled feeling of falling short of an objective, and the renewed dedication—for some, obsession—to "getting it right." For example, the twentieth-century artist Francis Bacon strove to best depict the "human cry." He began in 1944 at the age of thirty-five, and finally felt he succeeded in 1988 at the age of seventy-nine with his second version of *Tryptych, Three Studies for Figures at the Base of a Crucifixion.*

Those who demonstrate a *continuing* creativity are often still undergoing development in their creative endeavors, enabling them to make ongoing contributions in those fields. In such circumstances, time becomes an asset, allowing a person to acquire new perspectives and new information.

I think of the day a few years ago when I was approaching the National Library of Medicine, and briskly coming out the front door was Dr. Lucy Ozarin, in her mid-eighties and long one of my role models. Before there was an Internet, she was like one, in human form. Ask her a question, and you'd get a thoughtful response or good advice on where to get the answer, and you'd often get a question from her that would make you think very hard.

For as long as people could remember, Dr. Ozarin had always been that way, perpetually working hard at it, keeping up with the scientific literature, attending key scientific conferences, asking colleagues about their research and other goings-on in their fields, and *doing*—always doing—a variety of hands-on activities to provide her direct exposure to emerging issues in the field. For example, until she was eighty she participated on teams of consultants who visited various care facilities to evaluate them for quality purposes, keeping her up-to-date with the health care delivery system as well as the patients served by it. Presently, she chairs the Library Committee of the American Psychiatric Association (APA), and is active in organizing historical notes about the field of psychiatry. During the past several years she herself has written thirty-six notes about the history of the field in the APA's newsletter.

Sometimes to gain new insights about the "secret" of aging with creative energy, we need only look around at work or in our communities and take note of those men and women doing just that. I do. When I see colleagues in their seventies and eighties, enthusiastic, curious, asking tough questions, offering meaningful insights, I feel good, because I see that none of these desirable qualities need fall by the wayside. They give me hope and they give me evidence that that's the way aging and continuing activity, accomplishment, and creativity can be.

Creativity That Changes with Age

Some people display creative talents at a younger age and, as they grow older, they not only continue to be creative but may go on to fundamentally change the direction of their work or field of endeavor. Their career or lifestyle at age thirty-five might seem to have nothing in common with their work and life at age forty-five or sixty-five or eighty-five, but in truth, each career or lifestyle incarnation is a reflection of that underlying creative energy transformed by continued growth and expressed in forms of work or activity. Time also allows people to build confidence and helps cultivate a new courage. This constellation of factors empowers us to draw upon our life's work from a new vantage point and to speak about it with a new voice. The outcome is that time, aging, and continuity create new opportunities for our work to have an impact, to make a difference. The nature of the impact will, of course, vary; it can smooth rough waters in a new current of thinking, or it can cause new ripples.

The nineteenth-century English explorer and translator Sir Richard Francis Burton learned forty languages and dialects in his decades of travel and translated a great number of texts from foreign cultures. In his mid-sixties, however, during the Victorian period, Sir Richard risked prosecution and imprisonment by taking it upon himself to introduce to the West the sexual wisdom of the ancient East. For example, he secretly translated and had printed the *Kama Sutra of Vatsyayana*. Some people praised his translations for their honesty and robustness, while others called them "garbage of the brothels." The

James Hutton (1726–1797), a Scotsman, developed an interest in chemistry when he was young, then entered the legal profession, and subsequently became a medical doctor. From medicine, Hutton went on to devote himself to agriculture, and eventually, in his seventh decade, he focused on geology, where his extraordinary theories and discoveries earned him the sobriquet "the founder of modern geology." His noted work* A Theory of the Earth *was published when he was sixty-nine.

His work was revolutionary, because it not only challenged existing geological theory but it also provoked extreme reactions in theological thinking. Until Hutton's theory, most people believed the earth and its crust had formed through supernatural means some six thousand years earlier, shaped by such catastrophic events as the Great Flood described in the Bible. Hutton

showed how the earth was much older, how soils were formed by the weathering rocks, and how layers of sediment accumulated.

The effect of Hutton's ideas on the learned world at that time has been compared with earlier revolution in thought brought about by Copernicus and Galileo (when each of them was approaching seventy). His work later greatly influenced Charles Darwin.

praise won over the criticism, and he was knighted at the age of sixty-five.

Certain creative individuals may experience a growing tension if they find themselves in a given area for too long. Their restlessness is at times almost palpable. Odysseus, hero of Homer's epic poem *The Odyssey*, personifies these characteristics in his numerous wanderings and changing challenges—his personal odyssey—extending from middle age to later life. Here, too, we find personality interacting with one of life's major transitional periods in terms of inner psychological life. Middle age often triggers a period of reevaluation that can lead to crisis or more typically quest—a Ulyssean (Odyssean in Latin) quest.

While the circumstances surrounding Ulysses' odyssey often forced him to confront situations beyond his control, it was, as John A. B. McLeish said in *The Ulyssean Adult*,* his "questing spirit" that enabled him to survive these situations and return to his homeland and his beloved Penelope.

Another example is the Japanese master artist and printmaker Katsushika Hokusai (1760–1849), who continued to seek change in the same field and simultaneously in his life as a whole. Hokusai changed residences more than ninety times. He also changed his name, assuming a new *nom d'artiste* (Shunro, Sori, Kako, Taito, Gakyojin, Iitsu, and Manji) approximately once a decade; he had approximately two dozen other pseudonyms as well.

Meanwhile, the focus of Hokusai's art continued to shift, though always with excellence. He produced single-sheet prints of landscapes and actors, hand paintings such as greetings and announcements. He created picture books and picture novelettes, illustrations for anthologies of verse, historical novels, album prints, and erotic books, as well as figure prints and wood-block prints. But among his thousands of prints and books, his most notable works are the forty-six color prints he created between the ages of sixty-six and seventy-three, comprising *Thirty-Six Views of Mt. Fuji*. This body of work is seen as marking a summit in the history of Japanese landscape printing. Hokusai believed his art improved with his age, and longed to live to be over a hundred.

*John A. B. McLeish, *The Ulyssean Adult* (New York: McGraw-Hill Ryerson, 1976).

He did not make it, but the flames of his creativity burned long and strong until he died at eighty-nine.

Just as creativity commences with age for some because of a unique combination of time and developmental energy, those same factors in a different mix foster continuing or changing creativity. In midlife the inner drive to reevaluate our lives may generate a desire to continue along a creative path to bring it to some new level, or the powerful midlife tendency for quest, as reflected in one's Ulyssean quest, can set the stage for change. The Liberation Phase, too, with its greater freedom of time and resources, provides a supportive climate for changing creativity. Summing-Up energy may enable us to see the possibility for different kinds of creativity, supporting a desire for change. And in the Encore Phase, there may be a desire to make a final statement in an existing realm of creative expression or to take advantage of remaining opportunities to try a new form of creative expression.

The noted twentieth-century artist Helene Schjerfbeck was one of Finland's greatest painters. Her strongest work emerged when she was in her eighties, when her self-portraits underwent a metamorphosis into Abstract Expressionism. Her earlier work, through middle age, had been more traditionally representational. But she felt that what she was ultimately capable of expressing had not yet met its optimal forms, that is, until circumstances created a new art movement that Schjerfbeck intuitively experienced as a direction most congruent with her inner world.

DAVID BERG: WAITING A LIFETIME

As a young man, David Berg wanted to go to medical school. But circumstances conspired against him, he said. World War II broke out shortly after he finished college and before he applied to medical school, and he was drafted. By the time he finished his tour of duty, he was older than many of the students applying to medical school, and would have been older still because he had not met all of his science requirements and would have needed further courses before even applying to medical school. Moreover, his family was of very limited means and could offer him no assistance. Instead he prepared for the pharmacy exam, did exceptionally well, and began a career as a pharmacist in the Public Health Service for more than thirty-five years, until his early sixties.

David was an excellent pharmacist but found the heavy demands stressful and the lack of control over his job frustrating. A heart attack at age sixty-two led to his retirement. Free from the burden of his stressful job and under a new exercise and diet program, he made a very strong recovery and, two years later, at age sixty-four, felt stronger and

Daniel Defoe, author of **Robinson Crusoe** *and* **Moll Flanders,** *began working in the world of trade—especially with hosiery, wine, and tobacco. He later served his government as a secret agent, and subsequently turned to writing novels, a new literary form emerging in the eighteenth century as he was nearing sixty. His writing continued to diversify; between the ages of sixty-four and sixty-seven he wrote a three-volume travel book* (**Tour Through the Whole Island of Great Britain**)*, and at sixty-eight he published* **Augusta Triumphans, or the Way to Make London the Most Flourishing City in the Universe.**

healthier than he had in years. He decided to make a fundamental change in the nature of the work he had been doing.

While working as a pharmacist he had taken some continuing education courses on occupational health. For the previous year he had immersed himself in books on this topic and prepared to launch his own small business of consulting to both federal and private agencies serving employee counseling programs in occupational health. He started with a federal contact that he had made while in the Public Health Service, and this first consultation went exceedingly well.

Things gradually grew from that point, and five years later, at age sixty-nine, he had a thriving business in which he felt totally in control, allowing himself ample time off. He found his work highly satisfying. He also derived a new peace of mind about his missed career in medicine, sensing that his past—complete with its setbacks and frustrations—had brought him to a consulting career that was more fulfilling than any he imagined at an earlier age. Approaching his seventieth birthday, he was contemplating expanding his contribution to public health by developing and publishing a consultation guide for occupational health employee counseling.

Creativity in Connection with Loss

Contrary to the common assumption that loss, like a drop of ink in water, colors life with a grim shade of adversity, many survivors of loss offer a more encouraging picture of creativity in the context of adversity. The complex emotional effects of loss in life tend to be more subtle and gradual, more like rain in a cup of water: with each raindrop ripples form, but the water's color and consistency remain the same. We are able to deal with change in this manner because we are social animals, and we tend to go through change with social structures and people to help us. If a loved one dies, for instance, it is natural for us to experience what we call in psychiatry a "psychodynamic flux." On the one hand we can become overwhelmed by the sense of loss, while at the same time our spirit struggles to transcend the loss. This emotional tension or tug-of-war is captured in ancient Chinese wisdom, which reminds us, "In every crisis is an opportunity."

My point is not to romanticize loss, but to show that neither age nor loss necessarily shut down creative expression. This struggle to grow despite adversity reflects the most basic creative energy of life. In truth, many men and women experience creative expression despite loss—and at times, as the result of loss—in their later years. We'll explore this kind of creativity, and its healing and restorative power, more fully in Chapter 6.

Sarah Bernhardt (1844–1923) was the celebrated French actress who became one of the best-known performers in the history of the stage. She made her debut in 1862, achieving fame by age twenty-five in the role of Zanetto in Coppé's **La Passant.** ***In 1915, at age seventy-one, she had to have a leg amputated following complications from an earlier knee injury received when jumping during the last scene of*** **La Tosca.** ***Nonetheless, her acting continued, as playwrights found or developed roles for her that could be acted while seated. Her last role was in*** **La Voyante,** ***a Hollywood movie being filmed in her own house in Paris at the time of her death at age seventy-eight. Earlier that same year she wrote her treatise on acting,*** **L'Art du théâtre.**

BARBARA DAVIS: TO EVERYONE, EVERYTHING A SEASON

Barbara Davis was seventy-five years old when her grandniece, Lana, asked me to see her. Ms. Davis had been widowed nine years earlier, and four years afterward had lost her only child, her forty-eight-year-old daughter, who died from ovarian cancer. She had no grandchildren, but Lana, age twenty-four, was like a granddaughter. The loss of her husband had been difficult for Ms. Davis. She had looked forward to retiring with him after both had worked long and hard at their careers, he as a midlevel manager with the U.S. Post Office, she as an administrative assistant at a public high school. The loss of her daughter had been quite devastating and had taken a terrible toll on her; "it changed her," Lana said.

Ms. Davis had grown up in a close-knit family, the youngest of three sisters. Her father was a minister, her mother a homemaker, both very loving. One sister had died three years earlier; the other resided in an assisted-living facility several hundred miles away.

Lana lived in the same city as her great aunt and was her only local relative. Lana described Ms. Davis as always having been warm, open, and making you feel comfortable around her. The kids at the high school were very fond of Ms. Davis, and she was highly appreciated by the faculty. People liked her. She had always been very interested in her rich African-American family history, but more recently didn't seem very interested in anything other than her problems. She had become increasingly difficult to approach following the loss of her daughter, preferring to stay in her apartment by herself. She had become bitter and reclusive, both uncharacteristic qualities in her past.

Arthritis had become a problem, limiting her mobility, and Lana hired a part-time homemaker to help out. But the homemakers had a hard time with Ms. Davis, describing her as verbally hostile. One after another, caregivers came and went; they didn't want to work with her. Lana, after talking with her aunt at greater length, was concerned at the paranoid tone of her comments; her aunt believed the world was against her and the homemakers were stealing from her. Lana could not clearly document any theft and concluded that her aunt needed help. Although Lana asked me to see her aunt, Ms. Davis didn't want to see a psychiatrist and so refused to meet with me. I suggested to Lana that she explain to her aunt that she was concerned about her overall health and would like to arrange for a doctor to visit to see how she was feeling and doing. Lana did this, and Ms. Davis agreed to see me.

"A woman is like a teabag; you never know how strong she is until she gets in hot water."
—NANCY REAGAN

Our initial getting-acquainted meeting went well. In this first meeting, she let her defenses down somewhat and revealed some of the anger and suspiciousness that her grandniece had described. She also revealed some borderline delusional thinking. After talking about the toll of life events on her emotional wellness, I suggested we meet regularly and that she begin taking a medication that would relieve the delusional thinking, and ease much of the suspiciousness and hostility. She agreed to meet regularly, but was adamant about not taking any medicine. She said if she took medicine from a psychiatrist it would mean she was crazy. I said I would still be pleased to meet with her.

We met once a week in her apartment over the next two months, and at first things went very well. She was becoming more animated and interested in telling me about the rich experiences she had as a child growing up in a small Southern town where her father was viewed as a leader in his community. She was very proud of her family.

But then one day, following a poor night's sleep, she got into an argument with a neighbor about noise coming from the neighbor's apartment. When I saw her later that day, she had abruptly regressed in her behavior and was fuming. She said she didn't want to see me anymore because I wasn't doing her any good, that we had talked enough and that it was time to stop. She was adamant about it, and I left, but first told her that I would call her later that week to see how she was doing.

When I called, she said she felt better but still did not want to talk, and I agreed simply to call again the next week. The next time I called she was in an angry mood, said she didn't want to talk anymore and told me not to call—that if she needed anything she'd call me.

I knew that a visiting nurse came periodically to the building and saw Ms. Davis about her arthritis every few months. The nurse had once come during one of my visits and told Ms. Davis she was glad Ms. Davis was meeting with me. I contacted the nurse, explained the situation, and suggested that she might ask Ms. Davis if she wanted to see me again.

I was confident that medication would make a significant difference in the way she felt, and wished she would give it a chance; I felt our talks would further help her regain a more satisfying experience of life. I also knew that Ms. Davis's delusions fluctuated in intensity, and that during a more tranquil interval she might be more receptive to my returning. Indeed, she told the nurse she would be interested in talking with me again. During the next two years, we met intermittently and Ms. Davis kicked me out four more times, only to eventually invite me to come back upon the urging of her niece or the nurse.

On the whole, though, Ms. Davis's delusions were getting worse, and she was becoming more stressed. I again voiced my concern and the potential good of the proposed medication if only she would try it. She countered that her complaints weren't in her head—they were real. I suggested that her anxiety was real, too, and that the medication could at least help with that. She reconsidered and agreed to try the medication. She responded to the medication very well, and in the next year she became more like her "old self." She at last accepted the part-time assistance of a homemaker, showing appreciation, not abuse, toward the helper. At seventy-eight, her quality of life was improving.

On a subsequent visit Ms. Davis informed me that the recreation program in the building was launching an oral history program, asking for volunteers over age seventy-five to share their life experiences on audiotapes. The recreation coordinator, knowing about Barbara Davis's interest in African-American history, asked her if she would talk about

Gregario Marzan, born in 1906 in Puerto Rico, had lost most of his hearing by the time he reached his thirties. He worked at a job stuffing dolls and animals for a toy company; when the company switched to machine stuffing, he operated the machines until he retired at age sixty-five. Subsequently, he lost his sight in one eye; half blind and nearly deaf he pursued art, seeking his materials by walking the streets of Spanish Harlem for found objects to incorporate into his mixed media sculpture, which was included in a major traveling exhibit entitled "Hispanic Art in the United States: Thirty Contemporary Painters and Sculptors." One of his best-known works is **The Statue of Liberty,** ***which he created at the age of eighty-three; it is mixed media, with plaster, fabric, tape, glue, a light bulb, Elmer's Glue caps, and a wig.***

these experiences and allow them to be recorded. During the next six months, Ms. Davis participated in the project, deriving great satisfaction from it. I contacted the niece and encouraged her to keep her aunt going at this project, suggesting she might want to get a tape recorder and meet with her aunt periodically, perhaps once a month, to have her share her story for the family and future family members. They were both delighted with the project, which became ongoing for the next two years.

"Our energy is in proportion to the resistance it meets."
—WILLIAM HAZLITT

Throughout this period of several years I visited Ms. Davis once every other month, just to make sure things stayed on track. On one of my visits shortly after Ms. Davis turned eighty, she indicated that she had volunteered to become the "Floor Captain" on her floor of the apartment building. A floor captain's responsibility was to make sure each day that all the residents on that floor left a card on their door each night and took it in the next morning so others would know they were all right. But Ms. Davis took her responsibilities a step further, saying, "You know there are a few old ladies on this floor who are very lonely and would benefit from my periodically visiting them; some people are helped a lot by such visits." I nodded and savored the moment of her further branching out, trying something new at eighty—to help some of the "old" ladies.

Patients teach doctors a lot, not the least of which is humility. When I visited Ms. Davis on her eighty-third birthday, her best friend came in and she proudly introduced me—as her "podiatrist."

5

Creative Growth and Expression in the Context of Relationship

If a man does not make new acquaintance as he advances through life, he will soon find himself left alone. A man, Sir, should keep his friendship in constant repair.

—SAMUEL JOHNSON, 1755

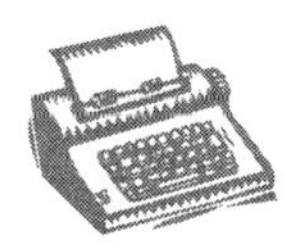

MARJORIE, AN ENERGETIC WOMAN with a husband, three teenage children, and a fledgling business making theatrical costumes, explained that she had recently dropped out of the women's book discussion group that she had attended for some years. She had always found the group enjoyable and stimulating, especially during the early years of motherhood when she felt starved for adult conversation. But recently several of the members had, in the course of literary discussion, made emotional disclosures of discontent with their marriages or choices in life, and Marjorie didn't like it. "They're dwelling on these painful personal issues, and I just don't want to spend time surrounded by negative energy," she said. "I'm too excited by my life right now, and all the really great things I have going,

Mary Barbara Hamilton Cartland, the English romantic novelist, earned a place in the **Guinness Book of Records** *for writing twenty-six books in one year, at the age of eighty-two (1983).*

to let myself get dragged down by that kind of conversation. I'm taking my life in other directions, new places."

Another woman in the group, Fran, acknowledged that she had lately begun to share with this trusted circle of friends her honest feelings about life issues that came up in discussion. This was part of her own new direction at midlife—one of self-discovery and a more forthright exploration of her inner emotional life. "I've kept a lid on my feelings all these years because it seemed like everyone needed me to be what *they* needed, and they all needed so much," she said. For the first time in her adult life, she said, she was now expressing the way she really felt, which sometimes included anger and sadness about aspects of her life. Encouraged in part by the other women in her book discussion group, Fran also had begun to write poetry, and one of her poems had been accepted for publication in a literary journal. "I'm starting to be more honest with myself about my feelings and express what I really think and what I really feel, and it's such a relief," she said. "I feel like a new person."

For both women, the book discussion group had been a stimulating environment for a number of years, but within the course of a single month the relationship had become a dead end for Marjorie, while for Fran it had opened new vistas of creative potential and self-expression. Each woman's individual needs had changed her experience of the group and the value of that social relationship in her life.

This is the nature of relationships and this is the way they influence our creativity as we age. Marriage, friendship, family, and workplace relationships each offer a unique context for creativity in our lives, an environment for personal growth and expression. Some relationships encourage our creativity, foster it, cultivate it, nurture it, respect it. Other relationships inhibit our creativity, limiting, discouraging, punishing such expressions of growing, changing individuality.

Most relationships have the potential to both encourage and discourage our creativity at different times; how we respond reflects the expectations, fears, and desires each of us bring to the moment. It is rare that two people are inspired at the same time in the same direction, but where partners are motivated, there are ways to close that gap, strengthen the relationship, and make it a sustaining one that stands the test of time.

For my Aunt Annie S. Greenside, "Nothing came easy to me at any time, and they continue on that track." Annie saw her job in her home as that of wife and mother, raising her three children (now all successful professionals) as full-time work. Annie was in her mid-forties when her kids started to put down their recorders and stop their music lessons, so she decided it was her turn, and she picked them up for herself, starting her own lessons. Like everything else, she reminded me, it wasn't easy, but self-enrichment was very important to her, and she began building a new social portfolio of personal activities, catalyzed by her changing role with the kids' going off to college. The first recorder group she attended she described as "consisting of a lot of engineers who could make their own recorders—too intimidating for me." So she sought out another group that seemed more like her peers. Turning

Most of us are sensitive to the need for planning to ensure financial security as we age, but we rarely think about where we'll be years from now in terms of our relationships. Wise financial planning involves putting your money to use in a variety of ways, creating a diversified investment portfolio designed to weather economic ups and downs while protecting and enhancing your finances. Just as important to our future well-being is a plan for social security, too, and I'm not talking about a government benefits program. When we invest in a variety of relationships, meaningful in different ways, we're investing in our creativity and our long-term emotional health. I call this a social portfolio, and we'll explore the idea later in this chapter, and in Chapter 9's creativity workshop, where you'll find the step-by-step instructions for creating your own. For now, it's enough to know that every relationship adds to our life experience, and in that way, to our creative potential as we age.

The Role of Relationship in Creative Development

Contrary to a common view that as we age we grow "settled in our ways," such that we can no longer grow or change, the second half of life offers remarkable opportunities for renewal through interpersonal relationships—new starts, new directions, and mid-course corrections. Charles Johnston, another contemporary psychiatrist who has studied creativity, talks about the way uncertainty and change infuse relationships with creative growth potential.

"When we risk feeling in relation to another, whether those feelings are tender or hostile, we never know ahead of time exactly what they will bring. The best we can do is to create rich potential spaces for what we think we want, and to step courageously into them. There is the possibility for living connection in the moment precisely to the degree we can let that moment be something that has not been before," Johnston writes in *The Creative Imperative.*

Relationship—whether it is marriage, friendship, family, or work-related—must incorporate change or weaken in the effort to silence or deny it.

eighty, she says she still has to work hard at the recorder, but it is fun, very rewarding, and quite gratifying when she participates in a periodic public performance.

A few years after picking up the recorder, she joined a singing group. As she entered her sixties, she felt responsibilities around the home continued to ease, and she joined two book clubs and a short-story group. Annie describes working very hard at understanding the nuances in these stories, but she finds the discussions to be very fascinating, often leading to people talking about their own situations, making the get-togethers very social. Upon entering her seventies, Annie felt she finally had time to devote more attention to physical fitness, always having been interested in athletics.

"To the degree that relationship is alive, it involves change," Johnston says. "In our fears of the unknown we may try to keep our relationships from changing, but even if we are successful, they don't stay the same; instead they become constricted and confined. In time, they simply die. Real relationship is an ever-evolving, shared creative journey."

When we engage in the creative work of relationship—and it is hard work at times—we not only gain in experience and insight, but over time we model the unique potential of continuing collaborative creativity in a way that can have powerful and positive effects on others. Enduring, loving marriages and friendships top the list because they model for others the ability to deal with crisis rather than dissolve with it. They also model the way in which relationships can grow, mature, and evolve with emotional intimacy, loyalty, and collaborative creativity. Intergenerational relationships—between grandparents and grandchildren, for instance—also offer rich potential for collaborative creativity.

Gloria Swanson (1897–1983), the glamorous American actress known particularly for her role as Norma Desmond in the 1950 film classic **Sunset Boulevard**, *married six times. In 1980, at the age of eighty-three, she wrote her autobiography,* **Swanson on Swanson.**

As we age, the network of our relationships expands—often in both magnitude and complexity. We typically have more acquaintances, colleagues, friends, and family over time, though closeness will vary with circumstances. In recent decades, marriages, in particular, have become more complicated because of the higher incidence of divorce, remarriage, and second or even third families. With a subsequent marriage, there may be children from both marriages who, as adults themselves, will marry and expand the family to include an impressive multigenerational mix of in-laws. Even the least sociable among us is typically part of numerous relationships in everyday life at work and in our communities.

We are shaped not only by each relationship but by the cumulative influence of them. The basic requirement of any relationship is to "learn" another person, or connect in meaningful ways, so with every relationship we add to our potential to see things from a new perspective, experience life differently, and respond in fresh ways.

This means that any change in one of our relationships has a greater chance to have a larger ripple effect when we are older than when we were younger. As we age, the growing mix and complexity of our social network results in new challenges and new opportunities in our relationships in general. The impact of these growing relationships is profound in their influence on both our inner psychological life and our outer world experiences—in this sense stimulating both *e*'s in our $C = me^2$ formula, enhancing our skills for dealing with people and our capacity to connect with our creativity.

Change in the second half of life comes on many different winds: change within ourselves, change in our significant others, change in our life circumstances, obstacles and opportunities, and change in social and cultural influences. Indeed, the network starts to look more like a galaxy in which shifts in relationships have a spiraling effect, affecting relationships seemingly far removed from the original point of departure.

For example, we've explored the human potential phases that emerge in the second half of life and offer us developmental opportunities to change from within—the Midlife Reevaluation, Liberation, Summing-Up, and Encore Phases. These same developmental phases are unfolding in the lives of others we know and love. A spouse, lover, friend, colleague, parent, or child experiences similarly profound changes. Situational changes—empty nest, retirement, second or third careers—also present opportunities for new challenges and growth.

Social and cultural changes also exert very important influences on our creative growth and expression within relationships. Men, in our own and many Western cultures, characteristically are more focused on the external world of work and achievement in their younger years, but often develop a greater interest in their inner life and personal relationships in later life. Women in these cultures more often begin with a focus on the inner world of emotion and find their explorations of the external world enhanced as they age.

The uncertainty, challenges, and opportunities that surround all these areas of change result in new possibilities, which show that our destiny has not been locked in by events in early development—no matter how powerful those events may have been—because these later experiences can be equally powerful. Uncertainty and change both are hallmarks of the second half of life, but how we respond to them is a matter of choice. At any time and at any age, we can choose to repackage what we have learned and experienced in previous decades, and modify the course set by early developmental events by taking new routes offered in our later adult years.

Baron Alexander von Humboldt (1769–1859), German naturalist and explorer, wrote his remarkable work* Kosmos *between the ages of seventy-six and eighty-nine (1845–1858). This book is regarded a landmark for popularizing science for the general public.

At the age of sixty-five (1948), Edith Clarke became the first woman elected a fellow of the American Institute of Electrical Engineers.

Creativity as a Catalyst for Growth in Relationship

"Creative minds always have been known to survive any kind of bad training."
—ANNA FREUD

One of the most exciting aspects of studying aging for me is the opportunity that such research provides to look at the human condition—its issues, struggles and opportunities—from a new vantage point. In any situation or field of study, whenever you can look at questions through a different window, you increase your chances of seeing something that has otherwise been missed. Historically, studies of human nature have focused almost exclusively on the early years and how they shape and predict an individual's outlook and behavior in the years that follow. That approach is limited, because there is so much about human behavior that we don't know; there are windows to understanding that we haven't even found, much less used to illuminate the subject. By using the second half of life as the starting point for the exploration of relationship and creativity we find new windows for observation and new questions to ask:

- How do our relationships influence our creative growth and expression in adult life?
- How do our creative growth and expression affect our relationships?
- How can we use creativity to support our individuality within relationships, strengthen relationships that are important to us, and develop new relationships to enrich our lives?

When we look at relationship as a context for creativity, we can see the rich potential for different types, particularly collaborative and social creativity. Creativity is not always a solo effort, remember; the combination of different personalities, experience, desires, and dreams offers a unique opportunity for personal growth through interaction with others. From the paired efforts of a composer and a lyricist in creating a musical to the mobilization of the team that put the first man on the moon, we know that creativity can be the unique product of a joint or group effort.

On a more everyday level, life is rich with opportunities for collaborative creativity, in marriage or any relationship of emotional intimacy, in friendships, in the larger family and in the community close and far. In adulthood, it is almost always possible for two emotionally committed partners to bring something new and valued into existence in ways that benefit their relationship and their own personal growth. Other relationships and social interactions offer ways to cultivate our creativity through exposure to new people and new ideas. Just as, in the biological realm, the brain's capacity to manage new information and generate new thoughts is expanded by new connections among billions of dendrites, our creative potential grows when we enrich our existing relationships and expand our circles of social interaction. This exciting potential exists for every one of us, regardless of education, income, or health status.

Sexologist William Howell Masters, M.D., of the Masters and Johnson team, at age seventy-one (1986) coauthored with Virginia Johnson (age sixty-one) **On Sex and Human Loving.**

As we move into and through the second half of life, not only does our number of relationships grow, but our relationship *experience* expands. In that process our ability to understand and deal with relationships generally increases. There is no pat formula for a successful relationship, just as there isn't one for creativity; both rely heavily on emotional chemistry that isn't fully understood.

However, just as special knowledge, life experience, and inner forces combine and synergize to spur individual creative growth, a similar synergy shapes creative growth in relationships. In some instances, the history of a relationship—shared interests, experiences, and emotional intimacy, for instance—grows more meaningful over time; we tend to attach more significance to the opinion or feelings of a friend who's known us for years than those expressed by someone we met yesterday.

In 1881, at the age of seventy-one, Phineas Taylor (P. T.) Barnum joined with his archrival James Anthony Bailey (age thirty-four) to found the famous Barnum and Bailey circus.

In other circumstances, however, history can hold us hostage to old habits and roles we have outgrown or wish to. If you are at a point in your life when the urge for change and growth is strong, a relationship heavily weighted by emotional history may feel confining. The challenge of relationship is to use its history as a foundation for creativity and growth rather than a walled fortress against change.

"Growth Gaps": Uneven Development Produces Tension

When one partner in a relationship is experiencing a dramatic growth in creative energy and the other is not, or has interests that pull in a dif-

Fanny Burney (1752–1840), the English novelist and diarist, was considered a forerunner of Jane Austen, whom she influenced in her portrayal of domestic scenes. At eighty she dedicated herself to the publication of her father's memoirs.

ferent direction, the result is a "growth gap" in the relationship that can either undermine the bond of emotional connection and experience or be used to strengthen it, depending on the individual responses of the partners. When a relationship is adaptable, these growth gaps can be stimulating as, at different times, one partner blazes a trail into a new territory of thought or activity that the other eventually comes to enjoy or appreciate.

When the growth gap is experienced by either partner as a threat to the relationship, reactions tend to grow adversarial, only adding to the challenge of moving forward together. As we age, our relationship skills and experience grow, enabling us to navigate these growth gaps toward stronger, or sometimes new, connections. However, in some circumstances, when the challenge of change is greater than the mutual desire to bridge the gap, the basis for relationship is lost. At that point, creative thinking becomes the tool for moving on to new opportunities and different relationships.

Ned and Nancy were in their mid-forties when the last of their three children graduated from college and the "empty nest" loomed large and inviting. Their children were well situated with jobs, friends, and busy lives of their own. Ned had some job security as a middle-level manager in a government office and looked forward to spending more of their free time and available income on travel. Nancy had sidelined her own career pursuits as a teacher eighteen years before to be a stay-at-home mother and now saw her opportunity to revive those interests. She had worked occasionally as a substitute teacher during their children's school years, but she wanted to return to school herself now and pursue an advanced degree in history, her longtime field of study.

In the early months of their newfound freedom, the most obvious changes were in Nancy's daily routine. She joined a gym and within six months had lost seventeen pounds, which motivated her to buy a new wardrobe. Feeling fit, she moved ahead with her educational plans to complete work for a doctoral degree in Eastern European History. She was like a kindling fire going to a full blaze the way she took to the courses and excelled. Before she knew it, one of the professors had asked her to assist him, teaching history to undergraduate students.

Now she was really aglow and was spending increasing time at the university preparing for lectures, meeting with students, and doing her own studies and research.

At first Ned was pleased for her, but as her enthusiasm grew, his dimmed. He felt left out. He was hurt that she could experience such newfound interest and excitement outside their relationship, without him. The situation grew worse as Nancy spent more and more time away from Ned. She was physically and fashionably looking so good, he began to feel it wasn't for him. Gradually their pleasurable conversations gave way to tense exchanges, beginning with Ned's irritability and nitpicking, and then made worse by his scheduling activities—obtaining theater tickets, for instance—on nights he knew she had an important school commitment. Nancy grew increasingly irritable and angry toward Ned. After one particularly heated exchange, they saw that the deepening rift in their relationship threatened their future together. They were at a standoff, Nancy pushing forward with excitement, Ned angrily digging in his heels, and the tension had strained their marriage to the breaking point.

How could such a promising period for Ned and Nancy disintegrate this way? Was Nancy supposed to set aside her promising new career and give up her dream of scholarship and leadership in her field of study? And for what? A marriage that confined her creative energy? A husband who seemed to resent her success? From Ned's point of view, with no clear vision of Nancy's inner life, everything seemed to have been working just fine, and he was puzzled—even stunned—by the magnitude of changes that had unfolded in a very short time. To heal the rift in their relationship would require considerable effort by both partners, collaborating to find new ways to understand each other and rebuild a shared life.

Another couple in trouble was Anne, forty-one, and Jason, forty-two, who had been married for eight years. It had been a stormy relationship from the start. They were both writers, which provided them much in common. But they were also very competitive. They were each working on their first book. In the interim Anne had had several articles published in different magazines, and they were very well received. Jason was receiving very little interest in articles he was writing and was

George Bancroft (1800–1891) published the tenth and final volume of his important work* History *at age seventy-four. Not satisfied with his* History *as a whole, he spent the next eleven years making revisions to correct the mistakes of earlier editions. His final revision was volume two of his* History of the Formation of the Constitution, *published when he was eighty-five.

Julia Ward Howe (1819–1910) was an American reformer, author, and lecturer best known for writing the "Battle Hymn of the Republic" in 1862 (when she was forty-three); it was published in The Atlantic Monthly. *She edited* Woman's Journal *from 1870 until 1890 (age seventy-one). At eighty-nine (in 1908), she became the first woman to be elected to the American Academy of Arts and Letters.*

becoming jealous of Anne. When she eventually received a lucrative contract for her book, while he continued to collect rejection letters, it was too much for him. He had an affair, didn't hide it, and made it clear he had no intention of making amends. He continued to vandalize the marriage, and eventually the two divorced.

Friends became the obstacles to creativity for Catherine, sixty-three, who had lived in the same small Midwestern town all her life. Her friends there were mostly the friends she had made when she was in grade school. She was widowed at sixty-one, after thirty-seven years of marriage to a wonderful man who didn't like to travel.

As she thought for the first time about life on her own, she reconnected with a long-dormant desire to see the world, and she began to investigate guided tours to foreign lands. Her friends didn't share her wanderlust, and initially teased her about it. When she persisted in exploring travel options and sharing her excitement, the teasing took a sharper turn, as her friends began to caution her about traveling alone "at her age" and criticize her for dropping out of leadership roles in community organizations to free up her schedule for travel.

With her first trip—a simple Amtrak train ride across the country—she discovered a world of friendly, interesting people who shared her delight at seeing new places. Back home she began to attend evening travel talks at the community library and became friends with a number of regulars like her. She shifted her volunteer work to the library, too, and joined a book discussion group that met there monthly. Bit by bit, she found herself busy with her new interests and warmed by the encouragement of new friends who admired her adventurous spirit and intellect. She didn't set out to lose her old friends, but they continued to be critical of her new choices, and over time she chose to see them less and less.

Nurturing the "Me" in the "We" of Intimate Relationship

Whether we express our creative energy in painting, teaching, farming, or philosophizing, whether it is big C public creativity or little c personal, our creativity offers the truest expression of our individuality. That true self can become overwhelmed at times by the demands or expectations of others, by a desire to please others, or by the power of someone else's vision of how things should be in a relationship. Is it possible to cultivate a "me" in a "we"? Are individual creativity and relationship mutually exclusive?

Martin Buber (1878–1975), the theologian and philosopher who published **I and Thou** *at age forty-five, published* **Between Man and Man** *at age sixty-nine and* **The Seventh Day** *at age eighty-nine.*

Love one another, but make not a bond of love,

Fill each other's cup, but drink not from one cup . . .

Give your hearts, but not into each other's keeping.

—KAHLIL GIBRAN

History and psychology tell us that while it may be a challenge at times to assert our individuality in relationships, many people find it easier to do so as they grow older. Why? They're more confident of themselves. They're less worried that they'll be judged harshly by those whose opinions are important to them. Sometimes certain pressures on the relationship have eased over time.

"When our children were all through college, without that financial responsibility I felt like I could finally relax and do the things I'd thought about for years but couldn't afford to risk doing," said William, seventy-two, a retired sales representative for a paint manufacturer. "I'd always wanted to learn carpentry, and even though my wife didn't have that interest, she didn't mind if I spent my time that way. She had her own things going."

When problems arise in expressing "the me" in a marriage or any close relationship, it most often is because one has not achieved that sense of autonomy, or self-awareness and self-direction, *before* the relationship. Many people, in the search to feel complete or to resolve feelings of inadequacy, marry or become dependent on others for that identity. Any relationship, but especially one of emotional intimacy, is an ideal place for discovering new aspects of ourselves *in relation* to a significant other.

If instead we have yet to establish who we are as individuals, this places a heavy burden on the relationship. The risk then is that with

Leonard Sidney Woolf (1880–1969), the English publisher who was married to Virginia Woolf and along with her founded the Hogarth Press, **wrote his** *autobiography, in five volumes, starting at age eighty:* **Sowing**, *1960;* **Growing**, *1961 (age eighty-one);* **Beginning Again**, *1964 (age eighty-four);* **Downhill All the Way**, *1967 (age eighty-seven);* **The Journey to the Arrival Matters**, *1969 (age eighty-nine), the year he died.*

feelings of wholeness or identity too heavily invested in the other person, the tenuous sense of wholeness is disrupted if major changes or a significant growth gap occurs. The dependent partner suffers inner emotional conflict that inevitably spills over into the relationship.

With aging, as discussed in earlier chapters, we more often have a better sense of who we are as individuals, and the issue of identity within the relationship begins to diminish. This positive psychological development, often overlooked in the stereotyped images of aging, is a tremendous boon to those who finally achieve a comfortable sense of themselves and are able to bring that to their relationships.

When a relationship is experienced in part as an opportunity for further self-discovery, adding to an established base of self-understanding, it provides both a loving and creative experience; through this kind of intimacy we discover something new about ourselves. The close sharing and interaction allow us to continue to thrive as individuals and as a couple at the same time. Maintaining the right amount of individuality on the part of both partners fosters a process of creative uncertainty and change that can keep the relationship vital.

Maintaining "the me" in relation to "the we" allows the ongoing exploration of both the me and the we—a double opportunity to be creative through discovering something new and bringing something new into the relationship either individually or together. Whenever we can look at ourselves in different ways, we increase the chance of identifying different aspects and establishing deeper understanding of ourselves. These are ways that creativity can help a relationship.

Mary Sherwood (1775–1881), nineteenth-century English author of children's books, wrote seventy-seven different works over her long career, including the popular* History of the Fairfield Family *series written over a twenty-nine-year period from age forty-three to age seventy-two.

The Role of Gender

In our experience of relationships as we age, the role of gender undergoes positive change. As alluded to earlier, one of the biggest issues in male-female relationships is the tendency for women to be more focused on the inner workings, while men characteristically focus on their activities and accomplishments outside. Women are commonly viewed as being more attentive to interpersonal issues, while men are typically seen as paying more attention to external actions affecting their career. Reflecting these patterns of interest and expression, women typically have closer, more highly developed relationships, while men typically have more activity-based, collegial relationships.

Cross-cultural research findings by gerontologist and professor of psychology David Gutmann have linked such gender differences in relationship to the traditional social training that divvies up parenting and other domestic roles and responsibilities along gender lines. By middle age these role differences begin to become less pronounced.

By late middle age and moving into later life, in many cultures, men become more interpersonally and relationship oriented, while women become more outer-world oriented and redirect interest in family growth toward personal growth once the children have matured. These changes bring husbands and wives closer together, revitalizing the relationship and bringing something new to it; husbands often approach the relationship with more emotional involvement, and women bring new dimensions of themselves based on self-discovery from personal exploration. This is valuable creative energy of a kind that becomes commonly available only in later adult life.

Snapshots of Relationships over Time

In my study of older persons doing well in later life, among the areas explored were relationships in general and marriage in particular. Here are some snapshots, depicted by persons in the study, of developments relating to relationships as we age. All the comments are by individuals age sixty-five or older. The positive comments should not be surprising in light of the very low divorce rate among older adults in general and because these were people doing well. But their perspectives, insights, and approaches shed some light on the way aging can change the climate of relationships and the support there for new growth.

"Now that I'm older I find that in my interactions with people I have fewer conflicts, fewer tensions."

Edward Jean Steichen (1879–1973), the noted American photographer who was director of photography at the New York Museum of Modern Art from ages sixty-six to eighty-three, published his celebrated work **The Family of Man** *at age seventy-six.*

"When we first married there were numerous arguments, but we worked it out."

"I find it easier to handle stress in my relationships now [in later life], especially since I don't have as many other distractions."

"I don't feel the same pressure to get even with someone now after a dispute that I did when I was young; I think more about working things out."

"In general I feel more calm, less stressed than when I was younger, and this certainly helps me deal with relationships."

"I have found that I am more tolerant of the failures of other people."

"The things that bothered my husband in the past don't seem to bother him as much now."

"My wife has become more spontaneous in activities we do together."

"We've grown closer. The bonds have strengthened in our marriage over time."

Alice Babette Toklas, known for her talented writing and legendary relationship with Gertrude Stein, published her famous The Alice B. Toklas Cookbook *at the age of seventy-seven (1954). The book is noted for its unusual mix of provocative comment, advice, anecdote, and, of course, gourmet marvels.*

"I am better adjusted now than twenty years ago; I can handle adversity better now; I get less irritated than in the past."

"Some of the sadness in life has brought us closer together."

"Grief is harder on the men, because they don't have as many best friends to help them handle the feelings."

"I find that I stand up for myself more now, and that applies to many other older women I know."

"I'm less cranky now than when I was younger; I'm more laissez-faire in relationships than in the past."

"In some ways marriage gets better; you settle the things you fight about."

"My husband's doing ironing now; that's been good for our relationship."

"My husband's starting to join me in more of the group activities I've always enjoyed."

"I have more self-assurance now than when I was a young mother."

"I'm more tolerant now, less demanding, less pushy."

"My relationship with my husband is better in some ways. He's more social now, and more active in everyday things. He also has more energy, not worn out from the three hours of daily commuting when he worked."

"As a couple we do more things together now; we're closer."

"We've been through some hard times, but we stayed the course. If it had been all smooth sailing in the past, it would be harder to deal with trouble now."

"Dealing with conflict with people is easier now because there's more time to deal with a misunderstanding immediately, before it builds up out of control."

"I find it easier to make friends now."

"Most widows wouldn't want to be married again, not wanting to cook."

"I'm not as shy now, and that certainly helps meeting people."

"I don't want to exist in a relationship, I want to live."

What stands out in these comments, and in others I hear frequently from older men and women, is the lessening of conflict in relationships as we age. For most people, age and experience give us greater opportunities to develop problem-solving strategies and skills. We're not only better equipped to deal with challenges in new relationships, but in established relationships of some duration, our experience bolsters our arsenal of tried-and-true options. Just as judges and diplomats bring that aged wisdom to their work, each of us is able to bring it to our own circle of relationships.

For many, especially those enjoying new freedom of time in retirement, the lack of pressure allows them to deal with a problem on the spot, "nipping it in the bud" or sooner than otherwise would have been the case. We learn to practice patience, to stand back, and especially in confrontational moments, let some of the passion settle before we impulsively respond. As we come to recognize the deeper value of rela-

Frank Harris (1856–1931), Irish-born American journalist, was an editor of feared talent, especially when he turned out scandal sheets. During his day he edited a number of important journals, including the* Saturday Review *(for which he hired George Bernard Shaw) and* Vanity Fair. *He has been described as being "the most colorful figure in contemporary journalistic circles, an incorrigible liar, vociferous boaster, and unscrupulous adventurer and philanderer, with an obsession with sex," which led to his autobiography's being banned for pornography. Indeed he is best known for his unreliable autobiography,* My Life and Loves, *which he wrote in three volumes from ages sixty-seven to seventy-one. Its sexual frankness was new for its day (1923–1927) and caused problems with censors in both the United States and Great Britain.

tionships, these problem-solving and coping responses help us maintain those connections, increasing the chance of building new bridges instead of burning so many behind us.

Billings Learned Hand (1872–1961) was a noted federal judge. Though he never served on the Supreme Court, he is generally regarded to have been a greater judge than all but a few who served on the nation's highest court. He served until his death at age eighty-nine. He published* The Spirit of Liberty *at age eighty and then updated it at age eighty-eight.

Conflict or Creativity: Five Arenas of Potential

Siblings quarrel and friendships hit some friction at times, but rarely do partners in those relationships seek counseling. So when we think of therapeutic strategies for understanding and mending relationships, it is most often in the context of marriage or a marriagelike relationship, generally accepted as the ultimate collaboration. In important ways, however, issues of creativity and aging follow similar patterns in many kinds of relationships. It would be a mistake to suggest that partners in a friendship, or any meaningful relationship, don't have the potential to significantly encourage or inspire one another's creativity; it would be just as mistaken to believe that friendship is somehow immune to jealousy, boredom, competition, and other obstacles to creativity commonly associated with marriage.

Because marriage is perhaps the most challenging of relationships, we can use it as a model for exploring the complex potential for conflict and creativity, and adapt key insights to strengthen our other relationships as well. Marriage, or any relationship between significant others, offers at least five *dynamics*, or arenas, in which we find that the mix of social, intellectual, or moral thought and action can contribute to either conflict or creativity. When there is conflict, examining each of these issues increases the chance of identifying the underlying problem. When seeking something new in the relationship, each of these arenas offers a potential starting point:

"Matrimony—the high sea for which no compass has yet been invented."
—HEINRICH HEINE

1. Dynamics in the interaction between the two spouses, or between two friends, family members, or other partners in a relationship
2. Dynamics going on within the husband (or one partner) alone

3. Dynamics going on within the wife (or other partner) alone
4. Dynamics between the husband, or one partner, and significant others outside the relationship, such as a child, parent, friend, lover, boss, or coworker.
5. Same dynamics between the wife, or other partner, and a significant other outside the relationship

If you're looking for the source of conflict that on the one hand causes tension in the relationship and on the other produces obstacles to creative growth in the relationship, this five-point review is a useful place to begin. If, for example, a marriage has stalled or tension is mounting, consider these points, which correspond to the five arenas listed above, in the same order.

1. Are the spouses being too competitive with each other?
2. Is the husband depressed and taking it out on the wife by being very demanding?
3. Is the wife anxious, bringing her irritation into the relationship?
4. Is the husband stressed at work because of an oppressive boss and unconsciously acting the oppressor (the boss) at home toward his wife?
5. Is the wife overburdened by family or other responsibilities and unconsciously acting out her exasperation by responding angrily to any additional expectations or requests made by her husband?

Pamela Hansford Johnson (Lady Snow), the English novelist who married CP Snow, wrote **The Good Husband** *at age sixty-six.*

For partners in marriage or any other relationship, any of the five arenas can be used to help target the point of conflict and develop more effective problem-solving strategies. At the same time each of these arenas reflects areas of creative potential initiated by one or both partners, and involving one or both. Creativity becomes a sustaining force when interactions and activities generate positive emotions and ongoing motivation to continue with them. I don't mean elaborate activities; I mean

"What counts in making a happy marriage is not so much how compatible you are, but how you deal with incompatibility."

—GEORGE LEVINGER

using creative initiative, including some thought about identifying activities that are satisfying in the relationship, making a commitment to doing them regularly, and venturing into some new territory together to explore other possibilities or expand on the tried-and-true ones.

If you want to recharge a relationship, or add to it, thinking or talking about it only takes you so far. You have to *do* something, find new creative interactions or activities. If you want the relationship to grow, you have to help it. Part of the fun and challenge can be a creative process in which partners explore together a new activity that either draws upon their complementary strengths or one in which they both have skills that when harnessed together could have a rewarding payoff. For instance:

- A joint, collaborative venture might be travel in which he takes the pictures and then she produces the text in creating interesting storybooks, or simple letters, for sharing with the extended family and friends.
- Individually, she or he might begin a course of study to develop background knowledge in a new area (preparation phase of creativity), and bring that positive energy back into the relationship.
- Either partner might become active in a local community effort that eventually draws the partner into that circle of activity and friendships also.

Through Conflict and Challenge: Mustering the Courage to Be Creative

Jerry, age forty-six, and Diane, age forty-five, had been married for twenty-three years. They had met when they were in graduate school at the same university. Jerry was completing his master's degree in business administration, and Diane was studying for a doctorate in psychology. A year after they married, Diane became pregnant, and she decided she would take a break from her studies to prepare for motherhood. She never did return to complete her doctorate, choosing instead to be an at-home mother for their family, which eventually included two children.

Over the years, Jerry derived great satisfaction from the opportunities that his job provided him to be creative in managing the finances of a rapidly growing electronics company, and he rose to become the company's chief financial officer. Diane at different times had wanted to return to school or work—at least part-time—but Jerry always discouraged her. He told her that she was such a great mother that he felt their children would benefit immensely if she devoted her talents to their upbringing rather than the impersonal workplace; he was quite sincere in these beliefs.

***Bishop Fulton Sheen (1895–1979), the noted Roman Catholic prelate and broadcaster, published many works, including, at age eighty-four (1979),* The Electronic Christian.**

Diane was torn about whether to divide her time between home and a potential career, but she loved motherhood and very much enjoyed seeing her children grow and blossom so beautifully. She was also sensitive to the downside risks of the two-career families she knew—too much stress, not enough family time, and children's needs sometimes lost in the rush of schedules. She decided to continue her full-time at-home mother status, and delay her career interests until the children were in college.

For the most part, theirs was a good marriage and they enjoyed a rich family and social life. In orchestrating the children's early activities, Diane made many friends. She had wonderful people skills. Her life was greatly enriched by these relationships, which helped contain her periodic resentment about giving up her studies and a career to stay at home. Even with Diane's sincere belief that this choice was the best for the family, she could not fully reconcile her situation with her own needs—to be out learning and working among her peers—and periodically her silent, smoldering disappointment about not finishing school would build up to the point of irritation, then anger and arguments with Jerry.

"I never hated a man enough to give him his diamonds back."

—ZSA ZSA GABOR

A good friend of the couple was the chief executive officer of a new multimedia company, and one evening when he attended a parent/teacher meeting at the school their children attended together, he became impressed by Diane's organizational and people skills. As a volunteer, Diane had coordinated and hosted the evening with singular finesse and great poise. Afterward, he suggested that she consider joining his company as a member of the public relations team. His company was planning a new marketing strategy targeted to a middle-age audience, and he felt that Diane, with the appealing presence she projected, would be a natural. Diane discussed this with Jerry, and he agreed that when their younger child went off to college there was no reason for Diane not to consider the position. He wasn't enthusiastic, but he didn't oppose the idea.

Alfred Pritchard Sloan Jr. (1875–1966) was an American industrialist who after restructuring General Motors became chairman of the board from 1937–1956 (ages sixty-two to eighty-one). Under his direction, GM became one of the largest corporations in the world. His autobiography, My Years with General Motors, *was written when he was eighty-nine (1964) and is considered a classic in management literature.*

It was not quite three months after Diane started her new job that Jerry came home distraught. His company's success had led to a distressing development for him. They were being bought up by a large company and as part of that merger the business would be moved halfway across the country. Jerry could stay with the company, but he would no longer be the chief financial officer, and he would have to move. Diane put her foot down firmly: absolutely not! She pointed out that she had stayed home all those years to help the children, and to create the home environment he so much appreciated, and now she finally was about to start a job far more exciting than she had ever imagined—a perfect fit. Furthermore, she felt their lives were enriched by the deep friendships that those years as an at-home mother had allowed her to cultivate. There was no way she was going to give up either. It was her turn, she argued, and besides, if Jerry didn't stay with the company he would get a separation package with a full year's salary, which she felt would give him the time to get another job. The two argued bitterly, but Jerry relented.

Over several months no breaks came Jerry's way; he became dispirited and increasingly unpleasant around the house, drinking a little too much, and was depressed each night when he came home. At first Diane was sympathetic, reminding him that this would pass. Meanwhile, her new career continued to flower. In addition to her face-to-face public relations work, her company was making a number of educational videos. When Diane was told that she had been selected to be the host of one of the films, she came home ecstatic—only to get a dour response from Jerry.

She became furious and let him have it, shouting her list of particulars: All those years he had come home boasting about his latest contribution or inspired idea at work, she had been the dutiful cheerleader, but now that fate had turned the tables, he didn't even have the basic decency to congratulate her. What kind of a partner was he? She reprimanded him further for feeling so sorry for himself. There was no need for it, she said. It wasn't an accident that he had done so well for so long; nothing about his skills had changed. Thanks to his previous success, they were in pretty good shape, and she now had a well-paying job. What was so different? They had always survived on only one salary, and hers was sufficient. There was plenty of time for him to find the right new job. "In the meantime, have some fun. Make some friends like you encouraged me to do all those years. Get a life!" she told him. She blew off years of steam.

They hardly spoke over the next two weeks, but then one evening when Diane came home she found roses on the dining-room table, which had been set for two with candlelight. Jerry had prepared a beautiful meal, and he apologized for having been such a downer for so long. He explained that he had initially resented her enthusiasm during a time when he was struggling. But he also had come to realize that she was right, that he had been selfish, and that it was not only her turn, but time for him to turn a new leaf as well. At last, committed to their mutual success, they began to work together on a plan to help Jerry find a new career path and get moving on it.

"The way I see it, if you want the rainbow, you gotta put up with the rain."

—DOLLY PARTON

This is the challenging inner work of change that awakens new creative energy and relies on it to make other needed and sometimes even more challenging alterations. What if one partner isn't able to change? Sometimes more discussion and working through the issues that are occurring, along with adjustment over a longer time, will foster resolution. At other times, individual or couples therapy may be needed to resolve the differences in expectations and experience of the relationship.

Family Roles: Using Creativity to Establish New Roles of Choice

Within sixteen to eighteen hours after hatching, a duckling will bond with whatever "mother" it experiences its first sensory contact, be it

William Harvey (1578–1657), the English physician and seventeenth-century discoverer of the circulation of the blood, which he wrote about at age fifty, later published a book on animal reproduction, **Exercitations Concerning the Generation of Animals** *at age seventy-three.*

visual, sound, or touch. "Mother" may be the mother duck, or in unusual situations, something else that was there instead: a child, another animal—even a broom. This is called "imprinting," and in certain species—chickens, turkeys, ducks, and geese in particular—it eliminates a lot of complicated thinking in determining who has what role in the family.

Fortunately, humans are wonderfully complex, and one of the benefits of this complexity is that, unlike the duckling, we are not overly vulnerable to one dominant influence or event. In our lives, nothing has such an unchangeable, immutable effect, even an extremely traumatic event. It is part of human nature to adapt, rather than to become irreparably traumatized, fixated, or stuck. Nonetheless, there are many factors that do influence us—our family, our environment, our experiences in life, crises, successes, and such—and these influences can be quite powerful. At times we can get into a rut that can be deep and long with fixed ideas and rigid behavior. But unlike the duckling whose destiny is shaped by imprinting, our destiny can be influenced by creative new insights or strategies that can enable us to get out of our ruts.

While the human experience doesn't include imprinting, we do "identify with" or develop strong associations or images regarding ourselves, our families, or others, and those can be positive or negative. An example of a positive image would be a story that the family has always told about a grandparent who was in his or her own way heroic or creative or innovative in the face of crisis. This person or his or her image may then become a model for us—in psychological parlance, an "ego ideal"—promoting positive feelings of identification and emulation.

At sixty-five (1998) Philip Roth won his first Pulitzer for his nineteenth novel, **American Pastoral.** *Set in suburban New Jersey, it examines the price of prosperity and respect and how a decent father can raise a daugher who becomes a terrorist to protest the Vietnam War.*

On the other hand, families sometimes shackle us with negative images that increase the chance for negative identification. The meaning of "like father, like son" changes depending upon who's saying it and what he or she is thinking. If "father" is a respected man, it's a compliment; if he is held in contempt, then the comment suggests guilt by genetic association. Family stories, family history, and the constellations of relationships and reputations in family life can play an important part in influencing the way we think about ourselves and our potential to learn new things and establish new patterns of behavior.

TIM: FORGIVING A FATHER, FORGING A FUTURE

Tim, forty, complained of anxiety that interfered with his work and sleep. He sought counseling when he became aware of a growing tension in various relationships at work, with women, and with friends. Tim described his growing-up years in which he was the oldest of three children. His mother, who had a drinking problem, worked as a salesperson in women's clothing stores, changing jobs periodically when her drinking interfered with her work performance. His father was a consulting engineer, involved in many international projects that often took him out of the country on short notice, and he would typically stay on these jobs unexpectedly long. Tim recounted many occasions when he had counted on his father to be at a key sports game or school or family outing, and was disappointed when his father, at the last minute, would be a no-show because of a new work assignment and the need to leave quickly. He also described many times when his mother was supposed to pick him up from a school event but would be late because she was intoxicated; one day, when he was seven years old, his mother had made a date with him to take him to a favorite museum, and he had waited for her outside his school for more than two hours. By the time she arrived he was trembling and in tears.

His mother resented her husband's frequent and long trips away from the family. And he made it clear he resented her drinking. Their mutual bad feelings toward one another mounted, and they finally divorced when Tim was ten. His father then moved overseas, remarried, and returned to visit only about once every five to ten years, and only briefly. Letters from his dad had been very few and far between, even though Tim, throughout adolescence and into his college years, had sent his father many notes. Tim continued to live with his mother until going to college, and he maintained contact with her even after moving out on his own. She continued to be unreliable, and whenever they made plans to see each other Tim never knew if she'd show up sober.

Ralph Waldo Emerson, American poet and essayist, wrote **Society and Solitude** *at age sixty-seven (1870) and* **Letters and Social Aims** *at age seventy-three.*

As therapy unfolded, we explored the connection between his anxiety and his trouble in relationships. It wasn't that the anxiety produced the trouble, but rather that when trouble would begin to unfold, anxiety overwhelmed him. As we looked more closely at his relationships, it started to become clear that Tim was doing subtle things, often unconsciously, sometimes consciously, to provoke the other person. He was a contracts coordinator at a large consulting agency, and sometimes at work he would fail to follow through on commitments and let things slide and miss deadlines; at times he turned minor misunderstandings into angry verbal exchanges. He had received a warning at work that if he failed to improve his performance and behavior his position would be in jeopardy; this was actually the event that precipitated his seeking out therapy.

In his relationships with women, he would often be late for a date, or even be a no-show. If a relationship was improving, he would start to find fault with it or provoke tension. With friends, too, he would often not honor key commitments, even flirting with a close friend's wife, causing considerable strain and the loss of a number of these friendships. As the intensity of therapy was building up he started to miss meetings and became quite delinquent in paying his bills. I asked him if he wanted to jeopardize this relationship, too; he was at first startled by the question, then realized that he had been blind to the potential consequences of his actions with me, just as he had often been blind about the impact of his behavior on others.

In 1086, Su Sung (1020–1101), the Chinese astronomer and inventor, was ordered at age sixty-six by the emperor to construct an armillary clock, far more elaborate than that of prior effort. At age seventy-four (1094) he completed a detailed monograph describing the construction and operation of the clock, from which it is known that it was housed in a tower some 10 meters high, driven by a waterwheel 3.3 meters in diameter, and was probably accurate to within 100 seconds a day, much better than many contemporary clocks.

Shortly after this discussion he got a letter from his father, now about to turn sixty-five, inviting Tim to visit him in Saudi Arabia, where he was working. An airplane ticket would be sent and all expenses covered. This was the first time in Tim's lifetime that his father had invited him to visit abroad. He also sent his son a beautiful gold antique pocket watch, and with the watch was a note that said too much time had gone by without their really getting to know each other; it was time to change. At first Tim was touched by the letter, the invitation, and the watch, and built up considerable enthusiasm about visiting his dad. Then his mood began to change, he became somewhat depressed, started to become anxious, and in an angry moment picked up the watch and smashed it outside on his concrete steps.

In therapy he recounted the sequence of events and sneered at the thought that after all this time, now that his father was getting on in years, turning sixty-five, he finally wanted to get to know his son.

Could Tim really trust this sudden expression of interest? Maybe he would travel to Saudi Arabia and his father would be a disappointment, or perhaps he'd go there and have a great time, only to return home to another ten-year wait between letters. Just thinking about it made him furious, which is what had prompted him to smash the watch.

The symbolism of his action with the watch and his predictable unconscious sabotage of relationships became apparent. He really loved the watch at first, but then associating it with his father, he unconsciously feared it would betray him—stop working. So he broke the watch before it could let him down. In his relationships he acted in the same manner; he valued them, but gradually began to fear something would go wrong and he would be left in the cold, just as his father had physically left him throughout his childhood, and just as his mother, because of her drinking, had left him in the cold emotionally. So unconsciously, he tried to end relationships before someone else did. He had felt so much pain time after time when his parents disrupted their relationship with him, he decided that if someone was going to disrupt a relationship, he would be the one; he would break the clock before it stopped.

Tim was able to see the pattern at work and he very much wanted to change it. Among the things I suggested he could do was to visit his father and to try to "reset the clock." It did seem as if something had changed about his father. Why not give it a chance? He did. The visit was wonderful. His father spent a considerable amount of time apologizing to him and said he had always been very proud of Tim even though he had never showed it. His father was also planning on retiring and was trying to decide whether to come back to the States. Tim took another big emotional step and encouraged him to do just that; it would be the best way for them to truly have a chance at a new start. His father agreed. Tim liked his dad's new wife, who assured Tim that his father was sincere in his desire—at last—to forge a relationship with Tim and his brother and sister. Tim's father, discovering at last in his own Liberation Phase the time and insight to value his children, was finally doing the right thing. Whatever issues had interfered with his commitment to meet his parenting responsibilities and enjoy relation-

If one is out of touch with oneself, then one cannot touch others.

—ANNE MORROW LINDBERGH

ships with his children, he was able to surmount them, liberate himself from those psychological shackles. His inner drive to do so had been given a boost by the encouragement from his second wife. She not only supported this effort, she had pressed him to retire and rebuild his relationship with his children in a new light.

Tim came back energized and determined to bring his new insights to bear on the troubled relationships in his own life. We also talked about his mother, and he decided to become personally active in getting her into a treatment program. She had tried at times in the past after Tim moved out, but he had never actively encouraged her to keep it up; he never thought she would, and he didn't want to be disappointed yet again by her failure.

But here, too, he was surprised when his age and experience enabled him to play his part differently. His mother was quite moved by his concern and agreed to give it another try. Tim remained a strong, supportive participant in her treatment program, and she succeeded in stopping drinking. She stayed in treatment, and Tim remained solidly involved in the process. Two years later, she was still not drinking and had become very active in volunteer work. For the first time in decades, he also enjoyed their visits together.

"The turning point in the process of growing up is when you discover the core of strength within you that survives all hurt."

—MAX LERNER

Indeed, across all his relationships, he no longer found it necessary to "break things" in anticipation of failure. Now he wanted to focus on making his relationships special, and he worked very hard to approach them in new ways. This creative process became a rich realm of self-discovery. He had mobilized his social creativity to begin to turn things around in his relationship with both his parents, his work, his social interactions, and most important, himself.

All in the Family: Changing Patterns, Revising Roles

We may grow up and out of our parents' home, but our place in the family travels with us forever and wherever we go. A family's comfort level with growth and change by any member of it depends on a number of factors. Key among them are the individual personalities in the family, the way they combine to create the inner emotional environment, and the external environment of circumstance and life events. Researchers who study the family as a system describe change in one member as having a ripple effect throughout the family as a whole and sometimes having marked influences on one or more specific other members. Let's look at three different scenarios with three different factors influencing change that require creative responses:

1. *Our sense of a unique role in the family can become altered.* An example: John always felt special, because among his three siblings he had the most education—a master's degree in public health and a master's degree in education. But then, after his sister Jane's children started elementary school, Jane returned to school herself and earned a Ph.D. in psychology. John felt a loss of self-esteem; his self-image was jilted. The way he saw himself and experienced himself underwent a fundamental shift, and it required some adjustments in order for John to regain his emotional equilibrium.

2. *Social changes can be upsetting or disorienting.* Grace, who just celebrated her seventy-fifth birthday, had felt very secure living just eight blocks away from her daughter Sally. But Sally's husband, Mike, got a job offer he couldn't refuse, a job five hundred miles away. Grace had felt very secure, but suddenly those supports were altered and she felt anxious, potentially in a more dependent and uncertain situation.

3. *Actual or feared financial changes can fuel anxiety.* George, an eighty-year-old widower and retired small retail store owner, had always been known as very independent and unpredictable. His wife had died from cancer fourteen years earlier, and he had never envisioned remarrying. After the death of his wife, he had retreated socially—unusual for him—but now he met someone with whom he felt he established a very close and quite comfortable connection. On the one hand, his three children were delighted with his new outlook on life. On the other hand, two of his children who were struggling financially wondered if he would still be able to help them out as much, and whether this would cause a strain in their relationship.

Ethel Percy Andrus (1884–1967), in 1956 at age seventy-two, was the primary force behind the establishment of the nation's first health insurance plan for people over sixty-five, the outcome of her advocacy efforts to obtain low cost insurance for members of the National Retired Teachers Association. In 1958, at age seventy-four, she founded and became president of the American Association of Retired Persons (AARP).

People change and forget to tell each other.
—LILLIAN HELLMAN

Just as the creative growth gap can create tension in a marriage, it can stress family relations as well when others lack the flexibility to see you in a new light. Their rigidity or negativity can become an obstacle to your creativity. If you are prepared for that backlash, and recognize the emotional undercurrents that erode family support for your efforts, you're in a better position to respond creatively and effectively.

In his early forties, while a partner in an East Coast law firm, Joseph developed a hobby of wine tasting and took up formal study of the making and bottling of wines. During many vacations, he would visit the most outstanding wine-producing areas and facilities in the world, enhancing his expertise. Two of his clients had owned vineyards. He had a dream of someday retiring and purchasing his own vineyard and making, bottling, and selling wine himself. Everybody always smiled at his plans, never thinking he would act on them. At sixty-two he went for his dream. He retired, purchased a vineyard in Oregon—a rapidly growing wine region and his and his wife's home state—and set up operations there. He aspired to bring one of the great new wines onto the market.

Anna Freud (1895–1982), pioneer of child psychoanalysis and the youngest daughter of Sigmund Freud, wrote* Beyond the Best Interests of the Child *at age seventy-eight (1973).

Joseph's family—his two children in particular—never thought he would do this. His son Donald, also a lawyer, had just joined his father's firm and had looked forward to his father's tutelage there for at least a few years. Donald worried about what would happen to his status there with his dad leaving, but his father assured him the other partners had the highest regard for him and were very eager to help him. Donald was also going to miss the companionship of his dad, who lived only thirty minutes away.

Donald and his sister, Louise, were very uncomfortable about what all this meant financially, because Joseph had invested virtually all his assets into this venture. His children were dismayed that he had not fully taken them into his confidence and discussed his plans with them, and they worried about what would happen to their parents' financial security if the venture fell flat.

Louise, though she lived farther away than Donald, was nonetheless very close to her parents, especially to her mother, Nora, who had always been very supportive during Louise's recent divorce. Joseph and his wife Nora also helped Louise financially, especially through financing her children's education. Louise wondered with their new investment whether this financial help would continue.

Nora had always been a free spirit, identifying with the Beatnik movement in her youth. She thrived on the new excitement. She was delighted to have her husband leave the law firm where he was becoming increasingly stressed and working long hours. She was excited at the prospect of moving to Oregon.

Joseph was very understanding. He was good as a problem solver in his work as an attorney, and he brought these same skills to this family challenge. He understood his children's concerns and dealt with them in a reassuring manner. But he knew his mind and his dream, and he asked his children's emotional support to help him realize his dream. Ultimately, they gave it.

The Social Portfolio: Investing Wisely

We are born into a world of relationships, a social milieu, and for the most part, the relationships that define our lives are the products of spontaneity and chance. We do what we do, some of it by choice and some not, but in that company of others we find our partners in work, community, friendship, and love.

When I first developed the social portfolio "planner" you see on page 167, it was to offer a visual description of the continuing potential for creativity through relationships as we age, no matter what our circumstances. Over the years, the Social Portfolio has proved to be an effective tool in therapy and beyond. It offers a way to evaluate your network of relationships, identify underdeveloped opportunities for creative development through social interaction, and go about strengthening the social fabric of your life.

A savvy investor plans a financial portfolio with four things in mind: liquidity, diversification, emergency funds, and long-term growth. You need to have some, but certainly not all, of your investments in a form from which you can easily withdraw funds. You need to have a diversity in your portfolio because at different times some assets will be better to draw upon than others. Similarly, you need to have

José Echegaray y Eizaguirre (1833–1916), the Spanish dramatist, began his career teaching mathematics. He subsequently participated in politics, then acquired literary fame through his many plays in prose and verse. He received the Nobel Prize in Literature at the age of seventy-one, then returned to politics as minister of finance at the age of seventy-two and also went back to science as professor of physics at Madrid University at the same time.

some of these investments set aside as a "rainy day" fund, in case you experience an unexpected disability, accident, or loss. Finally, you need to think about retirement long before you approach the real thing, starting at a younger age to save money and use the power of long-term growth and compounding interest to increase your savings.

The same four concepts apply to our lifetime investments in relationships and activities as an ongoing resource for creativity. You need to have *liquidity*—hobbies, interests, and relationships to which you can easily gain access. You need to have *diversification,* because depending on circumstances, some of these activities and relationships will be better developed to draw upon than others. You need to have *alternative resources*—emergency funds—with which to express your creative self, in the event that you suffer a physical decline or suffer the loss of a loved one with whom you shared social experiences. And finally, you need to think about *long-term growth* of your creative potential and purposefully expanding a curiosity or passion earlier in your life to cultivate through the years.

Englishman Donald McGill started drawing comic postcards at the age of thirty, and for the next fifty years, until age eighty (1955), drew an estimated five hundred cards a day. One of his postcards sold two million copies.

The Social Portfolio balances *individual* with *group activities, high energy* with *low,* and *high mobility* with *low mobility.* With these categories I have created a box with four groups: Group/High Mobility, Group/Low Mobility, Individual/High Mobility, and Individual/Low Mobility. The content of each category obviously varies greatly with the individual, but if you use the social portfolio as a basic rubric, or template, you can take a more active role in developing different relationship resources—true "social security" for your emotional life, and thus your continued creative growth and self-expression. While each category defines different types of activities, each provides opportunities for exploring new directions in current relationships as well as new relationships.

Elizabeth Gurley Flynn was a radical agitator who protested for labor reform and organization to benefit the working class. She joined the American branch of the Communist party (CPUSA), and at the age of seventy-one (1961) she became the first woman selected as National Chairman of CPUSA.

Group High Mobility/High Energy

This category is for anyone who likes to be around other people and who does not suffer from a physical ailment that limits energy or mobility. For example, if you have always been involved in civic and

THE SOCIAL PORTFOLIO

Tapping Creative Potential in Later Life

	GROUP EFFORTS	INDIVIDUAL EFFORTS
	Group/High Mobility	Individual/High Mobility
HIGH MOBILITY / HIGH ENERGY	• *Coordinate a new volunteer group in a neglected community* • *Take international folk dance lessons in host countries* • *Run for an elected office in your local community*	• *Create a neighborhood showcase garden* • *Create an annotated walking tour of your town* • *Photograph family mementos to create an album*
	Group/Low Mobility	Individual/Low Mobility
LOW MOBILITY / LOW ENERGY	• *Create best jokes and potluck dinner group* • *Create family newspaper with children/grandchildren* • *Host provocative novels book club at your home*	• *Create the "Secret Recipes" family cookbook* • *Create family tree with descriptive commentary* • *Create E-mail or "snail mail" letters to grandchildren*

political events in a small community, you may think about running for public office in later life. If you have always enjoyed watching birds feeding in the backyard, you might eventually set up a club for fellow ornithologists, possibly affiliated with a local or federal park service, that would offer the opportunity to take day or weekend trips. Or you could join the local chapter of the Audubon Society.

Rob, fifty-one, and his wife Alice, fifty, felt a growing sense of distance in their marriage which came into sharp relief when their accountant suggested they attend an investment seminar. After Rob came up with one lame reason after another for why he couldn't make the seminar, he finally told Alice that he frankly felt uncomfortable about the seminar because it was focusing on the future and he felt that with all the problems they were having in their relationship their future was uncertain. Alice confessed she experienced similar feelings.

Both were unhappy with the slow unraveling of their relationship

Dame Daphne Du Maurier (1907–1989), author of* Rebecca *and the short story "The Birds" (1952) that was later made into a Hitchcock film, wrote* The Rendez-vous and Other Stories *at age seventy-three.

and both wanted to revitalize it. However, both also had reservations about their ability to do it. In therapy, Alice spoke bluntly of the options: they could ignore the trouble signs and their marriage would likely fall apart; they could decide to get a divorce; they could continue with therapy; or they could try to make it work on their own.

They decided to try working on their own. After they each considered and rejected numerous suggestions, Rob suggested doing something physical together; maybe it would also warm up their sex life. Alice liked the idea, too, and both had suggestions: Alice suggested tango lessons. Rob suggested massage lessons, which they could then practice on one another. They did both. These were Group High Mobility/High Energy endeavors.

Marie Tussaud, better known as Madame Tussaud (1761–1850), learned the art of wax modeling from her uncle. Just prior to the French Revolution she was the art tutor to Louis XVI's sister, and was later imprisoned as a loyalist. During the Reign of Terror she was forced to make death masks from heads upon their being severed by the guillotine. Later she was able to return to making wax models, her collection consisting of both heroes and rogues. After touring Britain with her figures for thirty-three years she finally set up a permanent collection of lifesize wax portraits on Baker Street in London at age seventy-four (1835). Many of the original works of her noted contemporaries are still preserved, including Voltaire, Sir Walter Scott, and Benjamin Franklin.

Individual High Mobility/High Energy

This category of activity focuses on individual and fairly unrestricted effort and growth.

Jared was a fifty-three-year-old corporate tax attorney, very good at what he did. As he began to consider the prospect of retirement, he wondered whether he would be prepared. He knew things would be all right financially, but single and without other family responsibilities, he wasn't sure what he'd *do* without his work.

He liked his work, but he was beginning to feel in a bit of a rut in his job. He was becoming increasingly concerned about how much time he spent sitting inside consumed with numbers. He started thinking more and more about nature and wanting to spend more time contemplating ideas as opposed to dollars. On a plane ride, one of the magazines he skimmed through featured outdoor recreational pursuits, and he became intrigued by the pictures and the stories. He wondered what it would be like to hike beautiful trails.

The more he daydreamed about it, the more he wanted to look into it. He lived not that far from the Shenandoah Valley and the Appalachian Mountains, and he checked out a few library books on the region. He liked the idea of hiking alone, and after talking with some experienced hikers, he tried a few day hikes solo. He was hooked.

He eventually added photography to his hiking itinerary, and as he headed into the decade preceding retirement, he had already established a new path that he could begin to enjoy now, and continue to develop later. Jared's initial self-motivated interest in hiking reflected an Individual High Mobility/High Energy endeavor.

Individual Low Mobility/Low Energy

If you prefer independent activities and have a difficult time traveling or sustaining long periods of activity, there are always options for creativity that can fit the bill.

Veronica, fifty-one, was a landscape architect. She loved her work, but she started to be concerned that she wasn't doing much other than her work, keeping up with the professional journals, going to conferences, traveling to see what other landscape architects were doing. The traveling in particular helped her weave a little diversion into her work, but she began to feel that it wasn't enough.

She had only one other major interest, though it was a rich one: her family. Her father had eight siblings, her mother had seven. Veronica herself was married with three grown children, one of whom had just announced that she was pregnant—another generation on the way. All of this made Veronica think even more about family, and she grew curious about members of her family who predated her grandparents.

She discussed this with her pregnant daughter, who asked her if she had ever thought about having a family genealogy researched. Veronica hadn't, but as her daughter mentioned it she thought it could prove fascinating. She let her thoughts wander about on this, and decided to begin by researching the family history to establish the genealogy, with an eye to filling in the family stories in future years as a retirement project. She researched her project at the library and on the Internet, then bought a computer software program to help organize her effort. Veronica's activity, slow and self-paced, reflects an Individual Low Mobility/Low Energy endeavor.

Group Low Mobility/Low Energy

If you enjoy socializing in a low-key setting, these creative activities support social interaction with minimal logistic or energy demands.

I. M. Pei, the renowned Chinese-American architect, was born in Canton in 1917, became a naturalized American citizen in 1954, and at the age of seventy-eight designed the Rock and Roll Hall of Fame in Cleveland, where the term "rock and roll" was launched.

Selma Lagerlöf (1858–1940), the Swedish novelist whose storytelling was rooted in legend, became the first woman to receive the Nobel Prize in Literature, in 1909 (at age fifty-one). Her works drew heavily on the legends and traditions of her native Värmland of west central Sweden. She wrote her trilogy **The Rings of the Lowenskolds** ***when she was between ages sixty-seven and seventy.***

Mack Sennett (1880–1960), the Canadian filmmaking pioneer, is considered the father of North American slapstick comedy in the motion pictures. As a young producer/director he created the very popular Keystone Kops and is credited with discovering Charlie Chaplin. He is also famous for creating more than one thousand short comedy films and training many of the best comedians in the early days of motion pictures, including W. C. Fields. Much of this rich history is captured in his autobiography published at age seventy-four (1954), **Mack Sennett: King of Comedy.** *That same year he produced* **Abbott and Costello Meet the Keystone Kops.**

Some ideas would include group discussion or activity centered on reading, quilting, or other hand crafts.

Rosalyn, age fifty, was a psychiatric social worker whose practice had really grown and was starting to weigh on her. She very much needed a new diversion and wondered, too, whether she should be thinking about the future as well. She wanted some kind of activity other than her work to be fulfilling, something she could further develop over time.

She thought about her interests and things that she'd really like to do, and realized that she was a movie addict who loved going to movies with friends and analyzing the films afterward with them. Several of her friends had suggested she would make a good movie critic. She thought about it and sketched out a long-range, ambitious, but appealing plan for herself: she would begin by taking a course on the history of film, then a course on creative writing, and then another course on film criticism.

She enjoyed the stimulating discussions with others, and she felt that with the focused study behind her, she'd be ready to approach one of the small local newspapers and offer to write a column on movie reviews. She was excited about her long-term plan, but just as important, she enjoyed the course work and the many people she grew to know as she began her "understudy" phase. All of these related endeavors that she planned were Group Low Mobility/Low Energy.

Human Relationships: Creativity's Infinite Resource

An artist friend from a large city had moved to a beautiful suburb of new showcase homes, but after a couple of years decided he preferred the more diverse city environment. "I missed the texture," he said of his reaction to the well-groomed suburban landscape. "I like the old houses with unpredictable angles and spaces, and a town center where it seems possible for something interesting or unexpected to happen." His relationship with his surroundings was an important creative element for him, and he eventually returned to the nubbier texture of city life.

Speaking of architecture's powerful influence in our lives, Sir Winston Churchill noted: "We shape our buildings; thereafter they shape us."

Within the landscape of creativity and aging, we shape our relationships, and thereafter they shape us. No matter where we live, our creativity shapes our relationships, and our relationships then become the context for our creativity. It is important in our landscape that at times we are able to find structure and support, and at times wide open spaces for dreaming and experimentation. At best, where our age, experience, and creativity intersect, we will find in relationship those unpredictable angles and spaces and centers of activity where something interesting or unexpected can happen.

"Life is like a ten-speed bike. Most of us have gears we never use."

—CHARLES SCHULTZ

6

Creativity in Response to Adversity

Man is most uniquely human when he turns obstacles into opportunities.

—ERIC HOFFER, "REFLECTIONS ON THE HUMAN CONDITION"

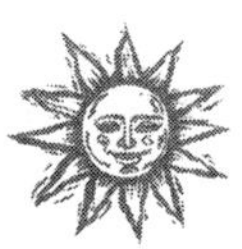

DURING MY TIME AS acting director at the National Institute on Aging (NIA), as I have mentioned previously, I had an interesting opportunity to interview George Burns as part of a series of public service messages with him. About to turn ninety-seven, he made a credible spokesman on aging. Upon my arrival at his office with my camera crew, the scene that we confronted was one that has remained with me ever since as the best picture of aging in the late twentieth century. In the weeks prior to our meeting, his agent had talked with me numerous times by telephone, going to great lengths to ensure a smooth meeting. Burns had agreed to fit our visit into a typically busy afternoon of work with his joke writer. When my crew and I arrived in Los Angeles and made our way to Burns's office, I expected

Mae West, still acting in her mid-eighties, pointed out, "When you've got the personality, you don't need the nudity."

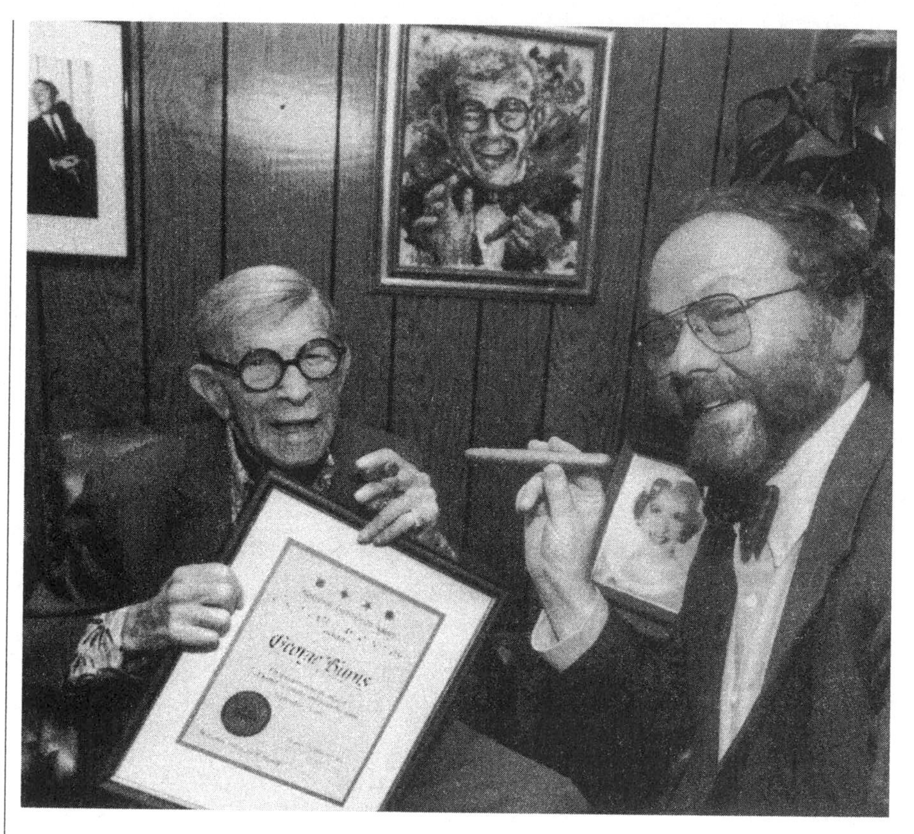

In the public service message that George Burns and I did for the National Institute on Aging, I asked him, "What does your doctor say about your smoking and your drinking?" With his inimitable timing and manner, Burns replied, "My doctor is dead." Burns then speculated on why he continued to endure as a successful comedian. He said that many performers over time don't act their age; they try to do things to look younger. "But Johnny Carson and I never did those things, and we continued to do well, even as we aged." Then Burns couldn't resist, "Come to think of it, I've always been old."

Burns's agent to be a protective sort, alert to his client's needs. I did not, however, expect the agent to be eighty-five, and Burns's joke writer to be in his seventies. This trio of undeniably, unabashedly old men gave us a hearty welcome.

One carefully planned piece of this visit was that I would present to Burns a certificate from NIA acknowledging his outstanding contributions on issues of aging with his humor. Burns had a plan of his own—a practical joke by the master jokester. As our cameras rolled and I made our formal presentation of the NIA certificate to him, a camera crew from television's *Entertainment Tonight* walked into the room (see picture of the two of us above).

"I have something for you," Burns announced, his gravelly voice light with mischief, and he handed me a cigar. It was irony that made the humor: This was during the height of the nation's surgeon general's campaign against smoking, and I was meeting with Burns as a federal

Public Health official. Further, President Clinton's recent comment deflecting criticism for alleged pot smoking in his younger days had become a public joke. With the cigar in my hand and the cameras in my face, the President's defense leaped to my mind: "Not to worry," I said, "I don't inhale." Quipped Burns: "Neither do I—and maybe I should run for President."

In our interview, I asked Burns whether he felt he needed to make any adaptations to aging. "Now I ask for my applause in advance, just in case. And I don't buy green bananas."

He told me later privately that he recently had developed back pain and was concerned that it would start interfering with his routines. He had discussed this with some colleagues. Their advice? "Sit down while you do your routines."

"How can I sit down," Burns sighed, "when all my life I've been a stand-up comic?"

He said he had thought more about their counsel, and eventually tried it. To his surprise and relief, he found that sitting had no negative impact on his routines. As for future lifestyle adaptations, he said after a pause: "And now, if necessary, I'll become a lie-down comic."

Burns demonstrated through his life and his humor that aging holds ample potential for creativity, and that even presented with new limitations, fresh thinking can enable us to continue to experience life, and contribute to it, in satisfying ways.

The life and work of William Carlos Williams advances our understanding of this idea further still. Williams was not only a great poet, he was also a respected physician. In his sixties, he suffered a stroke that prevented him from practicing medicine. Fortunately, the stroke did not affect his intellectual abilities, but it did affect him emotionally. He became so severely depressed that for a year, at the age of sixty-nine, he required psychiatric hospitalization. Nonetheless, he surmounted the depression and for the next ten years went on to write great poetry. His work *Pictures from Brueghel*, published when he was seventy-nine, was awarded a Pulitzer Prize. In his later-life poetry Williams wrote about an "old age that adds as it takes away." Through his life and his poetry, Williams showed us that aging need not be defined only as a steady accumulation of losses. Rather, as we struggle with loss and with change

Ethel Barrymore received the Academy Award for Best Actress for the film* None but the Lonely Heart *at the age of sixty-five (1944). From the age of sixty-seven to seventy-eight she appeared in twenty more films.

as we age, we encounter both problems and potential. Typically the problems become a catalyst for developing the potential.

In Greek mythology, the mortal Tiresias was walking through the woods, when his glance inadvertently caught the goddess Athena bathing in the nude. Enraged, Athena blinded Tiresias. But the other gods and goddesses asked Athena to reconsider, because Tiresias was a great man who had no intention of offending the gods. Athena did reconsider, but did not restore Tiresias' outer sight, instead giving him great inner vision, which grew as he aged. In his old age he predicted the plight of Oedipus. This ancient myth speaks to an old age that adds as it takes away.

Adversity comes in infinite variety—illness, death of a loved one, loss of a job or any undesirable change—any event or situation we experience as negative and that results in, at best, a sense of challenge and uncertainty. Under more severe circumstances more unsettling feelings include anxiety, despair, and helplessness or a sense of loss of control. Adversity is a powerful force in life, not only in terms of hardship but in the response it prompts from us. Our pride in accomplishments is often made all the sweeter by the knowledge of the obstacles we overcame in the process. What makes a hero but the context of adversity she or he overcomes?

What makes creativity such a powerful tool against adversity? Creativity is an emotional and intellectual process—a mechanism—that can, moment by moment, displace negative feelings, such as anxiety or hopelessness, with positive feelings of engagement and expectation. That emotional rise to challenge emboldens us with new ideas and the courage to try them despite obstacles or hardship. We see this in the resourceful relief worker at the scene of a natural disaster, the stroke victim who determinedly joins the mall walkers each day to "power walk," even at a snail's pace, or the countless others among us who struggle each day just to achieve the ordinary under circumstances that would deny even that.

Again we find the cycle of creativity and circumstance shaping our lives even as one imposes or inspires change in the other. Adversity challenges our creativity; it serves as a prompt for innovative thinking in that we instinctively seek relief from it. A creative response enables us to view our situation in a new way or do something different. This new response can ultimately change the circumstances of our struggle, as well. Creativity offers us a way to lift the emotional darkness of adversity, and may even contribute to physical healing, a phenomenon we'll explore more closely later in this chapter.

Creativity in the context of adversity has special meaning for me, not only through the struggle that I have witnessed in the lives of patients and others I have known through my work and community, but also through my personal struggle with the diagnosis of a catastrophic illness of my own, and later, my efforts to help my father, my family, and me cope with my dad's life and death from Alzheimer's. These shared stories contribute a powerful chapter to the literature on aging, reflecting both the struggle and the triumph of the human spirit. The two frightening dark chapters of personal experience provided me with new insight, and enabled me to tap the extraordinary life-affirming power of creativity in response to the kind of personal adversity we all encounter at one time or another.

Personal Adversity: Diagnosis Leads to Dark Days

In the fall of 1991 I suddenly found myself in a situation that changed the course of my life. Just a few months earlier I had been appointed as acting director of the National Institute on Aging (NIA) at the National Institutes of Health (NIH). It was at that time the high point of my career, a position I had hoped to hold before my return to academia. It was an honor and a major responsibility, managing a staff of approximately 550 and a budget of about $400 million. I felt on top of the world. But in September of that year, everything changed.

I began to notice some mysterious physical symptoms. My left calf muscle looked and felt noticeably larger than the right, and this was accompanied by increased muscle cramping. As a physician, I knew that in the list of possible explanations, a few were very serious, involving degenerative muscle diseases. I went immediately to get a physical examination and underwent a series of special laboratory studies. Two months later, following repeated abnormal electromyograms, I received the crushing diagnosis of a strong possibility of having Lou Gehrig's disease (amyotrophic lateral sclerosis, or ALS). As a doctor myself, I knew this was serious.

I was devastated. In times of personal illness, being a physician is sometimes the worst position to be in; you know too much. I knew that ALS was a progressive disease—one that got worse over time. Patients experience a gradual loss of muscle strength and control. The majority of people with this disease die within three to five years of diagnosis.

Nelson Mandela, viewed by many as "the world's most famous prisoner," gained his freedom at the age of seventy-one, after serving twenty-seven years of a life sentence on charges of establishing the military wing of the African National Congress (ANC). His release was welcomed by both black and white South Africans. With this strong support he led the negotiations with the South African government over a nonracial democratic constitution. In 1994, at the age of seventy-five, Mandela was inaugurated president in South Africa's first one-person one-vote election.

A profound sense of darkness, despair, ugliness, fear, and limited time descended upon me. My mind raced when I heard the news. What should I do? How could I tell my family? Should I take a lesser position? Resign? Go on a long trip to places where I had never been? As a psychiatrist, I recognized that my frame of mind was not conducive to clear decision making. I experienced denial—*maybe they were wrong about the diagnosis*. Then anger—*why me, why now?!*—though my medical knowledge reminded me that I was at an age at risk for ALS. I searched for hope—*maybe I would be one of that small percentage with an atypical slow course of the disease and would survive much longer and much better than expected, like physicist Stephen Hawking.*

"A man can be destroyed but not defeated."
—ERNEST HEMINGWAY

Influenced by that thought, I postponed telling those outside my immediate family and closest of friends. I decided I didn't want my parents to know, nor those with whom I worked, until the disease was clearly starting to take its toll with more or stronger symptoms. I felt I needed more time to know my own mind regarding what to do before everyone in the world knew and weighed in with their reactions and advice, potentially overwhelming me. It was a tough call, because this silence added greatly to the burden and loneliness of my situation. Then I began experiencing haunting dreams. I went through a series of "chase" nightmares in which monsters chased after me or I was stuck in a major calamity with a growing sense of an ominous outcome; I would awaken in a sweat. I realized that I needed to do something to alter the darkness and the dread that had invaded my life.

Soon after, one morning I awoke to what appeared to be an unusually beautiful day. The sky was a penetrating blue with pure white puffy clouds. It was uplifting. I studied the sky and wondered whether there was something I could do that would be fun and beautiful to combat the negative feelings and ugly images that had enveloped me. I started thinking again: were there things that I always had wanted to do in my life but never got around to doing? For good reason, I concluded it was now or never. I recalled that years earlier I had had an idea for a board game, but because of my commitments at the time, I had never been able to give it more thought.

Gradually, I was able to shift a good bit of my dark, negative daydreaming into thoughts about developing this game. A few months passed, and the concept of the game was really taking form in my mind. It was a visually dramatic game as I envisioned it, but complex as well, combining elements of language, spelling, strategy, and military concepts. I wanted it to have a striking design, something meaningful and memorable, but I am no designer. I didn't know whom to contact or even whether I could afford to hire a designer of the caliber I had in mind. My ideas stalled out, and my negative thoughts started to return.

Then a remarkable coincidence occurred. I had arranged a dinner party with a small group of friends, one of whom was my longtime friend Gretchen Raber, a gifted metal artist and jeweler. During the dinner, Gretchen commented that a gallery near her studio was hosting a national, judged exhibit of games as works of art. She lamented that she had always wanted to make game markers, but lacked the concept for a game. I couldn't believe what I was hearing! I piped in, "Well, I have the world's greatest game concept, but no markers!" We both got very excited and agreed that we would go for it.

"What doesn't destroy me strengthens me."
—FRIEDRICH NIETZSCHE

The only problem was that it was July and the deadline for the show was a mere two months away. Ordinarily, it would take at least a year to design and produce a finished sample of a game. But Gretchen was inspired and I was driven. We worked around the clock, totally consumed with this creative mission, and we managed to finish the prototype sample of the game the morning it was due. To our great surprise, it was selected as a finalist in the show and was then sent on to an internationally judged art competition, where it was again selected as a finalist. As a result, the game became part of a three-year, thirteen-museum traveling exhibition with the other selected art objects. It was later selected by *Fun & Games Magazine* as "Best Party Game of 1994–1995."

Edmond Hoyle (1672–1769), noted English expert and writer on card games ("according to Hoyle"), wrote his classic book on* Hoyle's Standard Games *at age seventy-six (1748).

As I look back on that period, I realize that it was my first significant personal experience of aging that "adds as it takes away." It was my most vivid experience of creativity transcending loss—in this case, the loss of my health and of any hope for the future. Unable to change my health condition or the grim prognosis, I had focused instead on something I *could* do—and with that creative shift in perspective I found new activity and new meaning in my days and was better able to cope with the uncertainty of the future.

A second long year passed—also an emotionally complicated and confusing year. My symptoms continued, the electromyograms showed the same abnormalities, but my overall condition did not appear to be getting worse. I began to think more about the possibility that the diagnosis might be wrong, but my doctors still could not give me a clean bill of health, and they were still very concerned. It could be that I was one of those with a slower course of the disorder. But how slow and for how long? I was still on an emotional roller coaster, but at least no longer in a frightening free fall. And, if indeed, the diagnosis was correct, for as long as possible I was determined it was not going to rule my life—at least not my emotions and actions. I was not going to let it jail me in an emotional purgatory.

Then, an interesting development occurred. The doctor who developed the standards for diagnosing ALS from an electromyogram was going to be at NIH as a visiting scientist for a couple of weeks. My doctors arranged for him to evaluate me. After another lengthy evaluation he met with me, shaking his head, saying it was most unusual, that everything so closely mimicked ALS, but he was pleased to conclude that based on the present findings and the lack of deterioration over the past two years it was likely that I did not have ALS.

"If we had no winter the spring would not be so pleasant: if we did not sometimes taste of adversity, prosperity would not be so welcome."

—ANNE BRADSTREET

My reaction was, in a sense, mixed. My predominant feeling was, of course, one of enormous relief. But I also felt some resentment that I had been misdiagnosed, that it had gone on so long, and that I had unnecessarily gone through so much. But I also knew from my own medical experience that such complicated cases occur and go this route. And as painful as it was, it had elevated me to a new vantage point in life in understanding myself and what I was capable of doing, and that was no small event. Meanwhile, all of my symptoms and an abnormal electromyogram test still existed, and my doctors could not explain them. They said they would need to follow me, and one of them left me with the following consolation: "May you live long and well with your interesting and benign symptoms." Fortunately, to this day, while my symptoms persist, they have not gotten worse and cause no new discomfort nor dysfunction.

As the darkness lifted, I felt a sense of awe that in the midst of my misdiagnosis, believing that such bleakness was ahead, I was able to not only cope with the dreadful forecast but actually emotionally transcend it through a creative process. I felt very fortunate that I was able to tap into this process and even more fortunate that I did not have ALS. And I was left with an even greater empathy for those not so fortunate, whose grave conditions do not go away. I also felt I would be able to help such individuals even more than I had in the past, because until my misdiagnosis was established, I had felt at one with them.

With my reprieve, I realized I no longer was looking at life and work in the same way. I had changed and felt the process of change was still in motion, and I was excited by it. I no longer faced the dark certainties of ALS, but my game had been launched, my passion for game development had been stirred, and I had no desire to abandon this new interest. I revised my career plans. Since I was a commissioned officer in the U.S. Public Health Service, I was allowed to retire after twenty years of active duty, which happened to fall on the eve of my fiftieth birthday. Though my work in the Public Health Service had been extremely fulfilling, my two-year misdiagnosis experience of emotional darkness, and deliverance through creative thought and activity, set me on a new course of exploration.

I accepted a position at the George Washington University to establish the new interdisciplinary research Center on Aging, Health & Humanities. Then I set up my own game company—GENCO—with an underlying mission to develop new ways to expand intergenerational creativity through games. My life was changed, and my new interest in games became a promising new piece in my personal social portfolio, as well as a tool for expanding my potential to "give back" and contribute to others in this second half of my life.

Loosening the Bonds of Adversity Through Creativity

Those who *commence creativity* with aging often do so because of a loss or other adversity. Loss also influences *changes in creativity* with aging, and can be seen as well in those who show *continuing creativity* with

At the age of thirty-nine, Sister Gertrude Morgan (1900–1980), in partnership with two other women, started an orphanage (Gentilly) in New Orleans. She devoted herself to this work, which she saw as her mission in life. The orphanage grew, thrived, and made a tremendous contribution to the community thanks to Sister Gertrude's efforts. But in 1965, when Sister Gertrude was sixty-five, tragedy struck—Hurricane Betsy swept through New Orleans, destroying the orphanage. Confronted with a devastating void in her life, Sister Gertrude began to do more of the painting that she had begun when she was fifty-six. In her seventies, her art reached maturity, and museums across the country began to exhibit it in recognition of her prodigious talent. Her work was included in the 1980 exhibit at the Corcoran Museum of Art, referred to earlier, on "Black Folk Art in America."

Jesse J. Aaron (1887–1979) was a descendent of slaves and a Seminole Indian grandmother. Before he completed first grade, Aaron's parents removed him from school and "hired him out" to do farmwork at seven dollars a month. He eventually worked as a baker, a field hand, and a cook—from his forties into his seventies. In his seventies he retired to care for his disabled wife and started a nursery. He was forced to sell the nursery to pay for a cataract operation for his wife, and for the first time in his life, at eighty-one years of age, he was unemployed; he later said that thereafter, "The Spirit woke me up and said, 'Carve wood.' " Inspired, Aaron carved human and animal forms from wood, achieved notice, and reached the exhibition circuit. He received a Visual Artists Fellowship from the National Endowment for the Arts at age eighty-eight.

aging. The creative life of the great American artist Grandma Moses exemplifies this synergy of creativity, age, and adversity.

Anna Mary Roberts Moses was born in 1860 in Greenwich, New York. She experienced an early interest in art, but the circumstances were not right for her to develop her talent with rigor. She did not even dream of obtaining formal art training. The closest she came to be drawn to art at an early age was in her geography lessons in the one-room district school she attended. She described it this way: "The teacher would give us maps to draw, and I would make the mountains in my own way, the teacher liked them and would ask if he might keep them." But Anna Mary's mother discouraged her from art, pushing her toward more practical things. At age twelve she was working as a hired girl on a neighboring farm, continuing this work for the next fifteen years, until she met a hired man, Thomas Salmon Moses, whom she married. She viewed their marriage as an equal partnership, but admitted, "I was the boss."

As her children grew up and left home, Mother Moses was able to dabble in art for the first time since childhood. Thrift governed her materials. Her husband, for example, who was supportive of her growing interest in art, once brought her an old window from a caboose, suggesting it could be painted on both sides. But the painting was still just a pleasurable aside, not moving yet to a serious commitment. Her primary commitment was still to helping her family make ends meet. She had once submitted a few pictures at a local fair along with her noted canned fruits and raspberry jam. She won a prize for the fruit and jam, but no recognition for the pictures.

The death of her husband when she was sixty-seven was a significant change and loss for her. Her daughter encouraged her to do some embroidery, and quickly this work revealed her considerable talent; requests for her embroidery grew. She continued this handwork until arthritis made it difficult to manipulate a needle. But Grandma Moses found it less painful and manually easier to paint. This launched her serious interest in painting at age seventy-eight. She was discovered shortly thereafter, leading eventually to fifteen one-woman shows in Europe. Her famous painting career continued to the age of 101, when she painted her last great canvas, *Rainbow*, a work rich both in the vitality of pictorial content and in the optimism of the mental imagery of its title. Even as a centenarian, her creative skills continued.

Mary Roberts Moses's development as an artist illustrates creativity that commenced with aging and changed over time; hers was old age that adds as it takes away. Adversity holds this potential for creativity for all of us, whether we use our creative energy to produce tangible works of art, activism that changes our society, or new perspectives that can change our lives. It is no romanticization of loss to say that whatever the nature of our hardship, in the transition and adjustment it demands there is also the potential for creative growth and gain.

Once we understand this relationship between loss and creativity, we can see it all around us, in the lives of famous achievers as well as those whose passions and accomplishments play in the softer light of everyday life.

SISTERS: HONORING LIFE THROUGH CONTRIBUTION

Helen, forty-eight, was very close to her sister, Susanna, forty-six. They were each other's confidante, and loved to talk on the phone together, to shop together, and to get together for family events. They both were married, had children similar in age and lived in adjacent communities. Five years earlier Susanna had developed breast cancer. Her treatment appeared to be successful for the first two-and-half years, but the cancer returned and had a rapid course despite further aggressive therapy. Susanna died just before reaching her forty-eighth birthday. Helen and the rest of the family were devastated.

Helen then dedicated herself to doing something special to honor the memory of her sister. She became active in a local cancer support organization and was so articulate as an advocate and so successful as a fund-raiser that national cancer organizations noticed her and sought her collaboration. Helen's skill as an advocate for combating cancer grew even more and she received a local award and national recognition for her highly creative and effective efforts in mobilizing family activism and influencing the commitment of policy makers in this fight.

Helen faced the terrible adversity of the death of a loved sibling,

Max Lerner (1902–1992), was a widely read, very influential and provocative syndicated columnist for the* New York Post. *He also edited* The Encyclopedia of the Social Sciences *and the magazine* The Nation. *He authored many books and articles and had numerous teaching appointments at prestigious universities, through which his ideas had significant impact, particularly on political and economic thinking. At seventy-eight he was diagnosed with cancer—first lymphoma, then prostate. His prognosis was poor.

Lerner later wrote, "After the shock and anguish, the stress and pain, the anxiety and fear, the bottoming out and slow ascent, I began to have the feeling of putting it all together." What followed was a late-life battle where the psychological mind and the human spirit joined forces with

creatively coping with it through enabling important contribution to accompany painful loss. The process not only created new meaning for Susanna's life; it created a new direction and sense of purpose and potential in Helen's.

medical treatment to combat serious illness.

Lerner then began to wrestle, "not with the disease alone, not with the doctors and their medications and interventions, nor even with the 'spite of Fortune.' It was with the unfathomable mysteries, with Jacob's angel, with the dark man who came in the night and stayed and left—the angel at once of death and life—the Angel of God."

Max Lerner lived another twelve years, until he was nearly ninety, writing, teaching, influencing. Along the way, in 1990 at age eighty-eight, he wrote* Wrestling with the Angel, *which he described as "A Memoir of My Triumph over Illness."

BRAD: CAREER DISAPPOINTMENT AND AN UNCERTAIN FUTURE

Brad, fifty-five, had worked at his company for thirty-one years and was a candidate for one of the top management positions that had opened up. He was almost certain he would get it, and all of his colleagues felt he was a shoo-in, given his high performance as a financial planner and long dedication to the company. But at the eleventh hour, complicated politics entered in, and Brad did not receive the appointment. It was a terrible disappointment for him, a blow to his self-esteem, and he became very resentful because of the unfairness of the decision. Further, that he had been passed over for the promotion was a clear sign that the internal power brokers had made their choice: Brad was out. He talked the situation over with his wife, Marla, sharing his impression that it was time for him to get out or get ready for worse.

Marla, fifty-six, was a clinical psychologist at a community clinic. Marla didn't want Brad to make a hasty decision he might regret, and she suggested he seek the help of a therapist to sort out his feelings and options. He came to meet with me. Meanwhile, Marla could see that it would never be the same for Brad at his company, and after they hashed over options between themselves for the next several days she asked Brad if he was up to doing something bold that would involve both of them in a new business partnership. She pointed out to him that they both were eligible for early retirement, and that income, along with their savings and some investments, would allow them to do something different—something she thought would be fun and very satisfying.

They had recently purchased a large old Victorian house along the coast of Maine that they planned on using for a summer vacation house. The building had previously been used as a mom and pop assisted living facility that ran into financial difficulties and had to close. Because of its previous use, it had been divided into individual units. Brad and Marla's original plan was to have an agency manage the house and rent out units, saving one for them when they vacationed in Maine.

But Marla was "thinking outside the box"—trying a completely different perspective—and she had a new idea: They were both ready for a career change, she loved to cook, and he loved to tinker and fix things, so why not run the place as a bed-and-breakfast during the summer and operate a small business the rest of the year that used their professional skills to run retirement-planning seminars? Between his financial planning knowledge and her understanding of psychological issues, they would make a great seminar team during the winter months, and during the summer they would enjoy applying their cooking and tinkering hobbies for fun and profit.

Excited by the prospect, they paused to review the risks and the benefits of the plan carefully. They couldn't help but note the growing trend of layoffs and downsizing in Brad's field and the vulnerable nature of employment anywhere in such a climate. But retiring from one's career and becoming self-employed were two major lifestyle adjustments—multiplied by two if they took the plunge together—and would require some emotional as well as financial risk taking. With a clear sense of their inner and outer resources, they stepped out of the "box" that had put a lid on Brad's career, and moved on to a new career together, excited by the challenge and the potential that lay ahead. What appeared at first to be a career catastrophe became instead an opportunity advanced by internal and external forces. Brad and Marla drew upon the human potential that lies at the intersection of the Midlife Reevaluation Phase and the Liberation Phase. Adversity was the external catalyst that prompted them to reevaluate their lives and eventually move in a liberating new direction.

Branch Rickey, manager of the Brooklyn Dodgers, at age sixty-six (1947) broke the color barrier in major league baseball by signing the first black player, Jackie Robinson.

SANDRA: REBUILDING A LIFE AFTER LOSS

Sandra and Stan, both in their early sixties, had planned on traveling during their retirement, making up for the years their heavy work and family responsibilities had forced them to put their wanderlust on hold. They were looking forward, too, to combining travel adventure with learning, and they spent many evenings poring over materials from various elderhostel study programs. They had been married forty years and had three adult children and two grandchildren of whom they were very proud. For those four decades, Stan had worked in construction, the latter half of his career as a building contractor for a large residential construction business. Sandra had managed their home and social activities, helping to make a happy life for her family.

Their home, a quaint turn-of-the-century house, required all manner of repairs year by year, and the upkeep was growing burdensome. They felt that retirement would be a good time to sell the old house and move to a newer, lower maintenance condominium. Stan seemed to adjust well to retirement, turning immediately to fixing up the old home to sell. But four months into retirement, repairing a gutter one day, he suffered a fatal heart attack. Sandra was overcome with despair. She felt all the more overwhelmed by, on the one hand, being alone in their house, despite all its wonderful memories, and, on the other, not being used to handling the maintenance responsibilities that Stan had overseen. Alone, Sandra was frequently tearful and terribly lonely. One of her daughters persuaded her to join a support group for widows and helped arrange it.

Ding Ling, pseudonym of the Chinese novelist and radical feminist Jiang Bingzhi, was imprisoned during the Chinese Cultural Revolution of the 1970s, from the time she was sixty-six until she was seventy-one. Following her release she published the novel Comrade Du Wanxiang, *based on her experiences in the Great Northern Wilderness, where she had been banished during an earlier period of disfavor from the Chinese government.*

Two years went by and Sandra was still struggling emotionally. She couldn't reconcile the suddenness and sense of meaninglessness of Stan's death. She felt her own life to be empty and meaningless, even though all three of her children constantly called her, visited her, and encouraged her to visit them. Meanwhile, the house was becoming too much for her to handle, and she sadly came to the conclusion that she would have to sell it and move into a smaller residence like the one she and Stan had planned to buy. She felt overwhelmed by her sadness, by the demands of the old house, and by the thought of leaving it and having to move to a new place. Fortunately, she got a call from a good friend, Grace, who lived in such a condominium complex, informing her that one of the units in her building, a two-bedroom condo that would allow family to visit and stay over, would soon be available on the market. Sandra liked Grace very much, and felt this would help with the transition. She sold her house and moved there. But the move was not easy. She continued to grieve and have limited motivation and spirit.

Grace was concerned about Sandra not being able to get out of her grief and saw an opportunity for her to occupy her mind in a different way. She hoped Sandra would be interested; it would involve Sandra drawing upon her earlier experience as an elementary schoolteacher. That had been many years before—before she and Stan had married—but she had used her skills later to help her own young son, who had suffered from a reading disability, and as a volunteer occasionally in her children's schools.

Neighbor Grace had another friend whose eight-year-old grandson had problems reading; she wondered whether Sandra might be interested in tutoring the boy. Grace asked Sandra if she would, strongly encouraging her to do so. After a little more encouragement Sandra consented and, as the boy's mother later remarked to Grace, "Sandra worked wonders."

Sandra herself was pleased and told Grace how she had always wanted to return to teaching, especially in reading. Grace had a brainstorm: it wasn't too late for Sandra to revive a career in teaching, and the demand for reading specialists was so great that with the right credentials Sandra could work as consultant, negotiating her own flexible hours. At first, Sandra was reluctant, feeling she was too old. But Grace persisted with her encouragement, and Sandra's confidence grew when another older neighbor suggested she lead a monthly book discussion group for grandparents and their young grandchildren. After two successful book discussion group meetings, Sandra felt motivated to take the next steps toward recertification and work in the schools.

With Grace's support, Sandra followed through, enrolled in courses, enjoyed the unanticipated intergenerational energy of taking classes with considerably younger students, did well, and received her certificate. A few months later she received a request to consult for a semester at a school where she had done fieldwork. Her new career was launched, and she came out of her grieving, experiencing a newfound satisfaction with herself.

Sandra's story is both a story of her own creativity in response to loss and of Grace's social creativity in helping a friend in need. Sandra's experience, like that of Brad's, Helen's, and my own, was one of creativity loosening the bonds of adversity.

Clara Barton (1821–1912), began her career as a schoolteacher. With the onset of the Civil War she organized an agency to acquire and distribute supplies for the relief of wounded soldiers. She came to be known as the "angel of the battlefield."

She became associated with the International Red Cross in Europe, and in 1881 (at age sixty), she founded the American National Red Cross, focused on providing relief not only in wars but also in natural disasters. She subsequently served in Cuba during the Spanish-American War in 1898 at age seventy-seven, and continued in the role as president of the American Red Cross until the age of eighty-three.

More on the Effects of Creativity on Health

In literature on health, the term *healing* is often used in two different ways that at times intersect. One use is that while dealing with the ravages of disease, people can take steps and become involved in approaches that heal their psyche, allowing them to cope with emotional pain and maintain human dignity while their disease runs it course, even to death. The other use is when healing refers to recovering from disease itself. The two roles of healing also intersect, as with those whose inner feelings are helped in the face of life-threatening illness so that they experience longer life before succumbing to their illness, in contrast to those not so healed. And there are reports, albeit much smaller in number, of those whose emotional and reflective life has been treated, enabling them to recover even from illnesses viewed as terminal. Most of these latter individuals have been described as recovering following a combination of traditional treatments and interventions aimed at healing their psyche, though there are some who have recovered where healing directed only at their inner world of thoughts and feelings has been reported.

American philosopher Susanne Langer, author of **Philosophy in a New Key,** *wrote* **Mind: An Essay on Human Feeling** *(three volumes) from 1967 to 1982 (ages seventy-two to eighty-seven).*

With both views of healing there has been considerable research—both behavioral and biological—aimed at understanding the underlying mechanisms that promote healing as a factor of one's state of mind. The behavioral mechanisms have been better documented. The biological explanations are presently much stronger in theory than in proof, though experimental findings are mounting and are quite intriguing. This research is referred to as "mind-body studies," investigations examining the interplay of mental and physical health. Both views of healing are interesting when we look at the influence of creativity on health. In reviewing the findings below, keep in mind what was emphasized earlier in the book—that later life is where research has shown the influence of the mind on the body and vice versa to be most robust.

Dame Mary Jane Gilmore, Australian poet, published six volumes of poetry from 1910 (age forty-five) to 1954 (age eighty-nine), reflecting a lifelong commitment to help the sick and the helpless.

Creativity as Activity: The Behavioral View

When we want to break out of a nonproductive pattern of thought or behavior, we can purposefully try new strategies designed to help us change those patterns and develop new, more helpful ones. These behavioral interventions, especially with creative dimensions, have been shown to have positive effects on the course of serious disorders. Expressive arts therapies stand out, in particular art therapy, dance therapy, drama therapy, and music therapy. In studies of behavioral factors that are associated with a worsening of physical health problems, among those most often implicated are *unexpressed emotions* and *learned helplessness*. Someone whose emotions are bottled up—whether they are positive emotions like love and joy or negative emotions like anger and fear—appears to deal with disease less well than those who express their emotions more freely. Expressive arts interventions help by creatively enabling individuals to express their emotions through a nonverbal approach when emotional expression in words is blocked.

People who feel that they have no control over their lives, and especially those who develop a persistent sense of helplessness, are also reported to have worse courses of illness than those who experience a higher sense of control over their lives. Here, too, expressive arts offer us opportunities to begin to experience a greater sense of control by first discovering that we can take control of our mental imagery by creatively expressing it via art, dance, drama, or music.

Support groups, spiritual counseling, and psychotherapy can all achieve similar effects, likely working along related pathways that permit us to express unexpressed emotions better and to discover ways to take more tangible control of our lives. Creative endeavors in general can have the same effect in that they typically are associated with a powerful sense of influencing our well-being, if not destiny; often, too, they tap into or free up one's emotions in the service of action.

Consider the role of humor, for example, as a form of creative expression. Humor can provide a shortcut for fostering creative, adaptive new strategies. Even dark humor—humor that arises from adversity—appropriately timed and applied, can be effective in stimulating supportive new perspectives and interesting new approaches. Like humor in general, dark humor or "black humor" gives us permission to consider options that we previously wouldn't have considered. Black

In 1172 A.D. the leaders of warring Venetia and Constantinople agreed to peace negotiations. Venetia sent its gifted diplomat, sixty-five-year-old Enrico Dandolo, to meet with the emperor of Constantinople. But the talks stalled when the emperor became too intimidated by the Venetian's intelligence, viewing him as a threat, and plotting his assassination. The emperor's guards posed as a band of robbers and attacked Dandolo on his return to Venetia. Dandolo somehow managed to survive, but not without losing vision in both eyes. Twenty-nine years later (1201), at the age of ninety-four and despite his visual impairment, Dandolo led the fourth Crusade and his country to victory over Constantinople. At ninety-seven, thirty years after seeking peace, he was appointed chief magistrate of Constantinople.

Comedian Phyllis Diller, in her book* The Joys of Aging—And How to Avoid Them, *published when she was sixty-four, wrote, "I'm at an age when my back goes out more than I do."

humor is also often described as laughter in the dark, humor in the face of despair, gallows humor, and from German, *Galgenhumor*, or "laughter from the edge of the grave." By any name, this is humor that acknowledges adversity without succumbing to it. George Burns was a master of it, as, in the story that opened this chapter, he quipped that he "no longer buys green bananas" and that he could, if necessary, shift from being a stand-up comic to a "lie-down comic."

Humor also helps us look at how relative age is when it comes to the human condition. American humorist Josh Billings, in the late 1800s, captured this relativity when he noted that "in youth we run into difficulties, whereas in old age difficulties run into us." In other words, old age does not have a monopoly on problems, just as youth does not have a monopoly on potential—a particularly important perspective for depressed older adults. Or, as George Burns saw it, "It's good to be a hundred, for very few people die after a hundred." And in an anecdote a 90-year-old patient of mine shared, she said she read a newspaper interview where a 105-year-old woman was asked the advantages of being over 100, to which the centenarian replied, "at 100, there is less peer pressure."

Creative Chemistry: The Biological View

Humor and other creative strategies have been shown to have positive effects on the immune system, underscoring the potential influence of your mind on your immune system in protecting your health. This is the psychoneuroimmunology explanation of mind-body effects as discussed by Candice Pert, Henry Dreher, and Michael Ruff in "The Psychosomatic Network: Foundations of Mind-Body Medicine."

A similar mechanism has been suggested to explain the positive biological effects of behavioral strategies offered through cancer support groups, spiritual counseling, expressive arts therapies, and psychotherapy. And it has been theorized that through these same lines of communication, repressed emotions and learned helplessness suppress the immune system and lead to adverse health effects.

In fact, studies by Yehuda Shavit and colleagues suggest that a sense of helplessness influences chemical responses in the body that cause chronic elevations of naturally occurring opioids, narcoticlike substances, which in turn depress natural killer (NK) cell functions in the body, potentially increasing one's vulnerability to certain forms of cancer. Others similarly theorize that longstanding repression of strong emotions also induces high levels of naturally occurring opioids, which in turn interfere with immune system responses involved in fighting infectious diseases and cancer.

One of the leading mind-body researchers, Candice Pert, Ph.D., professor of physiology and biophysics at Georgetown University Medical Center in Washington, D.C., has identified seventy or eighty chemicals known as neuropeptides that she views as biochemical mediators of emotion—the body's chemical communication system between mind and body, emotion and physical health. Based on her research, she suggests that a two-way communication exists between our brain and immune system, through which each influences the activity of the other. This two-way communication occurs between the brain and other organ systems of the body as well, she says. According to her studies, many of the above neuropeptides are released throughout the body, triggered by our emotions or influenced by psychological factors.

Pert believes that most of the organs of the body contain specialized receptor sites that receive the different peptides like locks accepting specific keys, with resulting health effects on these organs. Apart from the immune system, organs that contain these receptor sites include the kidney, pancreas, and the entire gastrointestinal system—from the esophagus to the large intestine. Pert theorizes that this neuropeptide receptor network along the gastrointestinal tract, for instance, is the scientific explanation for the common folk reference to "gut feelings," or the link between, for instance, anxiety and a churning stomach or "butterflies." Conscious and unconscious feelings, she suggests, are "root factors in health and healing." According to this theory, the highly engaged emotional state of creative flow would trigger the release of specialized neuropeptides throughout the body, producing beneficial health effects.

"All interest in disease and death is only another expression of interest in life."

—THOMAS MANN

My Father's Fate: Alzheimer's Painful Path

As the dark clouds of my own trying experience were passing, another very difficult period descended. My father was diagnosed with Alzheimer's disease. It was a tragedy and an irony. The irony was that I had made some of my most important contributions in research at NIH in the study of Alzheimer's disease. Now it was visiting my family; we knew hard times were ahead. For me, personally, thoughts about what would happen to my dad were very painful. I knew that he would progressively lose his memory, become increasingly incapable of doing things, suffer agitation, and eventually lose his ability to even recognize me. I felt terrible, too, for my mother and my brothers, but especially for my mother, who, after more than fifty years of marriage, would have to suffer the misery of watching her loving husband slowly deteriorate mentally, eventually having trouble recognizing even this most beloved woman who had been at his side virtually every day of those years.

Charles Henry Goren (1901–1991), noted expert and author on Contract Bridge, wrote **Goren's Modern Backgammon Complete** *at age seventy-three (1974). At age eighty-eight (1989), he started a new newspaper column, "Goren Bridge with Omar Sharif and Tannah Hirsch."*

In the early stage of the disorder my father was still able to do a number of things he had always done, but with increasing difficulty. He had also become physically frail, which compounded problems for him. During one of my visits in this early stage of the disorder I took out the cribbage board to play him a game. Cribbage is a 350-year-old card game. The game is very fast moving and is scored with pegs on a cribbage board. Cribbage has always been an intergenerational game, especially good for teaching number skills to children. It had always been my father's favorite, and I have many fond memories of the two of us playing the game together when I was a child in elementary school, then in high school. My dad worked long hours running a small hardware and housewares store, which limited the one-on-one time we had together; cribbage had provided a great opportunity for me to engage him in fun one-on-one experiences in the midst of his very busy schedule.

At the time of my father's diagnosis, I was in the planning stages of a second game that I hoped would set an example for industry that games or any products could be designed to better serve special-needs users without compromising looks or sales potential in the marketplace. Typically it is very expensive to meet the special needs of one par-

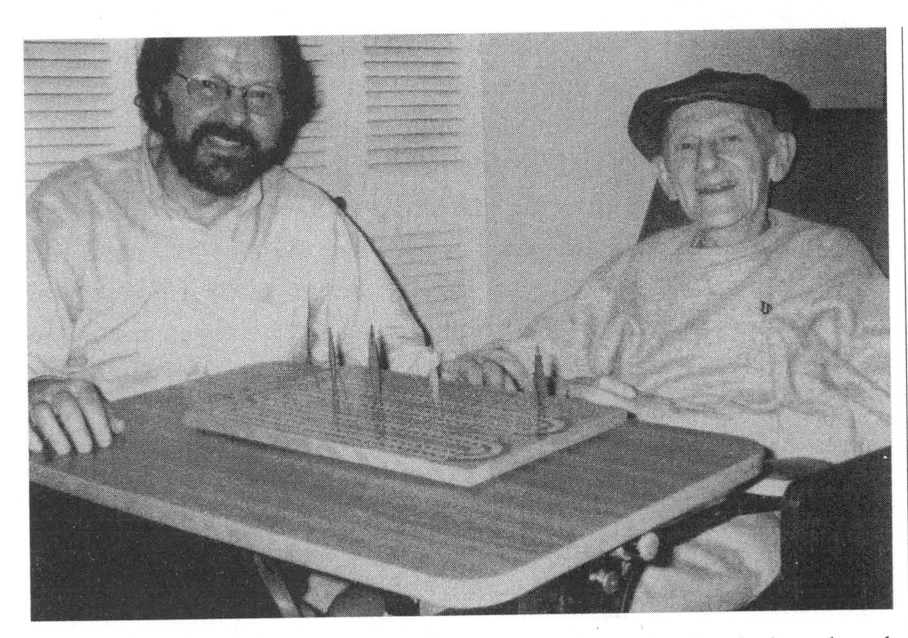

My father and I playing cribbage

ticular category of users because an adaptation must be designed and added to the original product. But when the "adaptation" is planned from the outset, design need not be compromised nor costs significantly affected. Experience also shows that special adjustments made to meet the needs of one group often benefit others. This is what architects refer to as "universal design," and you can see it in the sidewalks designed with a sloping curb for easier wheelchair—or bicycle, Rollerblade, stroller, or shopping cart—access.

The problem I had was finding the best game to use as an example. Then one afternoon, as I watched my father struggle to grasp the matchstick-size cribbage pegs he had once handled so easily, the sobering sight cast the entire game and its 350-year history in a completely different light for me and inspired my new project: the universal redesign of this classic game for the generations to come. As my father struggled to play his favorite game, the flaws in the standard design became clear: For older and younger hands alike, the pegs needed to be larger. If opponent pegs were shaped differently, and the board were reconfigured, then sight-impaired players could enjoy the game. My father's continued interest in playing despite the difficulty added to my motivation to make it better.

Altogether I made eight major improvements in the classic crib-

Milton Bradley's first game, the Checkered Game of Life, was introduced in 1860. It offered fun, education, art, and moral lessons. Movement was on a checkerboard, with a player's move being one or two spaces to the left, right, or diagonally. The path took the player from Infancy to Happy Old Age—the latter being the winning square. Landing on Bravery sent the player to Honor, Perseverance to Success, and Ambition to Fame. Gambling led to Ruin, and Idleness to Disgrace. If you did all the right things, you ended up in Happy Old Age.

bage set, and this "new, improved" GENCO version of the game became a success in the marketplace. I eventually secured a patent that did, in fact, make a statement to the industry about the value of creativity in product research and development.

More satisfying than the marketing success was the knowledge that the game made a difference in lives like those of two blind and elderly players who wrote to say the new design made it possible for them to enjoy an old favorite pastime once again. But my greatest satisfaction in developing the new cribbage board was that my father was able to enjoy the game of cribbage a little longer.

A Further Response to My Father's Illness

Benjamin Rush, the noted American physician and signer of the Declaration of Independence, wrote* Diseases of the Mind *(1821) when he was seventy-six.

Unfortunately, my father's disease continued to get worse, to the point that he could not play cribbage or carry out many other skills without considerable assistance from others. His memory and intellectual capacity had grossly deteriorated, to the point that his overall mental functioning was but a shadow of his former self. It was agony seeing him and contrasting his functioning to how he had previously been. I felt so bad for him, for my family, and for myself.

Alzheimer's disease (AD) is one of those dreaded disorders in which devastating effects on the patient and family caregivers bring profound stress to the family unit as a whole. I had long been concerned about the magnitude of this stress on Alzheimer's families—and now on my own—and had been thinking about an innovative intervention aimed at alleviating that overwhelming stress and gloom. It needed to be something that would offer families struggling with Alzheimer's disease to take a creative approach that ideally would have the same kind of beneficial effects that my game projects had had for me. My motivation now thrust into high drive. I was leaving NIH to return to a combined research and teaching position, a move that fortuitously freed more time to launch the project I had in mind. I called the project Therapeutic/Restorative Biographies (TR-Bios).* I

*My research on TR-Bios has been funded by the Helen Bader Foundation, Milwaukee, Wisconsin.

designed this project for families in general, as a response to the characteristic sense of loss and hopelessness that sets in when a loved one is stricken with Alzheimer's or some other debilitating illness. I offer my own family's experience not as a guide, but as a window through which to view the possibilities.

Finding a Place for Memories in Adversity: TR-Bios

Ere the parting hour go by,
Quick, thy tablets, Memory!

—MATTHEW ARNOLD

Basically, the TR-Bio project is aimed at preserving, restoring, and celebrating memories of the patient and the family for the benefit of the patient, family, staff, volunteers, and significant others in general. This is done through the creation of biographical stories about the patient and his or her family in video and yearbook formats—stories that humanize "the patient" and substitute for his own increasing inability to recall memories and to relate his own story. It is also an intergenerational intervention in that it can involve young volunteers—high school, college, and graduate school young people, many of whom are skilled in photography, film, computer imagery, oral history, and journalism. Their backgrounds bring ideal skills for helping families develop quality biographies.

TR-Bios are intended to offer quality time for the patient by providing engaging and accessible memories. At the same time, TR-Bios alter family members' experience of the illness in a positive direction, enabling them to feel less helpless by making a difference in how their loved one is perceived by others. The TR-Bios also attract visitors for the patients, because they provide a basis for interaction and reduce uneasiness on the part of others about how they are going to spend time with individuals who have a limited capacity to communicate.

In the case of Alzheimer's, TR-Bios can also bring pleasure and creativity into the course of an illness typically experienced as a wasteland of loss and despair. For example, in response to tendencies that families might have to sadly reminisce about good times they had ten years earlier, when the patient was doing well, meaningful moments are

For mem'ry has painted
this perfect day
With colors that never
fade,
And we find at the end of
a perfect day
The soul of a friend
we've made.
—CARRIE JACOBS BOND

created in the present, centered on positive events. The patient's birthday, for example, may provide the basis for a young "film crew"—often video-savvy grandchildren or family friends—to come in and record a day in the life of the patient interacting with the family during the birthday celebration. The filming and the high energy that surrounds it typically attract the interest of staff who see the patient in a much more personal and human light. It is not uncommon on some future day for a family member, friend, or staff member to recall the TR-Bios production day with pleasure, a welcome topic for conversation that simply did not exist before.

To illustrate creative opportunities, I'll share an experience involving my father. My father's memories that remained the strongest were those of when he was in the U.S Navy during the early 1930s; he had been selected as the poster sailor for recruiting others into the navy. So we went to work developing the story about this time in his life. In his scrapbook was a newspaper article that included a picture of the ship on which he had sailed. We zoomed the video camera in on the image so that the ship was all that showed—not the text from the article. Then we gently rocked the camera, which made the ship appear as if it were sailing. Finally, we used the microphone attachment to record a snippet of music—"Anchors Aweigh"—and showed these newly created segments on video to my father. His warm smile made the whole effort worthwhile and motivated everyone involved to be even more creative.

Three other episodes poignantly underscored the value of the TR-Bios to my father and my family. One day when I arrived to visit him, it was apparent that he didn't recognize me, though he initially enjoyed my company. Then his mood changed suddenly, he grew agitated and upset at my presence, and yelled at me to go away. I told him that I was his son, here for a visit. Quite angry, he yelled at me: "You're a liar—get the hell out of here!"

I figured it was time for a break in the action, and I told him it was good to see him and that I'd visit him at another time. I left his room, collected the file of yearbook-type images that we had developed of his time in the navy and came back into the room for another try at the visit. I entered, saying, "Benny, I have some wonderful pictures of when you were in the navy." He looked curious, and I sat down, showing him the images and telling him about each one. He was quite pleased and asked me if I had been in the navy with him. The rest of our visit went very well, and he hugged me before I left.

On another occasion, my father was sitting with my mother. He was looking at her with a puzzled look, clearly not recognizing her. She tried to help him make the connection: "Benny, don't you recognize me?" she said. "I'm your wife!" He still looked confused. Then she took out pictures we had compiled from the time she was dating him—in those navy days—followed by their wedding pictures. He studied them closely, then a wonderful grin spread across his face as he looked at my mother and exclaimed: "Oh, the love of my life!"

Thou comest as the memory of a dream, Which now is sad because it hath been sweet.

—SHELLEY

And finally, on yet another visit, my mother, my oldest brother Frank, and I were all sitting with my dad. He looked very glum, then said suddenly in an anguished voice: "Throw me in front of a truck. I'm worthless. I can't do anything!"

We responded, telling him that we wanted to show him something from a time when he had done some very special things. We showed him a segment of the videotape that included his time in the navy and commentary about his achievements there. When it was over, we asked him what he thought about it. He replied, with a pleased smile: "Gee, I must be special."

The TR-Bios work like clinical roots, reconnecting the patient and the family to fond memories in spite of the dreadful prognosis of the disease. They also enhance the dignity with which each family member lives through a very painful process. In the end, the biographical products that are developed become a profound exit gift from the patient to the family, wonderful recorded memories for the family that might otherwise never have been assembled were it not for the patient's and the family's struggle with a catastrophic illness. (See Chapter 9 for tips on how to create a TR-Bios tape or portfolio.)

"To live in the hearts we leave behind, Is not to die."

—THOMAS CAMPBELL

Inspiration from the Depths of Despair or Disability

However painful the adversity in our lives, and however we choose to respond to it, loss or other hardship undeniably adds to our experience in ways that inevitably provide new opportunities for growth. Again this is not to romanticize emotional suffering or to put a positive spin on pain. It is to say that when we recognize the complexity of the human experience in its entirety—the joy as well as the pain—we are better able to cope with it and learn from it. Our creativity equation—$C = me^2$—in which both life experiences, inner and outer, are such important factors—serves as a reminder of the significance of *all* life's experiences in expanding our creative potential.

John Muir (1838–1914), American naturalist, is considered the father of the modern environmental movement. His interest in nature developed after he nearly lost an eye in an industrial accident. Establishing himself as an authority on natural history and an eloquent writer, he advocated effectively for the federal government to adopt a forest conservation program. The establishment of the Sequoia and Yosemite National Parks occurred in 1890. Many others followed. His book My First Summer in the Sierra *was written when he was seventy-three (1911);* The Yosemite *was written at age seventy-four.*

In this chapter, the source of adversity was different for Sandra, whose husband died suddenly; for Brad, whose career and self-image suffered a painful blow; for Helen, whose sister died after a long struggle with illness; and for me in the dark days of my mystery illness and the even darker days of watching my father succumb to Alzheimer's. However, with our eventual creative initiatives, each of us was able to loosen the bonds of adversity.

We have explored ideas about creativity in the context of adversity in everyday lives, but sometimes I like to come back to artists for the lessons their stories can teach us, not just about art, but about seeing the potential of the moment differently. So often their great creativity as artists is chronicled, while the value of that creativity in responding to adversity in their lives is overlooked or forgotten.

Henri Matisse had long been fascinated with the vivid use of color, but by his early eighties Matisse suffered from heart disease, lung disorder, and gastrointestinal problems, all of which together sapped his energy, leaving him largely wheelchair bound or bedridden. He was no longer able to paint as he had before. But this loss of physical energy led to a new burst of creative energy that enabled Matisse to reroute his passion for color from the canvas to cutouts, removing the constraints that adversity had momentarily placed on his initiative and innovation. His new direction in art fit his capacities but did not compromise the quality of his work. Matisse created cutouts of pure color, and in the eyes of art historians he was viewed as closing the gap between color and form in a unique way.

Despite his physical limitations, Matisse remained determined to express his creativity visually. This same quality of determined cre-

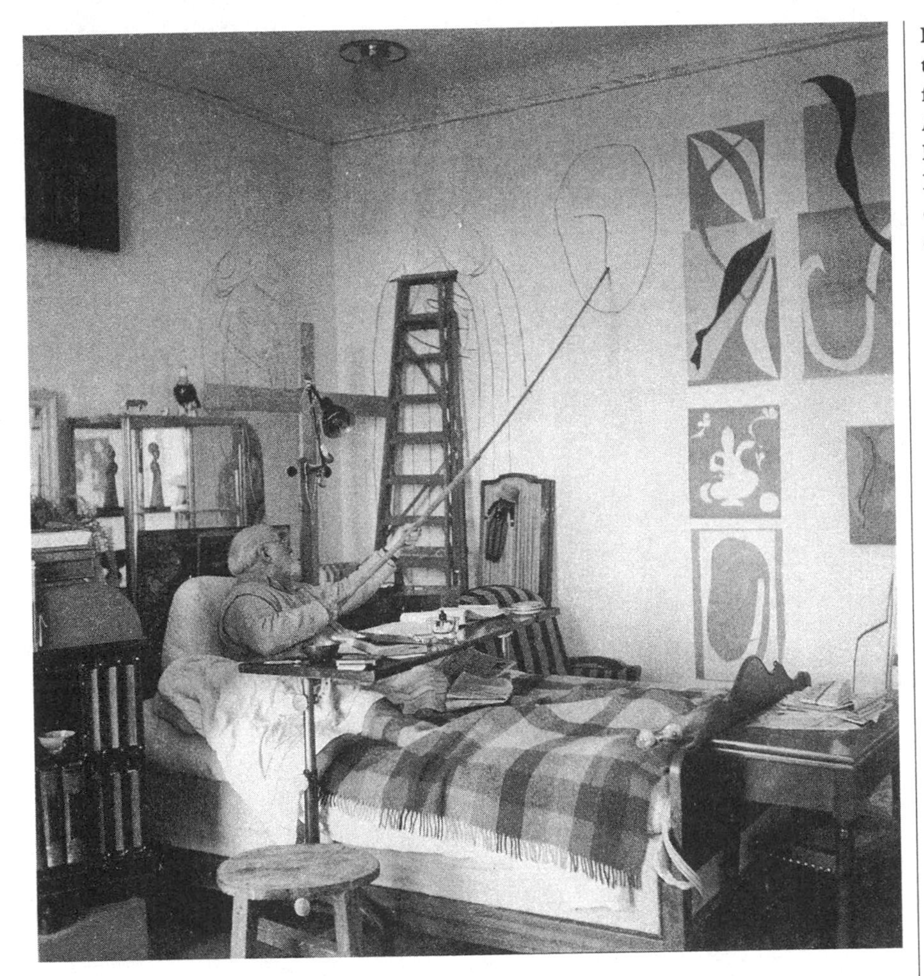

Matisse in his bedroom at the Hotel Regina, 1950, found on page 418 of *Henri Matisse: A Retrospective.* The Museum of Modern Art: New York, John Elderfield, curator, 1992
COURTESY W. CARONE, *PARIS MATCH*

ative thinking enabled Henri Matisse to change the direction of his painting following loss, and in the process provided a new page in the history of art.

The photograph above shows Matisse making sketches for such cutouts on his wall, using a pole while lying in his bed. In a keynote speech at a new state-of-the-art nursing home that opened several years ago, I showed this image. At first there was considerable exhilaration and some amusement in the room. But then, a growing restlessness began to set in. Finally, the subject of the hubbub reached me. Various nursing home administrators wondered whether I was advocating that nursing home residents draw on their bedroom walls like Matisse.

The great French painter Pierre-Auguste Renoir (1841–1919) was unable to walk as he neared seventy. His fingers were also no longer supple, but despite this he continued painting, attaching a paintbrush to his hand. In his final years he also took up sculpture, directing assistants to act as his hands; Venus Victorious *is a better-known example, exhibited at the Tate Gallery in London in 1914 (when he was seventy-three);* The Washerwoman *was created when he was seventy-six.*

The dry branch burns more fiercely than the green.

—ELDER OLSON (IN HIS MID-SEVENTIES)

I laughed, too, at first. But now I say: "Why not?" Creativity has the power to alter the darkness in our lives, whether we paint with it, draw with it, write with it, sing with it, work or play with it, or even just think with it. Considering the vast therapeutic potential, I can't imagine a better use for a blank wall.

7

Creativity and Community: Bridging the Generations

The proliferation of support groups suggests to me that too many Americans are growing up in homes that do not contain a grandmother. A home without a grandmother is like an egg without salt . . .

—FLORENCE KING, *REFLECTIONS IN A JAUNDICED EYE*

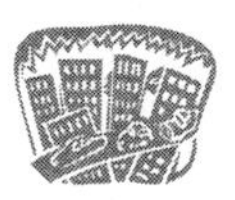

MRS. APPLEGATE, A WIDOW at eight-five, was a participant in my study of coping styles of older individuals. She lived independently in a retirement community with some housekeeping assistance. As a young woman, Mrs. Applegate had worked mostly as a housewife, raising four children, and occasionally as a substitute teacher. Mrs. Applegate and her husband had always liked to travel, so his death four years earlier had left her without a husband, traveling partner, and significant other available to help her should an unexpected problem occur.

"Women may be the one group that grows more radical with age."

—GLORIA STEINEM

Though she could get around fairly well on her own, she did have some health complications that gave her a concern about travel: She had a mild cardiac arrhythmia that had contributed to a few brief

Dame Freya Madeline Stark (1893–1993) wrote two dozen books based on her travels around the world. When she began, she journeyed to remote areas of Turkey and the Middle East where no European women were known to have traveled before. She later traveled to Asia, notably Afghanistan and Nepal, following which she published The Minaret of Diam *at age seventy-seven.*

episodes of congestive heart failure, which became well controlled with medication; she also had mild diabetes, controlled by diet. Occasionally, her left hip would bother her, making walking difficult, but she was able to compensate for it with the use of cane and medication. With her glasses, her eyesight was pretty good.

Despite these health concerns, Mrs. Applegate still wanted to travel abroad and, together with her eighteen-year-old grandniece Janice, worked out a creative plan. Mrs. Applegate proposed to her niece that the two travel abroad during Janice's summer vacations from school. But Mrs. Applegate and her niece worked out the plan so that Janice's freedom on the trips would be maximized.

Mrs. Applegate would sign up for a guided group tour arranged through the retirement community. The host country coordinator could respond to any minor problems that might occur, and others on the tour would provide companionship for Mrs. Applegate. But if any major problem occurred, Mrs. Applegate felt the coordinator could not be fully counted on to arrange adequate help. Hence, her niece's role was as emergency backup. Janice roomed with her aunt during the evenings, but was essentially on her own the rest of the time, remaining on call should an emergency occur.

For this insurance, Mrs. Applegate paid for Janice's trip. The plan worked beautifully. Mrs. Applegate could travel with peace of mind that if the unexpected occurred, she had backup on the spot; the family felt at ease; and Janice had the opportunity both to establish a wonderful relationship with her great aunt and to see the world.

Mrs. Applegate shared this successful scenario with an eighty-four-year old friend who was in a very similar situation, widowed and wanting to travel, financially able, but worried about potential health complications that might arise overseas. Her friend had a nineteen-year-old granddaughter who could serve in the same role as Mrs. Applegate's grandniece Janice. But Mrs. Applegate's friend's attitude became an obstacle to a creative solution; she insisted that if her granddaughter wanted to travel to Europe with her, and if their relationship was that important to her, the young woman should be willing to pay at least part of her own way. Three years had gone by, and Mrs. Applegate's friend was still not traveling. Her reluctance to use her resources—good enough health, finances, and family—in a creative way to enable her to travel left her indefinitely, and unnecessarily, homebound and discouraged instead.

I didn't work with Mrs. Applegate's friend, but her response was, sadly, a common one. Sometimes people simply have pockets of rigidity or fixed ideas about certain issues, money matters often being one of those. Sometimes the reason given is a smokescreen camouflaging certain fears or feelings of unreadiness that a person might have. To further explore the possibilities, we can gently ask if there are other reasons as well that might make the person uncomfortable with travel or unable to follow through on whatever the action under discussion might be. If the person expresses a fear or reason for unreadiness, then these offer opportunities to explore them further and perhaps to ease the discomfort or come up with a way to remove obstacles.

Advances in technology, community resources, and social awareness have created an environment that produces exciting opportunities for creative collaboration across generational lines. From E-mail and the Internet to community gardens and book discussion groups, the infrastructure for intergenerational creativity is in place. We are, as a culture, just beginning to realize the potential of the best-educated population of older adults we've ever had for contributing to the fabric and culture of society, be it through community volunteerism, philanthropy, or their own later-life occupational and artistic contributions. In the same way that we need some tutoring in computer technology in order to make full use of it, we also need to take a purposeful look around us for successful models of intergenerational and community collaboration and learn how to use them to enrich our lives at any age.

Research indicates that, especially in the family, intergenerational support has a health benefit at two levels: One is a psychological reward, similar to the positive mind-body effects of support groups in general. The second benefit is practical, in terms of the help that family members provide one another as they seek to protect their health and manage illness when it strikes. Whether intergenerational collaboration occurs within the family or within the community, the benefits often extend far from the origin of the collaboration.

When we look at the creativity equation, $C = me^2$, from an inter-

Graham Greene (1904–1991) the well-known and prolific writer, in his later years wrote many works, including* Travels with My Aunt *(at age sixty-five),* The Honorary Consul *(age sixty-nine),* The Human Factor *(age seventy-four),* Monsieur Quixote *(age seventy-eight), and* The Captain and the Enemy *(age eighty-four).

generational and community perspective, we see the elements of the equation charged with rich infusions from multiple sources. Intergenerational and community interaction can add tremendously to the new knowledge (*m*) and quickly besides, taking full advantage of the collaborative contribution of knowledge from a team, whether it's a team of two or more. At the same time there is that rich diversity of perspectives coming from various inner- and outer-world experiences—the e^2—of the team members. What makes the blend of different knowledge and experiences uniquely rich and motivating is the sense of togetherness and pleasure of being with one another that is fostered by an opportunity to work toward a common creative goal. Crisis has this effect; when there's a serious illness at home, or a natural disaster in the community, or war for a society, these crises may themselves inspire collaborative creative responses. But an opportunity to do something creative for the common good of a relationship or a community—whether it's public "big *C*" creativity or "little *c*" personal creativity—can be just as powerful in bringing people together in synchrony that results in something special. It need not be a crisis, it can be a creative quest.

Percy Wells Cerutty was the noted Australian sports coach and trainer who coached the great Australian runners John Landy (the second human to have run a mile in under four minutes) and Herb Elliot, who was never beaten at the distance of a mile or 1,500 meters. At age seventy-four (1969) Cerutty wrote his book **Be Fit or Be Damned!**

Understanding intergenerational creativity and collaboration is particularly important as we search for what is meaningful in these relationships to each of us and to our culture, and how to develop that quality in different ways in response to our changing cultural environment.

Lady Jane Francesca Wilde (1826–1896), the Irish poet and hostess and mother of Oscar Wilde, had a salon that was the most famous in Dublin. She published several works on folklore in later years, including **Ancient Legends of Ireland** *in 1887 at the age of sixty-one, and* **Ancient Cures** *(in 1891 at the age of sixty-five).*

The Changing Cultural Landscape: New Potential for Families and Communities

Fairy tales and folk legends are informative in how they reveal the way people have thought about intergenerational relationships over the centuries. Two generational themes dominate folk literature. First, there is the role of intergenerational relations between the old and their adult children and how they model respect for life and family among the grandchildren. This theme is reflected in the following nineteenth-century Grimm's fairy tale about the role of older persons as keepers of the kin. The second theme is the role of older persons as keepers of the culture, passing down wisdom for the greater good of the young, as portrayed in the eleventh-century Japanese folk legend following.

Grimm's "The Old Man and His Grandson"

There once was a very old man whose eyes had grown dim, his ears deaf, and whose knees shook. When he sat at the table hardly able to hold his spoon he'd spill soup on the tablecloth, and a little would even run out of his mouth. This disgusted his son and his daughter-in-law, and so finally the old grandfather had to sit in a corner behind the stove. They gave him his food in an earthenware bowl and not even enough at that. He used to look sadly toward the table, and tears would come to his eyes. One day his trembling hands couldn't even hold the bowl, and it fell to the floor and broke to pieces. The young woman scolded him, but he said nothing and merely sighed. For a few farthings she bought him a wooden bowl, and he had to eat out of that. As they were sitting thus, his four-year-old grandson was fitting some boards together on the floor. "What are you doing there?" asked his father. "I'm making a trough for Father and Mother to eat out of when I'm grown up," answered the child.

The husband and wife looked at each other for a while, finally began to weep, and at once brought the old grandfather to the table. From then they always let him eat with them, and they didn't say anything even when he did spill a little.

The Japanese "Mountain of Abandoned Old People"

In ancient times there prevailed a custom of abandoning old people when they reached the age of sixty. Once an old man was going to be abandoned on a mountain. Then a local ruler issued a notice to the people to make a rope with ashes and present it to him. The people tried to make a rope by mixing ashes and water but no one

Elias Lönnrot (1802–1884) was a Finnish philologist and folklorist whose major achievement was the collection of oral popular lays (short poems, originally for singing by medieval minstrels), which he organized into a long connected epic poem of ancient life in the far north, the "kalevala"—publishing the longer version in 1849 (at age forty-seven). He later compiled a great Finnish-Swedish dictionary, working from the age of sixty-four to until he was seventy-eight (1866–1880), which helped to establish a literary Finnish language.

could do it. Then two brothers talked about this to their old father. The father said: "Moisten straw with salty water and make a rope of the straw; then after it is dried, burn it and present the ashes to the ruler in the shape of a rope."

The brothers did just as he told them and presented the ash rope to the ruler, who was much pleased and said, "I feel very secure in having such wise men in my country. How is it that you possess such wisdom?" The two brothers explained in detail about their father. The ruler heard them out, and then gave notice to all the country that none should abandon old people thereafter. The two brothers returned home with many rewards, which delighted the old father.

Armand Hammer (1899–1990), the noted businessman who always had good relations with the Soviet Union, acted as a U.S. intermediary in negotiating the Soviet troop withdrawal from Afghanistan in 1987; he was eighty-eight.

In the background of both of these stories are issues, not unlike those of today, about the way in which we view ourselves as we age, and the way society views older persons when their problems present a challenge. Just as important is the way we respond to those views, and whether we use creative thinking to find new solutions and forge new opportunities to gain access to the moral and cultural resources that the older generation has to offer.

As a society, we have shrugged at America's distinction of being one of the world's least respectful cultures in our casual and systematic ambivalence toward our older population, though other countries cannot be held up as paragons of virtue—they all have their inconsistencies in how they relate to aging. Anthropologist Christie Kiefer has pointed out that compared with modern Western societies, the old in ancient China were more venerated, but there was considerable variation among Chinese families, depending on historical period, family finances, and local conditions and customs. Still, Confucianism, which was very influential in ancient China, advocated veneration of the old. Kiefer also describes the equivalent of intergenerational lessons that were part of Confucius's teaching, in which he is described as seeking "to produce social harmony by clarifying and beautifying 'natural' social virtues such as love between parents and children."

Similarly, historian Andrew Achenbaum points out that although times have not always been rosy for older persons throughout Western history, both the Old and New Testaments set the stage for positive attitudes toward the elderly and for desirable intergenerational relations. He illustrates this with the Fifth Commandment: "Honor your father and your mother, as the Lord your God commanded you; that your days may be prolonged, and that it may go well with you, in the land which the Lord your God gives you." The construction of the thought is meaningful, he notes, in that it describes the younger generation's own well-being "conditional upon ensuring the personal and social security of those who are presently aged."

We are, in our culture today, in the process of writing a vibrant new chapter in the story of intergenerational collaboration. Contrary to old "generation gap" stereotypes of our culture suffering from friction or conflict between old and young, there is ample evidence that individuals, families, and society on the whole have been moving in the opposite direction—toward communication and creative collaboration between generations, a burgeoning phenomenon I call *intergenerationalism*. This active, growing intergenerationalism is reflected in a number of demographic trends, in research findings, and in casual observation.

For instance, the number of four- and five-generation families is growing. A study in a Pennsylvania county, for example, found that 60 percent of women who died in 1988 had great grandchildren (four generations); 20 percent had great-great grandchildren (five generations). This is a simple demographic consequence of increasing average longevity; the longer a member of a particular generation lives, the more likely he or she will see subsequent generations born into the family.

Similarly, we are seeing an increase in the number of the "old-old"—those eighty-five and older—and the more visible rise of centenarians, including many who are functioning fairly well. The New England Centenarian Study, for example, in 1999 found 15 percent of their 169 centenarians still living independently, with a remarkable four out of five men who made it to one hundred in good mental and physical health; women showed greater variation.

These older, able adults are making more significant contributions to the support and well-being of younger family members, shifting the

Henry Brooks Adams (1838–1918) was an American historian and the grandson of John Quincy Adams. He wrote the monumental nine-volume* History of the United States during the Administration of Jefferson and Madison. *He later wrote his classic autobiography,* The Education of Henry Adams, *at age sixty-nine; the work was awarded the Pulitzer Prize.

Charles Greely Abbot (1872–1973) was an American astrophysicist who conducted important research on solar radiation. In his later years, continuing to be very active, he was regarded by many as the "grand old man" of solar physics in the United States. Just prior to his one-hundredth birthday, he designed a device for converting solar energy into power.

traditional relationship between older and younger generations in families from one in which the elders were viewed as needy to one in which they are viewed as part of the family support structure. In fact, studies show that older members of the family are increasing their rate of helping younger members faster than younger members are helping older ones. Further, we see the increasing role of older family members in helping adult children, especially among the growing number of single-parent households.

Marjory Stoneman Douglas (1890–1998), was described in Time *upon her death at 108 as the "ever vigilant empress of the Florida Everglades." Her crusade to preserve this treasured water wilderness spanned half a century. She had written the classic book* The Everglades: River of Grass *in 1947 (at age fifty-seven). In 1970 (at age eighty), she founded the Friends of the Everglades, also known as "Marjory's army." She had been interviewed earlier by* Time *when she was ninety-three, reflecting on her environmental work with the following comment: "It's women's business to be interested in the environment. It's an extended form of housekeeping."*

For instance, a growing number of grandparents are assuming significant "parenting" roles for grandchildren whose parents are struggling with divorce, unemployment, mental or physical illness, or other life circumstances that compromise parenting. It is interesting to look at this data during the 1960s and 1970s, when stereotypes were on the rise about the mounting burden of the elderly on society. In 1962, 60 percent of persons age sixty-five and older provided help to their children; by 1975, that percentage had increased to 71 percent. In 1962, 50 percent of persons age sixty-five and older provided help to their grandchildren; by 1975, that percentage had increased to 71 percent—*an increase of more than 40 percent*. Looking the other way, in 1962, 69 percent of adult children provided help to their parents; in 1975, the figure was essentially the same at 68 percent.

Health and economic factors have supported this generally more prominent role for the older generation. A more affluent segment of older Americans is providing financial support for their adult children, including housing, not only for single adult children, but often for divorced adult children and their children.

With the rise in the number of divorces from the mid to late twentieth century, grandparents have played an increasingly important role in helping young grandchildren adjust to their parents' marital breakup. A healthier older age group has been providing more direct support for unemployed as well as physically and mentally ill younger family members who move in or continue to live with them; and a generally well-educated and worldly older age group has followed traditional roles of providing sage advice to struggling younger members of the family.

With their contributions of energy and insight, this population of older adults is serving an increasingly important role as "kin and culture keepers," helping to hold families together, providing a kind of personal "social security" assistance for the family, and contributing in other ways to society at large.

Other trends reflect a rise in intergenerational experience and interest in intergenerational issues. Major marketing and product development initiatives are designed to attract older adults as well as younger consumers. For instance, planned residential and vacation communities rich with recreational opportunities, easy maintenance, and other convenience services and amenities attract retirees as well as affluent singles, couples, and families with children.

The news media are more energetically reporting trends reflecting the challenge adult children face in providing care for elderly parents in need of specialized housing, health care, financial management, or personal living assistance. Publications from *The New Yorker* to the *National Enquirer* bring the issue to life through news and feature stories.

Schools are taking a more proactive role in promoting intergenerationalism through projects in which students perform community service that brings them into personal contact with older adults through community performances, or volunteer work at senior centers, or seniors-only residential complexes or nursing homes; some high schools now require public service hours for graduation. A growing number of schools also recruit older adults to volunteer in the schools as readers, tutors, and assistants in the classrooms. Corporate business-education partnerships, too, are tapping the expertise of retired or other older adult professionals to help improve the quality of education and corporate support for education.

In institutions of higher education and continuing education, the generations are mixing routinely as an increasing number of older adults enroll in college and university courses, as well as recreational classes in the community. The U.S. Census Bureau reports that from 1994 to 1995, there was a 26 percent increase in college enrollment of those age fifty-five and older. From 1995 to 1996, there was a 14 percent

John Dewey (1859–1952), an American philosopher and educator, was a major influence on the progressive movement in U.S. education. Educational concepts that he helped advance included: the educational process should be built around the interests of the child; the learning process should provide opportunity for the interplay of thought and action in the child's classroom experience; the goal of education should be the growth of the child in every aspect of being. At the age of seventy-nine (1938), Dewey wrote **Experience and Education.**

Lope de Vega (1562–1635), also known as "the Phoenix of Spain," was considered the outstanding dramatist of the Spanish Golden Age. He authored more than 1,800 plays, still writing in the year he died at age seventy-two.

increase. Hence from 1994 to 1996 there was a *44 percent increase* in the college enrollment of those fifty-five and older in colleges. During this same time there was a robust but constant college enrollment among boomers, though from 1994–1996 there was approximately a 10 percent increase in graduate school enrollment by boomers. Among boomers in the oldest age group (forty-five to fifty in 1996, there was approximately a 40 percent increase in graduate school enrollment as compared to 1994.

This role of older adults as a national resource, despite its increasing presence, gets relatively little play in the news or film media, typically eclipsed by images of more dramatic but far less common examples of intergenerational tensions. As a result, our view of older adults and the value of their creativity is a jumble of contradictions.

The Myths of Generations Divided

An assortment of myths and misinformation about older adults and family interactions have perpetuated a sense that old and young are often at odds over issues of money, power, and cultural point of view. A more accurate picture acknowledges that the generations may find certain aspects of the intergenerational relationship to have its challenges, but that creative approaches to problem solving and community building are highly effective in bridging any generational gaps. For every myth, there is an underlying challenge begging for creative solutions. Three common myths that suggest negative feelings between the generations each present an opportunity to identify more clearly a challenge that can be addressed with intergenerational communication, collaboration, and creative problem solving:

Myth #1. "Kids don't care." The idea behind this assumption is that adult children gradually abandon their aging parents and go their separate ways. More often, in my work with older patients and my research and public policy travels across the country, I find that most people—no matter what their age—do care, but that, at times, too much distance or too little time compromise the extent and quality of time together. On the whole the popular view of that distance has been exaggerated—physically and emotionally. The telephone, for example, has enabled a highly effective modern-day approach to reaching out and touching from a distance, keeping older parents and adult children in close contact. Moreover, the actual contact between these family members is considerably more frequent than most people assume.

Myth #2. Help between adult children and their aging parents is one-way. This assumption is that the younger generation gives and the older generation remains always in the role of recipient. The reality is that interdependence is increasingly commonplace, at different times finding the younger generation providing support for elders or the elders supporting the younger generations. The data above revealed that research examining the prevalence of help in both directions found that over a more than ten-year period (1962 to 1975) the prevalence of older adults providing help to younger family members went up about 15 percent and was found in approximately 70 percent of families. Help from older relatives to younger ones was typically in the form of gifts (found in 69 percent of families), help with grandchildren (found in 36 percent of families), and help with housekeeping (found in 28 percent of families). Also, the number and percentage of grandchildren under age eighteen being cared for by grandparents is significantly on the rise. On the other hand, the prevalence of younger family members providing help to older ones remained about constant, though similarly high, in about 70 percent of families. Here, help included regular financial assistance, occasional gifts of money, and making medical payments.

A related issue of perspective comes into play when we look at the way that care provided by family members is examined—mainly in terms of burden. Only rarely does research address the positive effects of caregiving, for example, looking at how families are brought closer together by illness. Also uncharted is the way in which disease and disability in parents' lives influence the younger individual's appreciation of life and approach to living. As far as any "balance of payments" between the generations, your conclusion depends upon your starting point. Many adult children feel that their payments, more circumscribed in time, are paybacks for lifelong contributions to them from their parents. In this sense, there is no imbalance.

Dodie Smith (1896–1990), English playwright, novelist, and theater producer, wrote the classic children's book **The Hundred and One Dalmatians** *at age sixty (1956). She then went on to write three autobiographies*—**Look Back with Love** *(at age seventy-eight),* **Look Back with Mixed Feelings** *(at age eighty-two), and* **Look Back with Astonishment** *(age eighty-three).*

Sir John Floyer (1649–1734) wrote the first treatise on diseases of old age—**Medicina Gerocomica**—*at age seventy-five, in 1724.*

Myth #3 perpetuates the notion of the timeless generation gap. Research suggests that as successive populations entering later life become more similar in educational attainment, income security, health, and general social values, objective grounds for conflict between age groups diminishes. Consider the dramatic changes in educational level in older adults just since 1970. In 1970 the median number of years of schooling in America for those age sixty-five and older was 8.6 years—less than a high school education, meaning that there were just as many who never made it to ninth grade as there were those who completed most of eighth grade and on up through high school and college.

By 1989, less than two decades later, the median number of years of schooling had climbed to 12.1 years—meaning that a much higher percentage of the population has finished high school and at least begun college study. Much of the perceived gap between the generations, particularly depicted in the late 1960s and early 1970s and personified in the phrase "You can't trust anyone over thirty," had not so much to do with age, but rather with education and the great difference in formal education experience between the older and younger people of that era.

That isn't to say that the relationship between parents and their children doesn't suffer tension and conflict at times—and for some quite a lot of the time. However, the gap in understanding, or the conflict over it, isn't about age. It's about family dynamics and the struggles for power and for autonomy in the context of family. Even in families where parents and children have significant friction that might be considered a "generation gap," we often find that those children are open to meaningful relationships with other adults—grandparents, aunts and uncles, and other family, family friends, teachers, community leaders, and volunteers.

Michel Bréal (1832–1915), the French philologist and mythologist, founded the science of semantics—with his Essai de Sémantique, *at age sixty-five.*

It is their parents whom they feel they must struggle against; they benefit from the friendship and guidance proffered by other older adults, and often parents encourage these "outside" friendships precisely because of their value to the adolescent or young adult child. Family tension between parents and children only underscores the importance of social creativity and intergenerational collaboration that maintains the connection between the generations as a positive one.

Myths survive on the power of people's need to believe, and when cultural changes occur faster than people are prepared to adapt, they are likely to feel overwhelmed and will mourn their losses and find fault with the changes until they discover they have the inner resources with which to respond successfully. Myths also survive for cynical reasons: They attract attention in the media, and they are used by various policy makers to rationalize certain decisions. For example, if policy makers feel that the "kids don't care" they may develop legislation that in effect imposes new burdens on already overburdened, highly caring adult children of frail older parents. At the same time, many myths are or will be on their way out as models of intergenerational collaboration and creativity become more widely recognized in personal terms as well as in the broader impact that community action can offer.

Intergenerational Creativity and Play: Practicing for Life

Games or other creative play have always held a visible role in intergenerational activity. The time-honored image of the old man and young child playing checkers or chess comes to mind. I also think of a woman I know in her fifties who remains a devoted partner in games and puzzles with her children, not because she loves the games but because she loves the conversations that can grow from the unpressured and undistracted time together. Psychotherapists who work with children often use board games or toys as a focal point for therapy sessions because a game offers the child a neutral territory for social interaction. Direct questions about feelings can feel threatening—even to adults who aren't comfortable discussing their emotions—but a game is a good time. It also provides a context for conversation and, depending on the game or type of play, a nonthreatening experience of conflict and competition, or of collaboration and problem solving. In this sheltered

When he was sixty-five, Walt Disney saw his second Disney theme park—Disney World—under construction.

comfort zone of play, it becomes easier to express feelings, share ideas, solve problems, and enjoy the feeling of connectedness that comes from pleasurable social interaction. Whether the players are a therapist and patient, or a multigenerational assortment of friends or family, the therapeutic qualities of play help build relationships and provide successful intergenerational experiences for younger and older play partners. The fact that it's fun is motivational, too, boosting the interest level in intergenerational play, and continuing to build on the creativity that it generates.

My own decision to design a line of intergenerational games was motivated by the great potential I see there for relationship building and the other benefits of collaborative creativity those experiences provide. I'm concerned by what I see as a largely disturbing turn in games away from social interaction toward solitary play at the computer screen. Even when others "gather around the screen" to share the game experience, the fast-paced action adventure themes of so many computer and video games offer little or no opportunity for reflection, conversation, or meaningful collaboration. Inspired by the universal designs that have made our sidewalks, buildings, and so many other components of everyday life accessible to the able and handicapped alike, I have designed games that offer a similar universal design to exercise the intellect, encourage social interaction, foster creativity and collaboration, and encourage intergenerational and team play.

If we note the therapeutic qualities inherent in intergenerational play, we can see that similar qualities are there for us through intergenerational exchanges in other facets of life, as well.

Margaret Sanger (1879–1966) trained as a nurse and became one of America's leading birth control reformers. In 1952, at the age of seventy-three, she played a creative role in the founding of the International Planned Parenthood Federation, and then served as its first president.

TERI HAMILTON: INTERGENERATIONAL CREATIVITY AS A HEALING INFLUENCE

Teri Hamilton was seventy, a widow and retired nurse. She came to me for the treatment of depression. She was despondent, bitter, and had trouble sleeping. Her husband had died unexpectedly a year earlier from a heart attack. She said she could not get over his death. They had been looking forward to an eventful retirement; now everything had changed. They had had one child, a daughter, who had gotten involved in drugs as a young woman and died from a drug overdose more than twenty years earlier. Teri had never resolved her feelings about her daughter's death; she blamed herself, feeling she should have been able to get her daughter help earlier. At the time, she had, in fact, made several unsuccessful attempts to help her daughter.

One of the reasons that she was having trouble sleeping, was a return of disturbing dreams about her daughter, dreams in which Teri would argue with her daughter about the drugs, and her daughter would storm from the house. The month Teri came to my office was the twenty-second anniversary of her daughter's death.

Teri had grown up in the Northeast, the second of three children. Her father was somewhat distant but supportive. Her mother was very loving. Family life on the whole was good, and Teri always got along well with her older brother and younger sister. Following high school she went to nursing school and earned a degree. After graduation, she worked full-time as a nurse on a unit at a community hospital until she got married; then she cut back to part time. She also enjoyed teaching, and throughout her nursing career she gave a couple of lectures a year at the school of nursing or in continuing education courses on the role of a nurse at a community hospital.

Teri responded well to a combination of psychotherapy and antidepressant medication, and gradually pulled out of her depression. We continued to talk about the emptiness she felt in her life and began to explore options for meaningful social activities. Many suggestions fell by the wayside, but one that registered was supervising students at the local high school who wanted to carry out their community service at a local hospital or nursing home. I had become aware of the program through a friend whose daughter attended that high school and wanted to do her volunteer work in this area. It was a chance for Teri to become more outwardly active and to return to a facet of teaching.

Teri followed through and contacted the head of the community service program at the nearby high school, and the school was delighted to have her involved. Because there were several students who wanted to serve in this way, Teri was asked if she might run a special class for the students. Periodically, all the students involved in volunteering at a hospital or nursing home would get together with Teri to share their

"What nobler employment, or more valuable to the state, than that of the man who instructs the rising generation?"

—CICERO

experiences and get advice from one another about how to improve their volunteer work.

She was very pleased to do this, and the experience worked out well for all involved. It developed into a wonderful intergenerational relationship for them and a real community contribution to the hospitals and nursing homes that became the sites for the volunteers. Teri also shared with me that one of her fondest memories with her daughter was when her daughter had asked, as a sophomore in high school, if she could volunteer at the hospital where Teri was working at the time.

Teri's new activities not only brought her to rich new intergenerational relationships and the valuable community service that resulted, but also provided her a way to deal with the emptiness she felt following the loss of her husband. Further, this emotional growth enabled her to more successfully resolve the conflicted feelings she felt about her daughter. She later described to me that she felt her volunteer efforts were a memorial to her daughter who provided the earlier model for volunteering.

Peig Sayers (1873–1958), was an Irish Gaelic storyteller. She displayed remarkable ability to recollect traditional narratives, drawing the serious attention and deep respect of scholars interested in this heritage. Her deep cultural knowledge was recorded and preserved as prose in **Peig** *(edited by Máire Ní) at age sixty-three (1936) and in* **Machtnamh Sean-Mná** *recorded at age sixty-six (1939). The latter was translated twenty-three years later (1962) as* **An Old Woman's Reflections.**

Creativity Discovery Corps: Community Action to "Find" Creativity in Older Adults.

Almost without exception, whenever I give a lecture on creativity and aging, someone comes up to me afterward and says, "You just told my story." I remember one talk, in particular, in a public housing retirement community, when I shared the stories of folk artists who had discovered their artistic talents, or learned to use them, quite late in life. When the talk was over, a seventy-two-year-old man came up to me looking radiant. He said in a soft voice, "They are not alone." When I asked him to clarify his cryptic statement, he replied, "Those folk artists."

When I still looked puzzled, he said, "I'll show you," and walked away.

A few minutes later the man, Paul Carter, returned from his apartment upstairs with an extraordinarily intricate wood sculpture of a

Buddha sitting on a platform. The Buddha was set on a hinge that lifted up to reveal a compartment. It had a penetrating presence—a style and detail that reminded me of the work of William Edmonson. The craftsmanship, the precision of the carving, and the details were amazing.

"Can I show you more?" he asked. I was pleased to stay to see more.

An excited Mr. Carter returned after a few minutes with an eight-by-four-foot cardboard painting of a 1934 Chrysler, with brilliant yellow coloring and aluminum foil to simulate chrome on the body. It was absolutely striking! Next came a series of lifelike paintings of cowboys, from Hopalong Cassidy to Gene Autry. After that came two "pistols from the future" in stunningly crafted oversized holsters made from the leather of an old suitcase. The pistols themselves were eighteen inches long, carved from wood with simulated pearl handles.

For the next forty-five minutes, while people were still milling around the room, Mr. Carter brought down piece after piece—paintings and sculptures of mixed media. His works often combined wood, metal, leather, and other materials and were usually painted in bold colors. Most of the residents in the building had no idea Mr. Carter had this creative talent, but as he brought down the first of his artworks, a crowd had gathered around us to view these remarkable pieces. Mr. Carter had created art since childhood, but only after retiring from the police force a few years earlier did he have time to devote to his hobby. His apartment was wall-to-wall with art projects.

Over the years I would share inspiring stories like Mr. Carter's with colleagues. One day, a social worker named Barbara Soniat, with whom I was collaborating on a research project at George Washington University, invited me to lunch with two colleagues to share stories like that of Mr. Carter. Dr. Soniat and the two other social workers regularly encountered such people.

Over lunch, the four of us swapped stories about creative older people. Mr. Freddie Reynolds, for example, lived in an apartment filled with paintings, sculptures, family mementos, and objects that symbolized civil rights and his special idea of family. Then there was Ms. Dorothy Lewis, whose apartment was overrun with beautiful hats she had made between ages eighteen and eighty.

There were also examples of older people using their creativity to

Henri Breuil (1877–1966), the French archeologist and authority on cave paintings, helped launch the study of ancient Paleolithic art. His book* Four Hundred Centuries of Cave Art, *written at age seventy-five (1952), was a monumental contribution to this field.

fill the role as "keeper of the culture." Jackie Griffith, for instance, had collected an extraordinary number of artifacts and memorabilia about African-American life in Washington, D.C., that spanned more than eighty years. Ms. Griffith contributed many objects in her collection to a Smithsonian Institution exhibit entitled "Passing Down the Years," which captured the legacies of African-American families. Another example is Kingsley Gibson, a graphic artist who for at least half a century drew street scenes of the nation's capital. Finally, Ms. Ida Clark, now in her eighties, managed to collected scores of dolls from different countries, thus playing the role of keeper of many cultures.

Agnes Chase was a botanist who contributed significantly to advancing knowledge of grasses. At the age of 81 (1950) she published the revised edition of the Grasses of the United States. *At the age of ninety-three, with Cornelia D. Niles, she published the* Index to Grass Species.

All of these people displayed creativity in their own way and all of them came from varying backgrounds. Ray Ford worked for a family hauling business, a junk yard, and then a landscaping company. Upon retirement, he began to experiment with painting. His first canvas was an old pillowcase. Then he began painting on boards, mirrors, lamps, and chair backs. He is particularly interested in painting birds and gardens of flowers, because it allows him to use a combination of vibrant colors. Dr. Aurora Gordan, another example, turned to painting following a successful career as a pediatrician. Then in retirement, she enrolled in a pastels and watercolors class and continued to enjoy her exploration of painting as a hobby.

After entertaining each other with these impressive stories, Dr. Soniat, her colleagues, and I became even more convinced that the frequency of these types of inspirational stories is much higher than anyone, including the four of us, originally believed. We realized that there must be a large number of older people whose creative accomplishments are hidden behind closed doors, as in the case of my first example, Paul Carter. Most likely they were generally underrecognized or undervalued by their communities, like Vincent Van Gogh, whose work was not appreciated until after he died. We decided to form a group dedicated to discovering and promoting the work of talented older people. After some deliberation, we decided to call this group the Creativity Discovery Corps, composed of professionals, students, and other volunteers from a wide variety of disciplines, including the arts, humanities, gerontology, and social work, to name a few.

Our objective would be fourfold: to discover talented older persons in the expressive arts or those whose efforts contributed to our material culture, a term used to denote physical objects produced in traditional ways. Material culture embraces folk architecture, folk arts, and folk crafts. These headings can encompass diverse arts, including the construction of houses, the design and decoration of buildings and utensils, and the performance of home industries according to traditional styles and methods. The shape of fences, the making of sorghum molasses, and the sewing of quilts all fall under material culture. Third, we aimed to obtain life histories on these creative individuals, and finally, to identify other programs or practices providing opportunities for older persons to access their creativity.

Very soon after we formally organized the Creativity Discovery Corps, a twist in the story of one of our "discovered" elders assured us we were onto a good thing. We had arranged for Dorothy Lewis's hat collection to be in a group exhibit, an event that preceded the Black Fashion Museum's decision to acquire her hats, and we had just begun to interview her to develop the biographical statement to accompany her work. It became apparent that she was experiencing memory loss, resulting in gaps in her biography, and we had no other sources for information from her younger days. At the group exhibit that we organized in downtown Washington, however, a woman viewing Dorothy Lewis's hats gasped, "Oh, my God!" It turned out that she had been a high school classmate of Dorothy's, and had taken the same class with her some seventy years earlier on how to make hats. Dorothy's classmate remembered this early history in great detail and allowed us to fill in most of the gaps in Dorothy's biography.

Theodor Seuss Geisel, also known as "Dr. Seuss," author of **The Cat in the Hat** *at age fifty-three (1958), wrote* **You're Only Old Once** *at age eighty-two.*

The Corps also helped arrange for some of Freddie Reynolds' collages to become part of the holdings of the Smithsonian Institution. Ray Ford, the painter, continued to sell his artwork following two group exhibitions that the Corps arranged to show his work. Paul Carter, who came up to me to show his work after the lecture I gave in the building where he lived, is expected to have the first formal exhibit of his work at an upcoming exhibit held by the Creativity Discovery Corps. A national conference on Creativity & Aging was held by the Creativity Discovery Corps in December 1998. The conference highlighted the creations of many of the talented older persons we have discovered as well as showcasing best practices of exemplary programs in the Washington, D.C., area that have fostered creative expression on the part of older persons. The conference combined theory, practice, and performance. (For more specific information on how to start your own Creativity Corps, see Chapter 9.)

The story of Sergeant White is another interesting story from our Creativity Discovery Corps adventures. Washington, D.C., is the home of The Women in Military Service for America Memorial, located at the entrance of Arlington National Cemetery. The Women's Memorial has developed a biographical registry for women who have served in the military since the Revolutionary War. Sergeant White had served during World War II, but health problems kept her from acting to get her name on the registry. After being contacted by a social worker, the Corps helped her to complete this process, and, to her great delight, Sergeant White is now on the registry.

John Ericsson (1803–1889), Swedish-born American inventor and military engineer, during the Civil War in 1861 (at age fifty-eight) designed the ironclad **Monitor**, *the first warship with an armored revolving turret. His inventions are considered to have largely revolutionized navigation and the construction of warships; in 1878, at the age of seventy-five, he created the ship named* **The Destroyer**, *which could launch underwater torpedoes.*

But her situation resulted in yet a further contribution. When Creativity Discovery Corps volunteers initially approached the staff of the Women's Memorial about Sergeant White, the staff came to realize that they had an inadequate outreach program to find those like Sergeant White who had served but had difficulty contacting the Memorial or were simply unaware of its existence. Memorial staff, with technical assistance from the Creativity Discovery Corps, now have begun to plan an outreach program. Meanwhile, the Corps's own outreach efforts have grown through networking by social service and other community programs, word-of-mouth among Corps members and their colleagues, and techniques as simple as leaving flyers describing the Corps at talks on creativity and aging.

Finally, media stories about the Corps have drawn public attention, and inspired others to volunteer and broaden and strengthen the network. As word of the Corps has spread among others in Washington, D.C., increasing numbers of referrals are coming from service providers elsewhere in the city. Moreover, word is spreading among older persons themselves, particularly from those who participate in programs where Corps members work.

Once a candidate is referred to a coordinator, the process of reviewing the candidate's materials and preparing the biography becomes an intergenerational activity that further enriches the lives of those involved by combining their creative energy in a collaborative effort. The coordinator recruits a volunteer from the Corps's volunteer pool to get background information about the candidate so that the best possible plan of action can be developed to generate visibility for the candidate's work and life story. A number of oral history, art therapy, and journalism students have volunteered time—their tasks offering an appealing fit with their areas of study.

Through this program, and other community-sponsored activities that bring young and old together, the different energies and intellects of generations are able to connect in ways that enrich each differently, but all significantly.

The Marquis de Lafayette (1757–1834) sailed from his native France at age twenty (1777) to help George Washington in the Revolutionary War, where Lafayette was instrumental in the defeat of the British. In 1830, in France at age seventy-three, he commanded the national guard that helped overthrow King Charles X (who tried to eliminate freedom of the press among other liberties) and install Louis-Philippe on the throne.

Living Treasures: One Activist's Journey and Gift to Others

Mary Lou Cook is a living treasure. Born in 1918, she became increasingly active in social causes when she was young and taught arts and crafts, eventually contributing her time to Concerned Citizens for Nuclear Safety, Habitat for Humanity, and the Community Peace Forum as she grew older. During World War II, when she was in her twenties, she volunteered for the Red Cross as an occupational therapist. After the war, when in her thirties, she helped start a preschool nursery for blind children. She was one of the first recruiters for the Peace Corps in the 1960s. By her seventies she also had become a calligrapher, a book binder, a basket maker, a tree planter, a lecturer on creativity, a counselor, and an ordained minister and leader of a spiritual community in her hometown of Santa Fe, New Mexico.

Martha Graham reigned for more than half a century as the indisputable high priestess of modern dance. She continued to dance until she was seventy-five, choreographing her last work,* Maple Leaf Rag, *in 1990 at the age of ninety-six.

In 1984 she founded the Living Treasure program as a way to honor those mostly older adults in communities, schools, or the workplace who, through their work or lives, serve as models and mentors to others of all ages. The program was inspired by a Japanese practice of honoring venerable craftspeople and folk artists as "living national treasures." The founders were also influenced by Gandhi's wisdom that "You must be the change you wish to see in the world."

Cook was eighty when I first called her to find out more about her program, and I listened to a voice of uplifting vitality and enthusiasm. She explained that candidates for the Living Treasures honor are selected on the basis of the qualities they bring to community, such as "simplicity, wisdom, grace, cooperation, appreciation, trust, courage, authenticity, humor, humility, truthfulness, civility, constancy, kindness, serenity, and respect."

Twice a year, Cook and her coordinating group, Network for the Common Good, solicit nominees for a Living Treasures award that consists of a certificate and a community ceremony that honors the recipients. The program was an instant success, and in order to help other communities start their own versions of the elder honors society, Cook developed a sixteen-page "how-to" handbook on the Living Treasures.* In 1997 the group went on to publish a book titled *Living Treasures*, which features the uplifting stories and photos of ninety-three remarkable citizens of Santa Fe.

Cook founded the program because she wanted to help the community find a way to recognize the gift that elders offer in "providing inspiration with their hope, heart, and wisdom," she said. "They are folk heroes who live amongst us."

Cook herself has earned the title of folk hero and living treasure, using her creativity from an early age to translate the abstract qualities of character and beauty into concrete experiences, from intricate handcrafted baskets to community awards banquets celebrating the contributions of elders, to books and speeches passing on their wisdom—and hers—to a wider circle of communities and new generations of collaborators.

With the publication of his **Complete Poems** *at age seventy-two in 1950, Carl Sandburg was awarded a Pulitzer Prize. At age eighty-two, he wrote* **Harvest Poems.**

Living Treasures was a pioneering program in the field when it was founded in 1984. Since then, many communities have developed similar types of programs as part of their efforts to foster intergenerational dialogue and appreciation. The Santa Fe program's "living treasures" are mostly older persons—typically at least seventy years of

*To obtain the handbook, write Mary Lou Cook, 321 Calle Loma Norte, Santa Fe, NM 87501.

age—who live in the area. They represent all walks of life and are recognized for their participation and contributions to the life, heart, and spirit of their community. Since 1984, more than one hundred such individuals have been honored in ceremonies that take place twice a year, each spring and fall.

Who are some of the people designated as Living Treasures? In addition to Mary Lou Cook, the other Living Treasures described in the book represent great depth and diversity in their contribution to their community. For example:

Tino Griego:

Born in 1927, Augustine "Tino" Griego distinguished himself as an athlete during his adolescence, winning the Golden Gloves championship. Tragically, in his teens, he became crippled by arthritis and confined to a wheelchair for life. In 1947, he was offered a job as supervisor of a city youth center in his neighborhood. Reluctantly, he took the job as director of the Palace Avenue Youth Center for a one-month trial. Five decades later, he was still there, building up the programs of the center and encouraging and coaching thousands of young people who came to his center over the decades. He said, "I would never retire. I love the kids too much. I'll stay as long as I can push this wheelchair around."

Frances Tyson:

Born in 1912, Frances Tyson moved to Santa Fe in her mid-sixties with her husband, who was diagnosed with Alzheimer's disease. His illness altered their social activities, taking her into the new realm of environmental activism. Her career as an environmentalist took off after she attended a conference of the New Mexico Solar Energy Group.

"There I was with all these thirty-year-olds," she recalled. Gradually her involvement deepened, to the point of belonging to at least fifty environmental groups and engaging in considerable advocacy. She creatively practiced what she preached. In Santa Fe, she built a solar greenhouse. Then moving to Las Vegas following her husband's death, she constructed an energy-efficient house of her own design, using a

Solomon Lefschetz (1884–1972) began working as an engineer. But an industrial accident that resulted in his losing both hands in 1910 (at age twenty-six) forced him to give up engineering, from which he turned to mathematics. He became the leading topologist (the study of geometric figures that remain unchanged even under distortion, so long as no surfaces are torn) of his time in America. This work took him to the faculty at Princeton in 1925, where he stayed another twenty-eight years until he retired at age sixty-nine. However, he continued this work after retirement as visiting professor at Brown University.

wind generator and photo-voltaics to get heat and light from natural renewable sources.

At the age of seventy-five, the poet/writer Hilda Doolittle (H. D.) wrote **Helen in Egypt** *(1961), considered one of her two strongest works. It is a reworking of the Helen of Troy–Achilles myth.*

Norbert Kreidl:

Born in 1904, Norbert Kreidl trained as a physicist in Europe. He came to the United States in 1938 to escape the Nazis, and eventually become director of materials research and development at Bausch and Lomb. When he retired from that position at age sixty-four, he taught graduate students until he was seventy-two. He then moved to Santa Fe and began a new career as a traveling lecturer and consultant. One of his trips took him to Egypt, where he befriended another Ph.D. glass physicist. The two decided to make a different type of social contribution. They traveled to the small Egyptian village that had been the ancestral village of his new Egyptian friend. They went as technical assistance experts, asking the community how they could best help. Some fifteen years later, the village, through their help, has created ten cooperatives conducting work ranging from knitting to furniture making.

The village honored Kreidl by naming a library after him. He traveled back to Egypt for the ceremony, entering the village riding on a black horse, the first horseback ride of his life—at age eighty-four.

Rae Douglas:

Born in 1914, Rae Douglas in her later years became known as northern New Mexico's "Christmas Lady," after thirty-five years of volunteer trucking to distribute food, clothing, and household goods to the needy, especially at Christmas. She reflected, "Very seldom do I miss a day when I haven't taken care of someone." At the time of her award, she had already put 100,000 miles on the second van that the town had donated for her efforts. In 1994, at a church celebration of her eightieth birthday, the choir sang "I Ain't Got Time to Die." For Rae Douglas the sentiment was right on target, as she asserted, "I'm going to keep on going. If they lift the lid down, then I'll have to quit."

Allan Houser:

A Chiricahua Apache, Allan Houser was born in 1914. In 1934 he came to Santa Fe to study art at the Santa Fe Indian School and later developed a career as a sculptor, painter, and a teacher of art. He received a Guggenheim grant in sculpture and painting and went on to teach a whole generation of Indian artists. Robert Breunig, former chief curator of the Heard Museum in Phoenix, commented on Houser's work: "I think we can safely say he is the father of contemporary Indian sculpture." In 1992, at age seventy-eight, Houser joined the likes of Georgia O'Keeffe, Marian Anderson, Ella Fitzgerald, and Aaron Copland in receiving the National Medal of Arts. Allan Houser's philosophy: "You look inside. You experiment. You explore. You do things that are different."

Community programs like Living Treasures and Creativity Discovery Corps are changing in profound ways the experience of aging and creativity for older adults, as well as younger people with whom they collaborate or communicate in intergenerational activities. These programs, and the lives of those young and old who are touched by them, offer tangible proof of the power of community to celebrate the full spectrum of creativity and human potential.

Toni Morrison (b. 1931) won the Pulitzer Prize at the age of fifty-six for her book* Beloved *in 1987. The story follows a group of slaves, from before to after the Civil War, as they struggle to survive. Morrison's writing is rich in how she describes the experience of rural African-Americans. In 1993, at age sixty-two, she was awarded the Nobel Prize in Literature. In 1997, at age sixty-six, she published* Paradise, *which became an "Oprah Book Club" selection.

Medicare in an Intergenerational Context: History Forgotten

We have still with us today a powerful example of community creativity through public policy, but it is rarely viewed in so positive a light. In public debate over who will be the haves and who the have-nots, the history of the genesis of Medicare has become increasingly forgotten. The impetus for Medicare was not only coverage for older adults, *but protection for the family* who would have to foot the bill if their older members could not pay. Medicare was, is, and always has been a family-in-mind program—not a we/they, old-versus-young competitive resource distribution problem.

Peter Ferdinand Drucker, American management consultant, is credited with providing much of the philosophical and practical underpinnings for the modern business corporation. His later works on practical management have been particularly influential, including **Managing in Turbulent Times** *(1980), written at the age of seventy-one, and* **The Changing World of the Executive** *(1982), written at the age of seventy-three.*

"In real dollars," despite Medicare coverage, older persons pay more out-of-pocket for health care today than they did prior to the enactment of Medicare; this is caused by the significant costs patients are required to pay in copayments, the rise in poorly covered medication expenses, and from services or devices not covered under Medicare. Even with Medicare, they are not having an easy time. The economic situation of older adults as a whole also does not leave many with much wiggle room to assume more personal financial responsibility. While social security has helped keep many older adults out of poverty, the sixty-five and older age group still has the greatest percentage of individuals at near-poverty income levels, according to 1990 data. The percentage is yet higher for those most at risk for health care problems—hence, in need of coverage—the eighty-five-and-older age group. The rising cost for health care, in turn, places more of a burden on the family system as a whole, because the adult children are being called upon more to assist in payments.

In the table that follows, it is apparent that inadequate Medicare coverage for older adults cannot be compensated very much by older adults themselves—especially by those at an advanced age.

1990 BELOW 150% OF POVERTY AGE DISTRIBUTION

AGE GROUP	BELOW 150% OF POVERTY
<65	21.2
>65	27.2
>85	38.6

Note: The 1990 poverty level was $6,268.00 for single persons age 65 and older; the threshold for a two-person household with no related children was $7,900.00 The 1990 150% of poverty level for a single person age 65 was $9,402.00.

Data adapted from U.S. Senate Special Committee on Aging report on "Aging America—Trends and Projections, 1991"

In the absence of adequate coverage, older patients will either go without necessary care or families who are highly committed to the care of older loved ones could experience the return of excess burden that was historically relieved by the introduction of Medicare a generation ago.

I bring this up because it is an example of a disingenuous public policy discussion. Rather than going to the policy table with a full understanding of the issue in intergenerational terms and the commitment to be creative in solving the financing of Medicare, some attempt to divert the issue by framing it in an inflammatory way as a conflict-between-the-generations problem—giving resources to the old, denying them to the young. But history shows us that its intent was to protect the family and its intergenerational relations—something that would be undone by approaching Medicare with a budget-cutting ax.

Friedrich August von Hayek, a political economist, received a Nobel Prize in Economic Science in 1974, after writing, at age sixty-eight, on* Politics and Economics *(1967). He later wrote, at age eighty,* The Political Order of a Free People *(1979).

Creativity in Symptoms of Sickness and Community Response

Sometimes the benefits of intergenerational communication can be found in the simple things like a willingness to view someone differently. I'd like to share the story of a troubled man, an "odd bird" often ridiculed and rarely accepted. I share his story for two reasons: one is to offer an inside view of mental illness and an often misunderstood link between creativity and madness; another is to demystify the way in which a community can respond to these needy members with tolerance and compassion.

In history and literature, movies and myths, there is often a perceived relationship between madness—insanity—and creativity; I often hear expressed a misinformed, romanticized view of madness as a pathway to creativity. But there is nothing romantic about madness, which typically refers to psychosis, nor does psychosis provide a shortcut to creativity; typically it produces an impasse. There is another side, though, to the creativity and madness issue—sometimes the creative symbolism of psychotic symptoms can be a desperate plea for help.

The later films of the master of suspense, Alfred Hitchcock, included* Psycho *and* The Birds, *directed in his early and mid-sixties, and* Frenzy, *directed at age seventy-three (1972).

Symptoms have classically been viewed as signals of underlying trouble. Fever, for example, is a symptom signaling underlying infection. Psychiatrically, symptoms serve the same function of signaling underlying problems, but in the realm of mental rather than physical illness. At the same time, a psychiatric symptom sometimes contains

American poet, literary scholar, and critic Ezra Pound was regarded by T. S. Eliot as the motivating force influencing modern poetry. In 1945 he was indicted for treason following antidemocracy broadcasts he made during World War II for Fascist Italy. The trial did not proceed, however, as Pound was adjudged to be insane and placed in Saint Elizabeth's psychiatric hospital in Washington, D.C., from 1946 to 1958 (ages sixty-one to seventy-three. The general impression was that he had a paranoid psychosis. He was discharged and designated sane in 1958. During his hospitalization, and afterward, he continued to write highly regarded poetry, including his work Thrones: Cantos 96–109 *in 1959 (age seventy-four) and a collected work* The Cantos, *published at age eighty-five.*

symbolism that provides a clue to the conflicts with which the patient is struggling. Both psychiatric problems and their symptoms are painful, but sometimes the symptoms show how creative the *unconscious* mind can be in sending out clues, at times camouflaged, about the nature of inner emotional adversity. Consider the case of Terrance Newman.

I had just started consulting at an apartment building for older persons in 1971. The resident manager of the building said she would like to discuss with me problems of a bizarre older man whose behavior was frightening to many, including her. Basically, the resident manager wanted my concurrence that the man presented a danger to himself and others and needed to be evicted from the building. I asked her to describe him to me. She said he walked around the building with pennies taped to his wrist, carrying a Bible and a bar of soap, and spraying a deodorizer around him as he walked down the hallways. In this constant flurry of motion, he would alternately touch the Bible and a bar of soap to his lips.

When I heard the description, I agreed it was indeed bizarre, but I commented that it appeared that he did not physically threaten anyone; he was mainly a visual disturbance. The resident manager said that was true, although she had never thought of it that way. She had always thought of him as physically threatening even though he had never actually done anything threatening. I then suggested to her that what she described were perhaps desperate symptoms of emotional pain. I said if such was the case, then he needed help, and I felt that I could help him.

The manager seemed more open to this. I suggested that since she knew him, the next time she bumped into him she should tell him that she was concerned about him and wondered whether he might be interested in meeting with a new doctor who was coming to the building. If he seemed interested, she could give him my name and ask if he would like for me to call him. She did this, and I met Mr. Newman in the clinic of the building.

He displayed all the unusual behaviors that the resident manager had described. He was a retired cook, sixty-six, living in the building with his disabled wife. It quickly became clear that he was schizophrenic and suffered from delusions and hallucinations. He described vivid olfactory hallucinations in which he thought something was burning and smelled horrible. In his psychotic way he desperately tried to control the smells by spraying the deodorant around him.

In our next meeting, the meaning of the Bible and bar of soap that he would alternately touch to his lips also was revealed. Whenever he would have thoughts that he felt were not virtuous—feelings of envy or anger—he felt guilty and tried to cleanse himself by "washing" them away through his ritualistic handling of the Bible and the bar of soap.

The pennies that were taped to his wrist proved more difficult to decipher. During a subsequent meeting, I noticed that every time he talked about the horrible smells he experienced, he would rub the pennies. In psychosis unusual thought patterns occur where unusual associations result. Another name for a smell is a scent, the homonym for which is a "cent." Mr. Newman was trying to control the scents (cents) he smelled by trapping them under tape. Months later I gained yet a further understanding of why his hallucinations may have been in the form of smells. I noticed one hot day while Mr. Newman was wearing a short-sleeve shirt that he had burn scars on his upper arms. I asked him about them. He described that when he was an adolescent learning the skills of cooking from his father, oil on the oven caught fire and he suffered serious burns all over his back, shoulders, and upper arms; he could still vividly recall the horrifying smell of his own flesh burning. I believe this terrible experience influenced the nature of his symptoms, his hallucinations, when he later experienced the onset of schizophrenia.

Meanwhile, there was a crisis at hand. The manager still wanted him evicted from the building. I explained that his annoying behavior was a medical issue, and that I felt his symptoms would respond to special medication, the same way that diabetes, which was a chemical imbalance, could also be treated with special medication. Once the building manager had a better understanding of Mr. Newman's symptoms and the emotional pain he was experiencing, she was less afraid and more curious and compassionate. She agreed that he shouldn't be evicted and should have the opportunity for treatment.

I continued my work and longitudinal research at the building where Mr. Newman lived for the next twenty-five years. For the first

It was finally in his seventies that Colonel Harland Sanders (1890–1980) made it big with his "finger lickin good"* Kentucky Fried Chicken. *By the age of seventy-four, more than six hundred franchises in the United States were selling his chicken. He then sold most of his empire for a substantial sum, and received a seat on the board and a lifetime salary from the new parent company, for whom he continued to be an official ambassador for his famous chicken in commercials and ads right up until his death at age ninety.

fourteen years I continued to meet with and treat Mr. Newman. Though his symptoms improved they never completely went away, as is typical with schizophrenia. During that time, the management of the building changed six times, and each new manager initially viewed Mr. Newman as a menace because of his bizarre symptoms.

With each I explained Mr. Newman's situation as I had done before, and each of the new managers moved from fear to feelings of curiosity and to compassion, and finally tolerance of his behavior. It also became apparent that most of the people in the building had become tolerant of Mr. Newman as well, realizing that he was emotionally traumatized and meant no harm to anyone. Mr. Newman continued to live in the building, with his symptoms, receiving psychiatric treatment, until, at eighty, he died from cancer of the prostate.

Apart from the remarkable symbolism of his symptoms, Mr. Newman's story reveals the role of the community beyond that of the individual in determining how well and how long one can remain in his community while struggling with the effects of severe inner emotional adversity.

LUDY AND PACY LEVINE: A TRADITION OF INTERGENERATIONALISM

Robert Frost (1874–1963), the Pulitzer Prize–winning American poet, who had been referred to as "the voice of New England," in a memorable event presented his poem "The Gift Outright" at age eighty-seven at President Kennedy's innauguration. The next year at age eighty-eight, he published his work In the Clearing *(1962).*

Ludy and Pacy Levine, my wife's great uncles, probably should be designated an American institution for all that they did for themselves, their extended family, and their community. Articles about them in *The New York Times*, the *Boston Globe*, and *Yankee Magazine* have said the same. Ludy was born just before the start of the twentieth century, Pacy just afterward. They were close from the start to the finish, and those who knew them well referred to them as "the boys." Their father had opened a clothing store on Main Street in small town Waterville, Maine, that became, after L. L. Bean, the second best-known store that sold clothes in Maine. The store thrived for 107 years until it went the way of other small family-owned stores on Main Street America, closing not long after Ludy, nearing ninety-nine, had to retire. Their father, who had escaped czarist Russia, opened the store in the late nineteenth century. By the late 1920s, Ludy had left medical school and Pacy law school to help out in the family store. Their collaborative creativity as quality clothiers brought the store into a golden age where it thrived and served its community well. As the store's success grew, so, too, did Ludy's and Pacy's contributions to their community—helping the YMCA, the Boys' Club, and virtually every social service agency and club, church charity, the local synagogue, and cause that asked their assistance. They were also extremely loyal Colby College alumni, who became important benefactors to the college and provided numerous scholarships for needy Colby students.

They never married, and as they entered the second half of life, their community, in effect, became an important new part of their family with all the help they extended and all the love and appreciation they received back.

Ludy and Pacy became famous for helping young Colby students, whom they allowed to purchase clothes on credit without interest at the start of their college career and pay when the students graduated or earned enough money. No student ever failed to come through. They became so popular in their town that a local restaurant named burgers after them—a Ludy Burger and a Pacy Burger.

Their devotion to family was immense, and when they were in their mid- to late seventies, they renovated and expanded the family's summer camp into a substantial cottage by a beautiful lake to maximize the extended family's incentive for getting together throughout the summer—a very creative act as keepers of the kin. Ludy would say, "If you want the family to get together, you need a place for it to happen, where they would want to be together." On every summer Sunday at the camp "the boys" would hold court for the local family, and every Fourth of July scores of family members and friends would come by to visit.

"The boys" were also avid sports enthusiasts. They supported local Little League and football teams, bought Colby its new baseball scoreboard and its new football scoreboard, as well as contributed extensively to its new track. The Colby faculty and students were very fond of these elder boys. They would let Pacy sit on the bench during the football games. But Pacy was so enthusiastic that he would often run down the sidelines onto the field during the play of the game—

Cornelius Vanderbilt (1794–1877), an American financier, became successful as an owner of steamships, but in 1862 (at age sixty-eight), he sold his ships and entered on a great career of railroad financing. At age seventy-nine (1873), he turned to philanthropy and gave $1 million to found Vanderbilt University.

Connie Mack (1862–1956), the noted American baseball player and manager, holds the record for most years managing (53) and most games won (3776), winning the World Series for Philadelphia in 1929 and 1930 at the ages of sixty-seven and sixty-eight.

even in his late eighties—so the coach always assigned one eager player to tactfully accompany Pacy and keep him from running onto the field and potentially getting run over by the opposing front line.

By their eighties and nineties, a bench was placed in the store where they held their supreme court. Countless students, friends, and customers would come by to chat and seek their advice, sometimes even about clothes. This was social creativity in action.

When each brother died, his funeral was in the chapel at Colby College. Both times the chapel was packed, and both times what brought spirit to our souls and tears to our eyes was when the entire football team solemnly walked in to respectfully take their seats and pay tribute to two men old enough to be their great grandfathers but ageless enough to be their buddies.

In Erik Erikson's description of earlier-life stages of development, he associates the relationship between elders and young people as a context for learning about trust, a fundamental piece of emotional development. Trust, he says, quoting from the Webster's dictionary of his era, is defined as "the assured reliance on another's integrity." Children of any age continue to look for that integrity in the older generation, and they are strengthened by it in profound ways, as Erickson saw it, when he said, "Healthy children will not fear life if their elders have integrity enough not to fear death."

"A man finds his identity by identifying. A man's identity is not best thought of as the way in which he is separated from his fellows but the way in which he is united with them."

—ROBERT TERWILLIGER

Ludy and Pacy Levine, in their exercise of trust and creative responses throughout their lives, inspired young lives and engendered in those of all ages a feeling of shared purpose in community. The nature of their creativity changed as they developed new ways of expressing it throughout their lives, as young boys, as college students, as retailers, and as kindly, supportive members of a community. But their success in life through all those years arose from their ability to see things differently, think a different way, and look for the potential in every encounter—and every generation.

8

Identity and Autobiography: Life as a Work in Progress

People often say that this or that person has not yet found himself. But the self is not something that one finds. It is something that one creates.

—THOMAS SZASZ, *THE SECOND SIN*

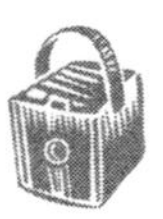

WE ARE ACCUSTOMED TO thinking of autobiography as the province of famous people—world leaders, movie stars, great authors, thinkers, and inventors—individuals who have left a significant impression on history and want to leave the story for posterity in their own words. Autobiographies or memoirs are also generally viewed as acts of literature, intended for publication and judgment on the basis of literary or historical merit. Beyond the bookshelves and arena of public lives, however, autobiography as an *emotional process* plays a much larger, though overlooked, role in our culture and in our lives.

***Harpo Marx (1893–1961), the silent harp-playing brother among the legendary Marx Brothers comedy team, at age sixty-eight wrote his autobiography,* Harpo Speaks.**

Autobiography—the telling of our own life story—can be especially meaningful for each of us not only as a contribution of tales to our family or community, but also as a highly personal journey inward that can lead to new self-discovery and creative potential in the days to follow. The external process of sharing our experiences and telling what we know enables us to combine qualities of creativity and aging to become *keepers of the culture,* the long recognized role of elders, passing on values, wisdom, and a way of life, whether in the culture of a family, a geographic community, or a people bound by ideology.

Perhaps even more important, however, autobiography illuminates a typically obscured internal process of identity development that begins in childhood and continues throughout the life span. What is "identity"? The term came into broad clinical usage from the work of Erik Erikson, and broad popular usage followed. I like psychoanalyst Allen Wheelis's definition that builds upon Erik Erikson's work:

> Identity is a coherent sense of self. It depends upon the awareness that one's endeavors and one's life experiences make sense, that they are meaningful in the context in which life is lived. It depends also upon stable values, and upon the conviction that one's actions and values are harmoniously related. It is a sense of wholeness, of integration, of knowing what is right and what is wrong and of being able to choose. A firm sense of identity provides both a compass to determine one's course in life and ballast to keep one steady.

It is this last point that emphasizes the psychological importance of identity as a compass or stabilizer in pursuing our course in life. Psychologically, our identity is the ultimate product of our creativity, reflecting as it does what we make of ourselves in response to a world of influences and experiences.

Much of our understanding of human emotional development has been informed by traditional theories that use early-life experience to predict and explain much of what follows later in life. Most of this theory development occurred in the absence of study or understanding of aging and what occurs and what is possible as we grow older.

To his credit, Erik Erikson, who has contributed most to our understanding of different stages in human development, pointed out

William Christopher (W. C.) Handy (1873–1958), altered the course of popular music by being the first to introduce the "blues," characteristic of black folk music at that time, to printed music with "Saint Louis Blues" in 1914 (when he was forty-one). Forced to publish "Saint Louis Blues" himself, he created a publishing firm that he continued to direct until late in his life. He produced anthologies of Negro spirituals and blues as well as studies of black musicians in America. Handy wrote his autobiography, Father of the Blues, *at age sixty-eight. He remained active in his efforts to promote the cultural role of African-Americans in the history of music until his death at age eighty-five.*

The great German philosopher Immanuel Kant, one of the most outstanding figures in the history of Western

that "identity formation neither begins nor ends with adolescence." However, because five of his eight defined developmental stages occur by adolescence, Erikson's theory suggests that he saw the largest part of identity formation having occurred by adolescence. His only hint at more was one stage defined for later life: "Mature Age."

With the growth of the field of gerontology we have discovered new windows through which to look at human psychology and behavior. We are just beginning to modify our theories to accommodate what we now can see from the vantage point of older age and a lifetime of emotional growth and development.

Continuing research on aging is advancing our understanding of both early and continuing psychological development. Classically, in the fields of psychology and human development, successful negotiation of adolescence has been seen as essential to be ready to take on the tasks of adulthood. The common view among many mental health professionals has been that the self-concept you have by the end of adolescence is close to the finished product, and if it's weak or flawed, then what follows is destined to be fraught with endless variations of trouble.

From my work in aging, it is apparent that we need to separate these concepts—"finished product by the end of adolescence" and "flawed product at older age" to make room for the changes that can and do occur. If one's sense of identity is not coherent or integrated with a sense of wholeness by the end of adolescence, one is indeed at risk for problems in handling the tasks of adulthood. At the same time, findings from research and the practice of psychotherapy show that this identity confusion and crisis can be healed—that change is possible. Studies on aging not only show the same, but they reveal that one's sense of identity is not a finished product by the end of adolescence. Erikson, himself, never said it was.

Fortunately, studies of the life cycle and aging point to many opportunities as the decades unfold for mid- and late-course corrections in the development of our sense of self and how we act on it in dealing with life. While our childhood and adolescent experiences are powerful forces shaping the landscape of our inner life, our capacity for continued emotional growth makes new understanding and new responses possi-

thought, wrote his most important works relatively late in life: **Critique of Pure Reason**, *at age fifty-seven (1781);* **Critique of Practical Reason**, *at age sixty-four (1788);* **Critique of Judgment**, *at age sixty-six (1790); and writing on political topics,* **Perpetual Peace**, *at seventy-one (1795).*

Anaïs Nin (1903–1977) emerged as a central figure in the new feminism of the 1970s. Her seven **Journals**, *written from age sixty-three to the time of her death at age seventy-four, provided a passionate and candid account of her voyage of self-discovery. Many women were influenced by Nin's intense autobiographical works in their own inner quests and autobiographical expression, through writing, art, and photography.*

ble at every age. With aging, the elements that comprise our sense of wholeness continue to evolve, as does their integration and coherence. You can experience change without jeopardizing stability or equilibrium; this applies to both our physiology and our psychology as we age.

Identity: Two Worlds in One

William Edward Burghardt (W. E. B.) Dubois, cofounder of the National Association for the Advancement of Colored People (NAACP) in 1909, continued throughout his life, into his nineties, to inform, sensitize, and challenge society about issues of race. Among his many important writings were **The Gift of Black Folk** *(1935), written when he was sixty-seven, and* **Color and Democracy** *(1945), written when he was seventy-seven.*

Identity is indeed a complicated concept because it has both inner-world and outer-world dimensions, much like the two *e*'s of experience that shape our creative growth and expression. Inner world aspects of identity reflect the development of a sense of stability and coherence while healthy, gradual change—reflecting ongoing psychological growth and development with aging—occurs. Outer world qualities involve how we relate to others and to cultural attitudes, ideals, and expectations that influence our role in the world. Identity involves this dynamic interplay between inner feelings of self and outer perceptions of role that combine to influence our overall view of who we are. When we are successfully able to integrate these diverse and complex influences and feelings, then we have a good foundation for creative exploration. Someone whose sense of identity has not adequately come together will spend more time struggling with identity confusion or crisis than pursuing creative expression.

Because in the past the predominant thought was that our sense of self is largely formed by the end of adolescence, Erikson's use of the term *identity crisis* was initially popularized in relation to this developmental stage. Erikson used the term *identity confusion* to describe one's psychological state when a coherent, integrated sense of self failed to develop. Identity confusion in turn could lead to an identity crisis resulting in adverse effects on one's self-view, relationships, activities, and perceived path in life. In truth, however, neither identity confusion nor identity crisis is confined to adolescence. As you can see in the two examples that follow, identity confusion can look quite different at different ages, but identity is no less an issue at either age.

Josh was eighteen, a high school graduate who never got help from his father when he felt vulnerable or in trouble. Worse, during such difficult times his father would typically reprimand him for not being able to get his life in order. His father was unconsciously repeating the physical abuse he received from his own dad in a psychological guise. When Josh turned to his mother, she would try to comfort him, saying his father really loved him but was often stressed from his work. Josh felt further diminished by his mother's efforts to sweep the problem under the rug. He developed a resistance to authority figures, feeling he couldn't rely on them when it mattered. As a result he began to challenge society's authority figures, only making matters worse as he increased his risk of getting into serious trouble with the law. His identity in relation to authority had not gelled, resulting in considerable confusion and inappropriate and risky behavior.

Barbara, forty-six, was a full-time homemaker for her husband and three children, and frequently volunteered for community projects that allowed her to use her natural talent for design and artistry. Married before she had finished college, Barbara had been too busy managing home and family to return to school or pursue her artistic interests. Her husband and family wanted her home and she was happy to feel needed, if not always appreciated. However, as she and her husband entered their forties, the children, two of them now teenagers, were increasingly critical of her in fairly typical teenage ways.

Then the marriage hit a plateau; her husband became more critical of her housekeeping and her parenting style, and more emotionally distant and indifferent. One day he stated flatly that he no longer found her attractive, no longer loved her, and found nothing in the marriage worth saving. Barbara was angry and emotionally devastated. She lost confidence in her judgment regarding even mundane life events and relationships.

With the prospect of divorce looming, Barbara felt at a total loss: unsure of herself, unsure of her or her family's future, and worst of all, unsure of how to respond to the dramatic turn of events. For Barbara, the crisis went beyond the marriage; she had put her husband's needs and family wishes first for her entire adult life, and now her identity and sense of self-worth were tied exclusively to her role as a wife and mother. With those relationships in turmoil, her deepest feelings about herself were thrust into crisis as well.

Fusaye Ichikawa (1893–1981), the Japanese feminist and politician, formed the Women's Suffrage League in Japan in 1924, and following World War II became head of the new Japan Women's League, which in 1945 secured the right for women to vote. From 1952 to 1971 (when she was age seventy-eight), she served in the Japanese Diet fighting for wider women's rights and battling different forms of corruption. After defeat in 1971 she triumphantly returned to parliament in 1975 (at age eighty-two), where she continued to serve until age eighty-seven.

With both Josh and Barbara identity confusion interfered with how they perceived themselves as individuals and in relation to others. The consequence for Josh was maladaptive behavior when interacting with others, while the result for Barbara was an inability to develop a sufficient sense of self or strategy for conflict resolution in determining a sound course of action.

When crises occur and fail to resolve in relationships with significant others, outside help in the form of therapy can make a difference. The therapeutic process can focus on providing corrective emotional experiences that improve self-image and our sense of self in relation to others.

Dolores Ibarruri, who went by the pseudonym "La Pasionaria" (the passion flower), became a legendary twentieth-century Spanish Communist leader and politician. She helped found the Spanish Communist Party. During the Spanish Civil War (1936–1939), while in her thirties, she became a national figure with her impassioned attempts to inspire the Spanish people to fight against the Fascist forces. Among her noted exhortations was "It is better to die on your feet than to live on your knees." With Franco coming to power in 1939, she escaped Spain for the Soviet Union, finally returning in 1977 at the age of eighty-one, following Franco's death, when she was reelected to the National Assembly.

Identity and Human Potential Phases: Timing Is Everything

More than two thousand years ago, ancient Chinese philosopher Confucius reflected on the continuing formative process of identity with aging. Confucius, who lived to age seventy-two (551–479 B.C.), wrote about his stages of life:

- At fifteen, I set my heart upon learning.
- At thirty, I established myself (in accordance with ritual).
- At forty, I no longer had perplexities.
- At fifty, I knew the Mandate of Heaven.
- At sixty, I was at ease with whatever I heard.
- At seventy, I could follow my heart's desire without transgressing the boundaries of right.

In this same way, the four human potential phases of adulthood that I defined in Chapter 3 become significant. These adult human potential phases, starting with the Midlife Reevaluation Phase, moving to the Liberation Phase, onto the Summing-Up Phase, then to the Encore Phase, speak strongly to the continuing sculpting of identity from within, which occurs with age.

Just as adolescence punctuates so strongly the sense of identity formation, the Summing-Up Phase similarly stamps out a strong statement about the course of identity across the life cycle. That desire to sum up one's life work, ideas, and discoveries and to share them with one's family and society increases with age across all fields of human endeavor. Storytelling by the older members of a family is perhaps the most universally recognized form in which such summing-up is expressed. And in more advanced age, the process of reviewing our lives may inspire the creative energy of the Encore Phase, in which we add yet one more distinctive chapter to our life story.

As we experience these developmental phases of potential with aging, the related writing or recording of autobiography, in particular, stands out in later life as a medium through which we can express ourselves, as well as discover more about ourselves. Autobiography represents a developmental form of creativity in the second half of life, *a form of creativity that emerges more strongly in later life* than in earlier adulthood. Not to overlook the obvious, *with age* both your store of information and perspective on life grow.

George Santayana (1863–1952), noted Spanish-American philosopher, poet, and novelist, wrote his remarkable four-volume philosophical work **Realms of Being** ***between the ages of sixty-four and seventy-seven. This work is noteworthy for elucidating extremely complex problems with remarkable clarity and succinctness. From ages eighty-one to eighty-nine, in a Catholic nursing home, losing both his hearing and vision, he wrote his three-volume autobiography,*** **Persons and Places.**

Autobiographical Authors Tell Another Story: Identity Development

If we look at the familiar form of published autobiography, we can see the ways in which the author's task mirrors the internal process available to us all. Typically, autobiographical authors reflect on who they are, where they have been, how they got there, and what it all means to them. They consider the meaning of what they have done in relation to others and society. In short, this summing-up process through autobiography reenacts the evolution of their identity—the continuity and change that they have experienced in their inner life and the roles and adjustments they have assumed in the outer world.

For students of psychology and human development the autobiographical products of these older individuals provide remarkable windows for tracing over the decades the influences that shaped their inner and outer lives. For all of us, they provide a wealth of material—from

Alex Haley, one of the great "keepers of the culture" created the blockbuster and best-seller **Roots: The Saga of an American Family** *in his second half of life, at age fifty-five. He was greatly aided by another keeper of the culture, his maternal grandmother, whose oral history provided invaluable background information and direction. Haley continued writing and researching until he died at age seventy-one, completing the novella* **A Different Kind of Christmas** *at age sixty-seven; it is the story of a plantation owner who rejects slavery.*

The work of American short story writer and novelist Eudora Welty draws heavily from her experience in growing up in Mississippi. Her writings combine psychological sophistication with humor. She has received

poor judgment and bad breaks to good choices and positive developments—from which we can learn and review in relation to our own life course. These autobiographies reflect social creativity in the sense that authors sum up their lives and share what they have learned with the broader community. These works also reflect the role of their authors as keepers of the culture.

But it is more than the identity of the authors that is being affected. For the authors, this process provides an affirmation or reaffirmation of their identity. But the identity of other family members is also being influenced, for the stories and experiences of the family elders become part of the modeling and lore for the younger generations and those that follow about their family roots. It is indeed a dynamic process revealing a further dimension of social creativity: that of influencing the family culture. In this sense, they are more immediately *keepers of the kin.*

The story of Laura Ingalls Wilder, author of the *Little House* children's book series, shows us the broader role of identity in later life and the way in which the individual's effort to get in touch with his or her identity—drawing upon all its roots—not only further influences the individual's sense of self, but the family's sense of identity, and each member's feelings about his or her roots. The *Little House* series, beginning with the first book in 1932, captured the pioneering quality and spirit that characterized the dominant American culture of the late 1800s, and in so doing, Laura Wilder's story goes a step farther—adding to the identity of her culture, helping craft a better sense of its heritage.

When Laura Wilder was in her sixties, her daughter strongly encouraged her to write down her childhood experiences because of their richness in portraying the spirit, independence, and values of family life on a Midwest farm in the mid- to late nineteenth century. As a young girl, Laura Ingalls had experienced the nature and rapid changes of American pioneer life, from the challenges and dangers of the wilderness, to farming, homemaking, and education, to the construction of frontier dwellings and towns and the establishment of railroads and progress in general.

Drawing upon all of these experiences and the inspired collaboration of her daughter Rose, she emerged as an author of children's books. She started with *Little House in the Big Woods,* which was published when she was sixty-five years old. This was followed by her immensely successful *Little House on the Prairie,* when she was sixty-eight. *Little Town on the Prairie* was published when she was seventy-four, and *Those Happy Golden Years,* when she was seventy-six. More than 40 million *Little House* books have been sold. A highly successful, long-running television series based on *Little House on the Prairie* followed in the mid-1970s, and a prize for children's literature has been named after the author. Hence, Laura Wilder's autobiographical writing not only influenced her own sense of identity, but also that of her kin and her culture.

In the same way, our own autobiographical activity is highly meaningful, though generally to a smaller, more intimate and informal audience.

two Guggenheim fellowships, three O. Henry Awards, the Pulitzer Prize, and the National Medal for Literature. Her autobiography,* One Writer's Beginnings, *was published when she was seventy-five (1984).

Autobiography as Creative Therapy

Most immediately, the autobiographical process can be health promoting or even therapeutic for the storyteller. Sometimes it is only when we tell our whole story or get it all down on paper that we are able to "connect the dots"—literally connect the dendrites—to gain a meaningful view of ourselves and our lives. In the process of taking stock of one's life—the disappointments and joys, the failures and accomplishments—we make a journey toward self-knowledge, understanding, and acceptance. Beginning with perhaps only an elusive sense of meaning, continued exploration of our life stories can enable us to appreciate ourselves more fully and our experience and contribution to life in the broadest sense.

Psychiatrist and gerontologist Robert Butler, who heads the International Longevity Center, developed the concept of the "Life Review" in the early 1960s and put it to therapeutic use with individuals. Butler describes the life review process as one "characterized by the progressive return to consciousness of past experiences and particularly the resurgence of unresolved conflicts that can be looked at again and rein-

Eleanor Roosevelt (1884–1962), humanitarian and wife of President Franklin Delano Roosevelt, was chairman of the UN Commission on Human Rights from the age of sixty-two to sixty-seven. She wrote the book* On My Own *at the age of seventy-four and her autobiography at the age of seventy-eight, the year she died.

tegrated. If the reintegration is successful, it can give new significance and meaning to one's life."

LARRY CARPENTER

A. Philip Randolph was an American civil rights activist and labor leader. He built the first successful black trade union in 1937 (at age forty-eight) to deal with the Pulman Company. In 1948 (at age fifty-nine), he influenced President Truman to desegregate the armed forces. In 1957 (at age sixty-eight) he became vice-president of the AFL-CIO, forming the Negro American Labor Council within it in 1960 (at age seventy-one). In 1963 (at age 74), he directed the great march on Washington, where at least 200,000 protested against continuing discrimination against blacks; it was the largest civil rights demonstration in American history, culminating in Martin Luther King's famous "I Have a Dream" speech.

I met over a period of two years with Larry Carpenter, seventy-seven years of age, divorced for thirty-three years, and retired from a career as a contractor. He expressed a number of regrets, including never being involved in work that was ultimately satisfying, suffering the end of a painful marriage and not being able to marry again into a better relationship, and experiencing tension with his daughter and son, but especially his son. He had a long-standing drinking problem and was starting to drink again, feeling his life was a failure.

The youngest of three brothers, Larry had outlived both his older brothers; they both had died in the previous five years. He recalled his childhood as characterized by a strictness on the part of his parents, without many toys, but one where there was a lot of fun, frolic, and mischief with his brothers and playmates. His mother, a homemaker, had been loving, but stern. His father had been even more stern, and had very high standards for the behavior of his children. His father had worked as a laborer in a shoe factory, earning relatively little money. He had a drinking problem, was emotionally distant, and was most likely to punish his children when intoxicated. Sometimes he would "discipline them"—hit them—with his belt or a strap.

Larry graduated high school, but while in high school had already started working at small jobs, learning how to repair roof shingles, make cement walkways and blacktop driveways, and do brickwork. As we talked about this, he realized that this home building and home repair experience had really helped him in his later contract work, which proved to be something he could do well.

After high school, he juggled a variety of jobs, from delivering papers, to delivering milk on a milk truck, to working as a chauffeur, to assisting in the construction of houses. Then he entered the army for four years, and learned considerably more skills that prepared him for his work as a contractor, as he assisted army engineers in a variety of construction projects. Upon leaving the army he got a job with a contracting group and quickly moved up to assistant foreman.

Just before turning thirty he married and, motivated to make a better living, formed his own construction company. He built a solid reputation for his company, specializing in making driveways, taking subcontracts to construct swimming pools, and accepting subcontracts in the construction of civic buildings. The quality of his work brought him a lot of contracts for municipal construction projects, but much of his dissatisfaction came from the constant stress over working to meet low budgets with quality work and still earn a profit.

Physician and social reformer Alice Hamilton at age eighty (1949) published a revised edition of her 1934 textbook,* Industrial Toxicology, *originally published when she was sixty-five.

Meanwhile, Larry and his wife had two children, and he began to respond to them with the same pattern of fathering he had learned from his father: sternness, emotional distance, and unreasonably high expectations. He also started to drink too much, and this led to a stormy marriage, and then divorce when his children were twelve and ten. They were very upset with him and not very sympathetic. He continued his work as a construction contractor until he retired at age sixty-five. The children had moved in with their mother after the divorce, and though Larry continued to visit them and take them out for special occasions, relations deteriorated when his children became adults and they had children of their own. The result was that he rarely saw his five grandchildren.

His own grown children had made numerous attempts in their earlier years of parenting to foster a relationship between Larry and his grandchildren. The problem was that on too many occasions when one of his children would visit and bring the grandchildren, Larry would be under the influence of alcohol; it soured the visits for all concerned and only increased the emotional distance between Larry and his children. His drinking problem also interfered with his sustaining any meaningful relationships with women; over time, he gravitated toward women who also had a drinking problem, only making matters worse.

In reviewing his life Larry came to appreciate how truly good a contractor he had been, recognizing that he had earned a reputation as a master problem solver on tough jobs. In so recounting, he began to develop a new respect for how well he had done and how highly others regarded his work. We then talked about his family and how his grandchildren were starting to grow up without knowing him.

When we discussed the possibility of his inviting his children to visit or his visiting them, he felt discouraged with their hesitance. He understood that they didn't want their grandchildren to see him drunk, and they couldn't count on him to be sober. In our discussions he would typically grow edgy, become self-righteous and speak with his father's sternness and exaggerated standards, saying that this was not the way he brought them up to be, and that if that's the way they wanted to be, so be it, they just wouldn't see him anymore.

The French novelist and diarist André Gide (1869–1951), who won the Nobel Prize in Literature in 1947 (at age seventy-eight), wrote his famous* Journals *over a sixty-two-year period from age twenty to age eighty-two.

I suggested the loss would be everybody's, including his, and that he might consider setting into motion two strategies: Strategy #1 was to start writing letters to his grandchildren, drawing upon the remarkably rich range of working experiences he had in high school and thereafter. It would be a way of letting them get to know him better, stir their curiosity about him, and perhaps encourage them to get together with him. He might start with a letter titled "When Your Grandfather Was a Teenage Shingle Layer," moving on to "When Your Grandfather Was a Teenage Cement Layer," then to "When Your Grandfather Was a Teenage Bricklayer," etc., addressing all his interesting work experiences.

Sir Francis Galton (1822–1911), the English scientist, in 1892 (at age seventy), devised the system of fingerprint identification, publishing* Fingerprints *that year.

In his discussions with me, he often recalled fascinating or entertaining anecdotes, like the time when, just after laying a cement walkway, the owner's two huge Irish wolfhounds darted out of the house, racing each other across the wet, unhardened walkway, leaving a trail of large dog prints in the cement. I told him that these letters and stories would likely become family treasures, which I suspected would also arouse the curiosity of his adult children.

Strategy #2 was to be implemented along with the letter writing; he had to get into an alcohol rehabilitation program. When he felt he was far enough along that he could make a commitment with certainty to be sober for a visit, then he could initiate a plan to get together with his family. I felt that when he shared the evidence of his commitment with his children, they would be amenable to the visits. Larry opted to try both strategies, and began the letters and the rehabilitation program at the same time. He made significant progress.

His daughter agreed first to have him visit, and following its success, she called her brother, who then invited Larry to visit him. Larry was very pleased. His new family connection—both to his children and his grandchildren—helped motivate him to steer clear of the bottle. The visits and the letters continued and became a source of considerable satisfaction and new self-esteem. Three years later, Larry suffered a heart attack and died. In our talks during that previous three-year period, however, Larry had expressed with deep feeling that for the first time in his life he felt whole; he had found a new sense of pride in his life and in the stories he was able to pass on to his family.

Opening Old Wounds for Healing: Sharing the Burden of Painful History

Exploring our past is almost always beneficial, but the prospect of doing it can be daunting or painful, even when the subject is someone else's life, as in the therapeutic/restorative biography (TR-Bio) activity I developed for my own family in response to my father's Alzheimer's disease. Another Alzheimer's family wanted to create a TR-Bio for the eighty-two-year-old father, Sam Rodman, who had recently been diagnosed with Alzheimer's disease. Sam's wife and daughter were very interested in the TR-Bio technique and were looking forward to reconstructing highlights of his life on film.

One of the student volunteers helping me knew that Sam's son had died five years earlier from colon cancer and that his death had been very difficult for the family. The student asked how we should deal with the son in making the TR-Bio; would his memory be too sensitive an issue and should we stay away from it? When we gently asked Sam's wife and daughter, they paused momentarily, then both stated an unequivocal desire to include the son in the TR-Bio. We then asked Sam, and without any sense of conflict he, too, said yes.

What we later discovered was that in making the TR-Bio video, Sam's wife and daughter felt very good about seeing the son on film—reliving many fond memories—as long as he didn't show the effects of

The great twentieth-century Abstract Expressionist painter Willem De Kooning (1904–1997) developed Alzheimer's disease in his late seventies. But for the next few years, into his early eighties, De Kooning continued to create museum-quality paintings, demonstrating the capacity for preserved skills despite the decline typical of Alzheimer's.

Federico Fellini (1920–1993), winner of four Academy Awards for Best Foreign Language Films, directed* Ginger and Fred *at age sixty-six and* Voices of the Moon *at age seventy.

the illness. The simple solution was to not have any pictures of him on film in which he looked sick. Sam, too, reacted very well to the video and to seeing his son on it. If any scene made Sam uncomfortable, all we had to do was edit it out.

The gifted playwright Lillian Hellman (1907–1984) came before the House Un-American Activities Committee in 1952 during the McCarthy era and expressed the celebrated phrase "I can't cut my conscience to fit this year's fashions." She subsequently described this low period in American politics in her memoir, Scoundrel Time, *written when she was sixty-nine in 1976.*

When there has been significant conflict in a person's past, the life review process should not be taken lightly and is best done with a therapist, since memories of the conflict may be overwhelming and lead to feelings of regret, guilt, despair, or a sense that life has been a waste. The worst-case scenario is that the individual had been barely successful in keeping painful memories buried, and inquiry about them throws the person into anxious despair and suicidal thoughts. It is no coincidence that elderly white males represent the group most at risk for suicide. My own clinical work and research in aging over the past quarter of a century, though, tells me that many of these suicides result from conflicts that have been carefully hidden and not discussed, and which eventually overtake the individual like a festering untreated infection.

However, it is a mistake to assume that a painful history is best buried without any eulogies. Some people may feel compelled to suffer alone; some may hope that someday someone will be interested; and others who are not initially comfortable or ready when first approached, later reconsider. Depression is also a common cause of retrospective distortion, removing gray zones in ambiguous situations, making them look predominantly black, especially when they occurred some time ago. For example, if in the past one's marriage had provided many good times, including some memorable vacations, but it also had included some strong bouts of anger and bitterness, depression would incline one to filter out the positive moments and focus instead on the negative ones as the true indicators of how one's spouse *really* felt—even if the angry and bitter moments occupied but a minority of the time. It is important to alleviate the depression in order to allow a life review through a more neutral lens.

With appropriate support through the inward journey of a life review, however, even troubled individuals can come to terms with the sources of their long-standing emotional pain. That relief, and sometimes resolution of the conflict, frees the mind to go on to new thoughts, new responses, new experiences of life. Each step of the process reflects creativity in action, illuminating new opportunities for inner growth and self-expression.

This was the case with Gerald Williams, whose daughter asked me to see him.

GERALD WILLIAMS: PERSONAL HISTORY

Gerald Williams was seventy-five, a widower with one child, a daughter. His son had been killed at age sixteen in an automobile accident. Gerald blamed himself because he had given his son the car as a birthday present, and because it was secondhand, he later assumed, though without basis, that there may have been something wrong with it. At the time of his son's death, the death of significant others had already become a major traumatic theme in Gerald's life. His father had died from a ruptured cerebral aneurysm when Gerald was only eleven, after which he worried about unexpected tragedy happening to those close to him. The death of his son years later brought this sense of tragedy to a more intense level.

Gerald was a devoted husband and father, and did well in his career as an accountant. But he was always serious and a worrier. His wife and daughter were very effective at being able to lift him out of himself with their humor, but this changed when his wife died from a stroke—another sudden and unexpected death of a loved one who had appeared to be in very good health. In the three years since the loss of his wife, Gerald had become increasingly withdrawn and unwilling to talk to most people; he feared they would discuss his painful memories. His whole focus on life had become fixated on avoiding these memories and fearing new tragic events.

He was no longer able to have pleasant recollection of any positive events that had occurred with those close to him who had died. Whatever special role he had cherished in the lives of any of his deceased loved ones also never received any consideration. Beyond helping him with his depression, my goal was to help him reconnect with these other snapshots of his life before he summed things up with a totally negative picture and closed the book.

After several visits, when he told me that his son would be around

John Cheever (1912–1982), the short-story writer and novelist who has been called "the Chekhov of the suburbs" for his ability to capture the sadness and poignancy of emotions in his characters by revealing the drama that lies beneath seemingly insignificant events, was awarded a Pulitzer Prize at age sixty-seven for his work **The Stories of John Cheever.**

Jorge Luis Borges (1899–1986), the Argentinian writer, by age fifty-six had become totally blind owing to a hereditary condition. He then went on to do his most noted work. After 1961 (at age sixty-two), when he and Samuel Beckett shared the prestigious Formentor Prize, Borges's tales and poems were increasingly acclaimed as classics of twentieth-century world literature. By the time of his death (at age eighty-seven), the nightmare world of his "fictions" had come to be compared with the world of Franz Kafka and to be praised for concentrating common language into its most enduring form.

my age if he were still alive, I knew that we were starting to make progress for two reasons. First, it was a big step for Gerald to bring his son into conscious discussion, and second he was beginning to demonstrate what we call in therapy *transference*—transferring feelings that he had or imagined he might have had about his son, if he had lived, onto me. Both dimensions provided pathways to exploring his emotions.

Further discussion of his son did follow. It was filled with much sadness and tearfulness, but there was also the start of talk about some of the better memories he had about his son. In our next session, though, he was morose and reluctant to talk freely again. For three nights after our earlier discussion he had recurring nightmares about his son's auto accident. He feared that our continued discussion would overwhelm him with the negative memories and was reluctant to open up again. I reassured him, though, that these were emotions that had built up for nearly thirty years and as painful as they were, our talking about his feelings would gradually lift an enormous burden off him.

Gradually he was able to talk about both his son and his wife, without nightmares. There were occasional setbacks, but each time with gentle encouragement he was able to resume talking about them. He began to bring up more and more memories of happy or interesting moments he had with both his son and his wife. His net picture of life was beginning to take on some color again after being so black.

Another turning point was when he finally accepted his daughter's invitation to join her for dinner along with her husband and two sons, who were coming home from college to be there for him. He had completely shut all of them out after his wife's death, rationalizing, with the distorted thinking characteristic of deep depression, that he needed to distance himself from anybody close to him who might in some way get hurt. He finally began to realize that they wanted to bring him into their lives more so that he could begin to make a new one for himself.

World History as a Context for Autobiography

We are all children of history and carry its imprint in our emotional lives. Survivors of this country's Great Depression in the 1930s emerged from that period with deeply held convictions about work and money that defined their lives ever after. Every war veteran carries emotional scars from his war experience, whether from personal losses or those of others. Often, it is only with age and the passage of time that any of us are ready to look at our past lives more objectively and learn the lessons there for us.

After nearly a half a century since World War II, many Holocaust survivors are beginning to share their stories in schools, in community halls, and sometimes even in their own families for the first time. What is striking about these survivors' public appearances or published accounts is the frequent remark that they kept silent all these years because the experience was painful beyond words, and because they felt no one really wanted to hear about it. They themselves often wanted only to put the experience behind them, to forget it; impossible as that was on an emotional level, many succeeded in moving forward simply by silencing the past, refusing to give it a voice in their new lives. And yet, decades and sometimes generations later, with an invitation and encouragement to speak at last, they were able to do so, and do so in painful eloquence.

Now frequently sought out, by schools especially, to tell of their experiences, they often are quite emotional in describing the effect the sharing itself has had on them. They are moved by the discovery that their communities care, especially the young people, and by the invitation to share the terrible stories that they have carried alone for decades. They are often surprised to hear their telling of personal history hailed as something important; that by sharing their remembrances as keepers of the culture, they deny a victory to those who claim the Holocaust never occurred. They also make a contribution of historic proportion in chronicling the past and educating a new generation. One old man spoke of his experience for the first time before a group of junior high school students. As he told of the loss of his family, he cried, and many in the young audience cried, too. When the program was over, he told a reporter that it was the first time he had ever spoken of the trauma of those years, and it was the first time he had ever confronted the depth of his sadness and cried. All this at about age seventy!

Sir Winston Churchill (1874–1965) was sixty-five when he began his five-year "walk with destiny," as Prime Minister during World War II, heroically guiding the British people through a terrifying period with dignity and glory. At the age of seventy-one he lost reelection, but again become Prime Minister at the age of seventy-seven, finally laying down high office at the age of eighty-one (1955). Meanwhile, he received a Nobel Prize in Literature in 1953 (at age seventy-nine), most particularly for his six-volume work, **The Second World War,** ***which he wrote from ages seventy-four to seventy-nine.***

"Because I remember, I despair. Because I remember, I have the duty to reject despair."

—ELIE WIESEL

Akira Kurosawa (1910–1998), the noted Japanese film director, directed a long series of classic films: Rashomon *in 1950 (at age forty);* The Seven Samurai *in 1955 (at age forty-five); his Academy Award–winning Best Foreign Language Film, the Siberian epic* Dersu Uzala *in 1975 (at age sixty-five);* Ran *in 1985 (at age seventy-five);* Madadayo *in 1993 (at age eighty-three).*

The power of autobiography to open emotional wounds for healing—even when the story is someone else's—was apparent in the overwhelmingly positive public reaction to moviemaker Steven Spielberg's film *Saving Private Ryan,* widely hailed as the most realistic and painful portrayal of war and its emotional casualties. Following the movie's release, a flurry of media stories brought attention to the real-life "Private Ryans" and opened the door for many of them to talk about their war experiences in the ways they had never been able to do before. Many of these veterans remarked that the movie spoke for them and enabled them to take the next step in speaking for themselves, expressing their own feelings.

As with the Holocaust survivors, the next wave of media stories found these veterans invited to schools and lecture halls to share their experiences within their own communities, and act as keepers of the culture. At a personal level, this process of autobiography enabled many veterans to share this emotional burden of history at long last and move forward in their own lives with a new perspective on their past and new potential for intergenerational and community connectedness.

ANNA DREW: PIONEER ON A DIFFICULT FAMILY FRONTIER

In her sixties, Mary McLeod Bethune (1875–1955), the civil rights reformer, created the National Council of Negro Women (NCNW), formed by uniting the major national African-American women's associations; she continued to direct the NCNW until the age of seventy-four.

The distance of years often enables us to confront the past and develop a new view for the future within the culture of our own families, as well. Mrs. Anna Drew was a depressed eighty-year-old widow when her daughter asked me to see her. Her daughter loved her very much and was very concerned about her. Since Mrs. Drew had also recently suffered a stroke, her balance was impaired, making it difficult for her to leave her apartment, so I saw her at her home.

She was a woman of small physical stature with a powerful presence, despite her depressed state. As an aside, I have always been intrigued by this larger-than-life effect some individuals convey, and in that way, she reminded me of the anthropologist Margaret Mead, whom I met for the first time when she was a visiting scientist at the National Institutes of Health. I had gone to Mead's office to escort her to a seminar I had arranged. As I approached the building where she worked, I met her coming down the stairs wearing a black cape, and my initial impression was that she was a towering giant. As she came closer, I suddenly realized she was a full head shorter than me. In the same way, when I entered Anna Drew's apartment, she rose slowly to welcome me, and her presence conveyed that of great strength of character. She immediately took control of the situation by telling me that my shirt collar was not folded properly. I paused to fix it.

Anna Drew had never had a psychiatric problem before, and in fact her depression was not caused by psychological factors as such, but because of her stroke. Approximately 50 percent of those who suffer a stroke are at risk for depression because of all the turbulence caused among the neurotransmitters in the brain that influence mood. This was immediately comforting to both Anna and her daughter. I reassured them that we could expect the depression to run its course, especially since Anna already seemed much better than she had even a few days before when her daughter had initially called me. Her balance was also improving, and her overall intellectual function was intact. As she told me about her life, I quickly came to understand the depth of her daughter's feelings about her, for Anna Drew was indeed a tower of strength and stability for her family.

Anna was the oldest of three siblings growing up in a small Southern town. Hers was a very loving family, and she was especially proud of her father, who became the first African-American dentist in the county where they lived. She was very close to her mother, who managed the home and brought in extra money as a seamstress as well as winning awards for her sewing at county fairs. Anna was also very close to her two younger sisters, helping them with homework, chores, and adolescent problems when they were growing up. She was still very close to her sisters when I met her, talking to them long distance at least weekly, ensuring that the family remained close-knit.

After high school, Anna went to college to become a teacher, going on to teach third grade until she retired at age sixty-five. She met her husband-to-be after she started teaching. He was a teacher, too, at another school in the same town. They married when she was twenty-five. They had two children—two daughters—four years apart. Family life was good, but eleven years after her second daughter was born,

***Anna Howard Shaw (1847–1919) became one of the most influential leaders of the women's suffrage movement. At the age of thirty-three (1880), she became the first woman ordained as a Methodist minister. At the age of thirty-nine (1886) she graduated from medical school, but decided to devote herself to the work of women's suffrage. From her late fifties to late sixties, she served as president of the National American Woman Suffrage Association. At age sixty-eight, she published her autobiography,* The Story of a Pioneer.**

Anna's husband developed meningitis and died suddenly. The family was in shock, and the younger daughter, Darlene, was especially traumatized. As an adolescent, Darlene had experienced a lot of emotional difficulty and much trouble getting through school. The older daughter, Dorothy, was an excellent student and went on to college.

Without Dorothy's help during the university academic year, Anna had considerable trouble with the younger Darlene. Anna also had to take on extra work to pay for Dorothy's tuition and make ends meet. Having learned sewing from her mother, Anna worked after school, out of the house, as a seamstress; like her mother, she proved to be very talented.

***Elizabeth Sanderson Haldane (1862–1937), the Scottish social-welfare worker and author, was the first woman to be a justice of the peace in Scotland, appointed in 1920 at the age of fifty-eight. The year she died, at age seventy-five, she published a book of her reminiscences,* From One Century to Another.**

The older daughter, Dorothy, did very well at school and went on to become a teacher herself, and then a junior high school principal. She married and had two children. Family life for Dorothy was very good, and she lived in a town adjacent to Anna's, maintaining contact with her. The grandchildren became very close to Anna, particularly because she sewed them some of the "coolest clothes with the coolest colors and coolest designs" that attracted much admiration from their young classmates. When I met Anna, these two grandchildren had graduated from college; one had just completed law school and the other was working as a program planner at a government agency.

Meanwhile, Darlene, also living nearby, had continued to have a very difficult life. She graduated from high school, but did not go on to college. Worst of all, she had turned to drugs, which only added to her emotional instability and difficulty holding down a job. Anna was successful in getting Darlene into a drug rehabilitation program and she remained stable for three years, marrying a man she met in the recovery program. She had kept this relationship a secret until after she married, knowing that her mother would have serious misgivings. Darlene then became pregnant, giving birth to a healthy boy, Arnold. But then trouble flared up again. Darlene's husband went back on drugs, got involved in an armed robbery, and was killed by a security guard in a shoot-out. Arnold was only two. Shortly later, Darlene was back on drugs. She seemed overwhelmed by the responsibilities of being on her own, despite Anna's financial and emotional support. She did agree, though, to let Arnold live with Anna.

Just a toddler, Arnold joined the escalating number of children in

America under age eighteen being cared for by grandparents. After almost a year had passed, Darlene again entered a rehab program under Anna's guidance and encouragement. She responded well and even accepted Anna's offer to learn sewing from her; Darlene discovered that she, too, had a special skill in this area, and sewed a rather artistic toy animal for Arnold. It became his favorite. But then very bad news again arrived. Darlene was diagnosed HIV positive. Infected during a time when treatments were not as good as today, Darlene died four years later. Arnold was seven, Anna was sixty-two.

Anna raised Arnold with the help of Dorothy and her family. His favorite stories were those of his grandfather—Anna's father. Anna had many wonderful stories about her dad, about how good a fly fisherman he was to how he got a scholarship to go dental school. Anna also worked hard at reinforcing the positive memories of Arnold's parents. There weren't many, but Anna was determined to have these few dominate over the tragic rest. There was a very special picture taken just after Arnold was born, with both of his parents holding him, together, and looking very proud. This, along with the beautiful toy animal that Darlene had sewn for her little boy, were on a little table dedicated to their display in Arnold's room. Arnold was an honors student in high school and went on to college. It was difficult for both him and Anna when he went off to school, for this was the first time that they had been separated since Arnold had come to live with his grandmother.

Anna's time in therapy was very productive. Through her physical rehabilitation program, she completely recovered from her stroke and, also through our work together, her depression cleared entirely. But she asked if we could continue to meet for a while. She said she was getting a lot out of our visits, and she found it very heartening the way we were navigating her life story. Without her saying it, I knew, too, that she had long been conflicted about the rough time that her daughter Darlene had experienced growing up, and felt some guilt about it, as if she were somehow to blame.

We talked about Darlene's plight and how an unfortunate confluence of circumstances had occurred that were beyond Anna's control. The death of Anna's husband, which had created a crisis for Darlene, was certainly not Anna's doing. It was also not Anna's fault that Dar-

Karl Landsteiner 1868–1943) was the American pathologist who discovered the four major blood groups (O, A, B, AB) in 1901. He received the Nobel Prize in Physiology or Medicine in 1930 (at age sixty-two). In 1940, at the age of seventy-two, he discovered the Rhesus (Rh) blood factor.

***Ralph Ellison (1914–1994), the American writer, as a young author wrote* The Invisible Man *(at age thirty-eight), an acclaimed semiautobiographical account of a young African-American intellectual's search for identity. At the age of seventy-two he published a group of essays, titled* Going to the Territory.**

lene's troubles overlapped the turbulent time in our society in the late 1960s and early 1970s, when drug abuse and emotional turmoil in young adults were both unusually prevalent, making it an especially hard time to be an adolescent or young adult. Despite the ongoing struggle, Anna had remained a steadfast source of love and support for her daughter; she had done her best.

I also pointed out that Anna honored her daughter's memory and her motherhood through the remarkable job she did raising Darlene's son and how well he turned out. Anna was comforted by this discussion and was able to come to terms better with the idea that Darlene's fate was influenced far more by factors outside Anna's control. She was able to go through a summing-up process in reviewing her life that allowed her to better appreciate the depth of her role in helping her family through her ideas and inspiration.

I was especially glad that we did continue for a while, because I had the great fortune of making one of my visits to Anna when she got a very excited call from Arnold. He had passed his exam to practice dentistry. Anna's pride and tears were infectious. We hugged, both of us with watery eyes. Anna Drew had truly been a keeper of the kin for her family, providing an identity bridge that linked generations, from her father, through her, to her grandson.

Dame Millicent Fawcett, the English suffrage and educational reformer, was president of the National Union of Women's Suffrage Society for twenty years, until age seventy-two. At seventy-three she wrote **The Women's Victory—and After.**

She was indeed a very special person who personified the strength that many older persons manifest holding themselves and their families together through calm and storm. Hers was a social creativity that increased with age, adding to the cohesiveness of the extended family and helping to rescue her young grandson from a terribly traumatic family life compounded by potentially very negative role modeling on the part of both of his parents. And she helped preserve the cultural tradition of her family that was shaped by her father—devotion to scholarship, human service, and community.

Exploring the Past for Strategies for the Future

"Autobiography is never entirely true. No one can get the right perspective on himself," wrote the famed American trial lawyer Clarence

Darrow in his 1932 autobiography, *The Story of My Life*. Darrow's purpose in writing his life story at age seventy-five was, he said, simply to provide "a plain unvarnished account of how things really have happened . . ." These were the thoughts of a preeminent keeper of the culture nearing the end of a historic courtroom career. True to character, he viewed his autobiography as an adjunct to history and wanted to leave an honest account for the record.

But what is often most valuable to us in reflecting on our own life story is not the historical facts or events, but the journey of self-discovery it offers. Just as important as our search for "the right perspective" on our past is the way we use that insight to illuminate fresh potential for our future, finding patterns, clues, and the motivation to create strategies for taking our lives in new or more satisfying directions.

Clarence Darrow (1857–1938), at age sixty-eight, defended John T. Scopes of Dayton, Tennessee, who had broken state law by presenting the Darwinian theory of evolution; this was the infamous "Scopes Monkey Trial." The next year, at age sixty-nine, Darrow won acquittal for a black family who had fought to protect itself against a mob trying to expel it from its residence in a white neighborhood in Detroit.

TARA DONLEY

Tara Donley was a forty-four-year-old unmarried government employee. Her work for the past twenty years had involved various aspects of administrative oversight of programs focused on helping youth. She had derived great satisfaction from this work, and she had received several awards or certificates of commendation for her efforts from the different government offices where she had worked. But her success had brought her greater responsibility that was accompanied by increased time demands, though these demands had come to be more and more self-generated.

She was already feeling the buildup of pressure that she hadn't experienced before at work when her mother, who had been suffering from multiple sclerosis for nearly thirty years, took a decided turn for the worse, developed a serious infection, and died from its complications. Everything suddenly seemed very meaningless to Tara, and she felt she needed to do something very different. She no longer felt the same about her work, which now made her feel far removed from the real world, with no hands-on contact with the young people her programs were designed to help. She was at a loss about what to do and, upon a recommendation from a friend, entered psychotherapy with me.

Tara was the oldest of five children. Almost from the start she

Pearl Buck (1892–1973), the noted writer and author of **The Good Earth** *in 1931, which led to her Nobel Prize in 1938, later turned to writing about the American scene and issues of family life. At the age of seventy-five she wrote the moving children's story "Matthew, Mark, Luke, and John."*

Peter Mark Roget began his career as a physician in England. In 1834 at the age of fifty-five he wrote **On Animal and Vegetable Physiology,** *but became best known for his later work in an entirely different field, writing at the age of seventy-three his* **Thesaurus of English Words and Phrases.**

seemed mature for her age. She was very close to her mother, who was a nurse. While her father was clearly fond of her, he was not that close, in part because he worked terribly long hours directing a new foundation focused on educating the public about the environment and was also engaged in some advocacy. Tara was fourteen when her mother, who was only thirty-seven, was diagnosed with multiple sclerosis. Initially, her mother's course was mild and things operated fairly normally at home. During her summers throughout high school Tara went away to camp, and after her first year of college she got a summer job at the same camp as a counselor. She was a very good counselor and worked especially well with the kids, so much so that the head of the camp assigned three of the most troubled young girls to Tara's cabin. They responded very positively to her, and this experience launched Tara's interest in helping youth.

Upon finishing high school Tara went to college nearby in order to remain close to her mother. She came home quite a lot to help her mother, especially during flareups of the illness. She also assumed much of the responsibility of her younger siblings. By the end of her second year of college, her mother was having more trouble, and Tara felt she could no longer continue to go away for her summer job at camp, getting summer work close to home instead. Upon completing college, Tara remained in the area and went on to get a graduate degree in public administration. Though she dated regularly, she hesitated to commit herself to a deeper relationship, feeling that her mother was increasingly relying on her help. She stayed in the area after completing graduate school, again to be close to her mother, and got a job in a government agency supporting programs for youths in need of special education. She became increasingly immersed in her work and increasingly involved in helping her mother, despite both parents encouraging her to get on with her own life. But this was her life as she saw it, and she gained a great deal of gratification from her job at work and job at her parents' home.

When she started therapy, she felt empty and directionless, and was convinced that continuing her present career path would be an utter waste of time. She exhibited the most energy when she talked about her family. She was proud of their commitment to helping others and her place in upholding a family tradition of service. I commented that she probably wasn't surprised then that she ended up in a career helping young people. But Tara said her work was different, because it wasn't hands-on. I commented again that her father's environmental work was very important, though not hands-on. But she corrected me, pointing out that he got involved himself with a lot of the teaching about the environment that his foundation promoted. She said she felt that she and her father shared a common trait in their devotion to work and willingness to work long hours.

I asked her then whether she thought about or daydreamed about other work that was hands-on. She said she tried, but never got that far, perhaps fearing at one level that change might make it more difficult to help her mother in the manner to which she had grown accustomed. I then reminded her about how well she had done as a counselor and how appealing that experience was for her—one that was very hands-on. A warm smile spread across her face as she thought back on it.

"What was it that most appealed to you about that experience?" I asked her. She said it was the way she was able to help the children and "get them moving onto the right road again."

Was there something she could do now that would bring her similar satisfaction?

"Yes," she said, adding with a tone of defeat that she would have to go back to school, and she was forty-four.

"Don't you know anybody else your age going back to school?" I challenged her. "More and more people your age and older—*much older*—are doing it today."

"If you think you can, you can. If you think you can't, you're right."

—MARY KAY ASH

Then another smile came across her face.

I asked her if she would share the secret behind the smile. She replied that it had just occurred to her that her mother's mother took up social work at age forty-eight upon the death of her husband.

With that opening, I asked her if social work appealed to her, and she nodded; she felt that it could. After all, she had been a social worker for her mother for nearly three decades.

"If you did pursue social work, would you want to work with all age groups or any particular one?" I inquired.

She paused, and, thinking out loud, said that while she had helped her mother a lot, her whole career had been with young adults. They would be the logical focus of any transition to a new hands-on career.

Tara did go on to earn a master's degree in social work, subsequently landing a job at a clinic for adolescents where she had done one of her social work student rotations. Five years later, because of her new clinical skills and her long-standing skills as an administrator, she was asked to apply for the job of director of that program, as the present director was about to retire. She was very flattered, but suggested instead that they involve her as a part-time assistant administrator, because she wanted to devote at least 50 percent of her time to being in personal contact with the children.

Tara's story illustrates one of many factors that can thrust an individual into a midlife reevaluation of where he or she is and where he or she wants to go. Embarking on an exploration that brought her back in touch with personal interests and strengths that she had not previously developed and in better touch with a family identity of helping others, her own midlife identity confusion resolved and took her to a new path that was now right for her.

Like Dante, as described in the lines of his poem in Chapter 3, Tara experienced the same feelings of "straying into a dark forest midway through life's journey, with the right path appearing not anywhere."

"How many cares one loses when one decides not to be something but to be someone."

—GABRIELLE (COCO) CHANEL

For Tara, the possibility of change, her creative potential to transcend circumstances, was enabled by the developmental potential that accompanied the midlife reevaluation phase. By examining her past, she was able to find windows to her future. Motivated to take action, she used her creative energy to reshape her sense of identity, wholeness, coherence, and direction in life.

9

Creativity in Everyday Life: Letting It Start with You

The journey of a thousand miles begins with one step.

—LAO-TSU

PART I: EVERYDAY ACTIVITIES

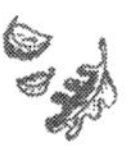

THE QUEST TO CHEAT time—extend life and enhance our bodies, our brains, and our sex lives—has been the driver of fortune as well as folly throughout history and in every culture. Today's antiaging wonder cures have their roots in a culture of denial that reaches back to the beginning of recorded history. In primitive societies recommendations for altering aging included recipes using the internal organs of young animals, with the idea that the new youthful viscera would impart renewed vigor to the patient's own aging parts. Ancient Hindu antiaging strategies touted the ingestion of tiger gonads—testicles—as a cure for impotence. The early Greeks endorsed similar efforts, such as eating the bone marrow of lions to gain courage. During the early part of the twentieth century, the flamboyant Russian-

"I don't want to achieve immortality through my work . . . I want to achieve it through not dying."

—WOODY ALLEN

born surgeon Serge Voronoff updated the ancient practice of eating animal gonads for virility and modernized it by grafting monkey testicles to older humans in attempts to restore youth and vitality to the men. In the 1960s, the Cryonics Society promoted the notion of freezing people immediately upon their death or, if legally permissible, just before they died, to preserve them for a later time when medical breakthroughs might offer them renewed health and longevity. And in the decades since, the search for the "fountain of youth" has taken gullible consumers through a wide assortment of remedies, from herbs to hormones.

Despite hope and hype, these "magic bullets" for extending life or reversing the effects of aging have all proven to be nothing more than blanks. There is no miracle product you can buy to cheat time or alter your age. There is, however, one proven, scientific way to alter the effects of aging and boost the quality of your life as you get older. That "miracle product" is your innate capacity for creativity, your ability to think a new thought and to act on it.

The planning strategies and practical exercises that follow are designed to build upon the different uses of creativity that we have explored throughout *The Creative Age: Awakening Human Potential in the Second Half of Life.* Whatever your age and whatever your circumstances, whatever your talents or skills, your dreams and desires, whatever you see as your limitations, these avenues of creative expression can boost your energy and outlook, improve your relationships, and help you get more out of every day.

Think of this chapter as a menu of options, but with *no* restrictions. You can do any of these activities at any time and in any order, and gain new insight and energy from each experience. If possible, use a designated notebook or file folder to save a paper trail of your thoughts and ideas. From time to time, review that paper trail, and I assure you that you'll find new paths to explore.

Let's get started! In the following creativity workshop material, I'll use the illuminated light bulb icon to designate a very simple activity to "turn on" creativity (see example at left).

Dreams are among the best reminders of our inner creativity. Their form and content are the essence of creativity. Write them down or draw them. Develop a dream journal.

Define Your Desires, Recognize Your Resources

Jump-start your creative energy by thinking about your interests and desires, and recognize that you have untapped additional inner resources—*different kinds of creative energy*—that will support your efforts. By doing this, you begin to position yourself in a take-charge role that enhances the way you feel about yourself and energizes you for exploring new directions.

Do you want to build upon what you have done before, and bring it to a higher level?

This is *continuing creativity,* a recharging process that knows no endpoint with aging, and one that will remind you of the depth of your potential and your capacity to access it.

- Reexamine what you have done in what has been your primary area of interest in accomplishment. Ask yourself, What are the next steps for growth? What remains unfinished?
- Talk to others who are doing related things; learn from their experiences.
- Look for new ideas. Explore books or popular magazines relating to your interest. Surf the internet for resources, contacts, and conversation.
- Look around you for inspiration. Tune in to the growing numbers of people your age or older who are actively engaged in new or challenging endeavors. You don't have to "measure up" to them, but only join their ranks through your own journey of enrichment and self-discovery.

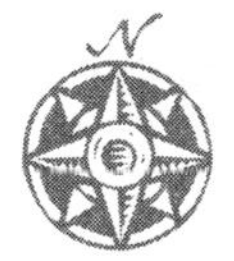

Do you want to change direction, either still drawing upon what you already know or moving into a very different direction?

This is the energy of *changing creativity.* It provides a wonderful opportunity to discover new aspects of yourself.

- Identify strengths you have that are underdeveloped, or interests you have long set aside.
- Explore a new pursuit just as you might experiment with a new recipe or travel to a different vacation spot.

- Empower yourself. Have confidence that you are capable of learning and growing.
- Others are doing it. You can, too!

Do you feel that you haven't done anything particularly creative, but now's the time to start?

Tap your capacity for *commencing creativity.*

- Ask yourself, "If not now, when?" And go for it—now!
- Visualize the beauty of "late bloomers" in the garden and see your own potential as ready to flower.
- Cultivate connections to the world of ideas and action. Look upon every conversation, movie, book, stroll—every ordinary experience—as a bridge to new opportunities for thought and action along a path of self-discovery.

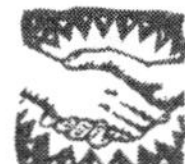

Do you wish you could join others in a meaningful or simply enjoyable project or activity?

This is *collaborative creativity* guaranteed to provide built-in encouragement and community. Sharing ideas and experience expands the creative potential of any moment in a special way, with rewarding social context and the satisfaction of contributing your ideas and energy to others.

- Enlist friends to share in a new activity, enriching your history together and opening the doors to new interests.
- Volunteer for a special project underway in your community or workplace as a way to meet new people and broaden your experience.

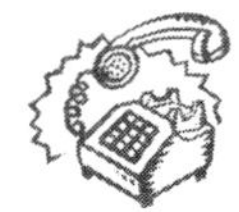

Does your circle of friends include those younger and older than you?

Broaden your exposure to new ideas with *intergenerational creativity.*

- Invite intergenerational diversity into your life. Look at older and younger people as a source of lively friendships and fresh, varied perspectives.
- Strengthen your family relationships by spending time actively involved with your children and/or grandchildren, or older members of your family, and their friends.

Are you looking for a sense of inner peace, purpose, and satisfaction?

You can enhance your inner life through personal creativity, or *"creativity with a little c."*

- Reflect on the significance of the unremarkable "little things" in life. Consider it a creative challenge to freshen your perspective and work toward an active appreciation of the smallest wonders.
- Recognize in the complexity of life the infinite opportunities for new ideas and interactions, and the power of small changes to bring about larger ones.
- Watch your language! Just as athletes "psych" themselves for victory with positive words and imagery, our habits of expression can psych us "up" with creative energy or psych us "out" with negativism. Language alone can marshal more creative energy to a task. A "problem" feels like an obstacle. A "challenge" is an invitation to success through innovative thinking. Take the challenge!

Do you want to do something more public-spirited for the community?

This is public creativity, or *creativity with a "big C."* Your contribution of time, talents, or other resources are critically important to the health of your community.

- Share your ideas for enhancing the quality of life in your community. Conversation is a catalyst for change, and every idea shared plants a seed for community growth.
- Be an activist in ways that work for you. Volunteer as a leader, a vocal supporter or a helping hand, offer to host a meeting or in other ways support a project or activity that you feel is important.
- View yourself as a community "treasure" and share generously of your unique experience, insight, and talents. This cycle of connectedness to community and the affirming self-view it produces becomes a continuing source of creative energy.

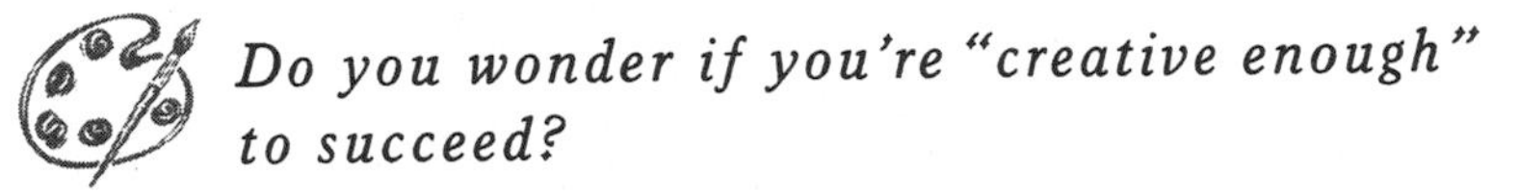

Do you wonder if you're "creative enough" to succeed?

You have what it takes. Don't limit yourself to the stereotyped view of creativity as "for artists only." We are each an artist of our own life. No matter what your life experience or circumstances, you can bring forth new thoughts and grow through new experiences that express different forms of creativity.

- Sign up for an art, music, writing, or craft class that introduces you to your ability to create or appreciate these art forms.
- Call an acquaintance, a friend, or a family member and take the initiative in setting up a time to get together for a pleasurable activity or simple visit. Offer your support in a project of theirs or invite them to join you in an activity of your choosing. This is *social creativity* and these connections strengthen your relationships and contribute to your own emotional resiliency.

Put the Creativity Equation to Work for You

Creativity = me^2

Remember the simple "math" of creativity with our equation: $C = me^2$ or creativity equals the *mass of what you know* multiplied by your *life experience* in two dimensions—your inner life or emotional experience, and your outer, or external, life experience.

- Where are you with the *m*—the knowledge base that you need to take the next step? Do you need to read, travel, talk with others or perhaps take a course or two to understand more about a field of interest?
- Think about the two dimensions of your life experience—inner and outer—as equally valuable resources that are renewable with each new experience.
- Evaluate your outer, external life and ask yourself: "What experiences do I have that I can draw upon to set the stage for new creative ventures?"
- Reflect on your inner world of emotional experience past and present. Do you feel psychologically ready to start on this new venture? If you feel uneasy or anxious about any aspect of it, discuss your concerns with good friends, attend a support group or consult with a therapist for short-term support or continuing help if needed.
- Tap into the additional psychological energy of the four developmental phases of adult life—Midlife Reevaluation, Liberation, Summing-Up, and Encore. Each phase offers a natural booster of motivation, insight, and emotional energy upon which to draw.

Invest in Yourself: Start Your Social Portfolio

It's never too late to start or build upon your Social Portfolio and to identify new opportunities for creativity through new and existing relationships (Refer again to the Social Portfolio idea below that was introduced in Chapter 5).

- Conduct an audit—strictly for fun! For each Social Portfolio category, list the activities, friendships, or other relationships that are already part of your life. What portion of your time is spent in solo activity? Group activity? With close friends? Family? Coworkers or new acquaintances? How much of your activity is low-energy or low-mobility, and how much of it requires more of you? If your list under any particular category is thin or empty, that's the type of activity or relationship you need to build.

THE SOCIAL PORTFOLIO

Tapping Creative Potential in Later Life

	GROUP EFFORTS	INDIVIDUAL EFFORTS
	Group/High Mobility	Individual/High Mobility
HIGH MOBILITY / HIGH ENERGY	• *Coordinate a neighborhood plant-a-new-garden group* • *Create a new sports group—e.g., a swimming-with-new-strokes club* • *Create a dinner and dance group, with a goal of learning new dances*	• *Create a descriptive walking tour of statues in your town* • *Hike a nature trail with the goal of creating photos or poems* • *Develop an exercise routine accompanied by select music*
	Group/Low Mobility	Individual/Low Mobility
LOW MOBILITY / LOW ENERGY	• *Create a dinner and video discussion group at your home* • *Coordinate a sit-down art class for complete novices* • *Learn a new game that can be played with family and friends*	• *Find an interesting area to volunteer via phone work* • *Learn about a new topic through library or internet research* • *Create a "story of my family" book with text and illustrations*

Read. Expand your reading to include a wider variety of books, magazines, and newspapers.

- Create a reserve of ideas by listing several things you do well, several other things that interest you, and several things you would like to do. Expand your options. Be bold. You don't have to skydive like President Bush did in his 70s, or go bungee-jumping off a mountain in New Zealand like my son Alex did when he was nineteen. But beware of limiting your options based on your past or on the wishes of family and friends. Be open to the idea of trying something new.
- Aim for diversity and balance in the way you invest your time and energy among those people and activities. Depending on the nature of social interaction that is under-represented in your current portfolio, develop opportunities for group and solo activities, low- and high-mobility options, and low- and high-energy options.
- Take action. Call local colleges and universities—including community colleges—as well as community centers and other resources for programs you might attend to advance your learning or experience in an interest area. For a variety of national resources for adult education programs see Creative Connections on page 274. Call a friend. Recruit company from among those you believe will make your venture more enjoyable or simply less daunting.
- Make the commitment to yourself. Whether you choose to develop a solitary interest or attend a class or travel to socialize in some other way more often or with different people, follow through with your plan. Look for ways to get the most out of the experience by investing your time and attention in the activity and in any new relationships it offers.
- Be adaptable. Have a rainy-day plan should there be an unforeseen change in your social network of significant others and/or your physical health status.

Social Portfolio
Marriage/Relationship Enrichment Tracks: A Context for Collaborative Creativity

Use collaborative creativity to strengthen your relationships and deepen emotional intimacy or connectedness. The following exercises are designed to expand creative experience and the opportunity for personal growth for both partners in a serious relationship. These kinds of positive experiences enhance self-esteem and satisfaction with each other and the relationship. To set the stage for your relationship work:

- **Begin with a better understanding of your relationship's beginnings.** Think about the basic internal and external forces at work in your marriage. People marry for different reasons: love, intimacy, sex, companionship that is close and enduring, having a soul mate, personal identity and a sense of completion in the marriage partnership, having children and cultivating a family life. What brought you together? What has kept you together? What more or what difference do you desire in the relationship?
- **Identify aspects of your relationship you feel need improvement.** Too often, personal dissatisfaction with one's own situation is taken out on the marriage. Sort out the issues that undermine emotional intimacy and connectedness. Are there warning signals that you can identify that are followed by behavior on your part that you later regret? Once those signs occur, can you stand back and ask yourself if you're going to act in the same predictable manner or try a different approach? Do you notice any connection between your level of anxiety or depression and anger or conflict that then is directed toward your partner or friend—blaming them when things in general aren't going well? Are there problem-solving strategies or therapy that you could use to stop "exporting" your tension or unhappiness to those around you? Do you place most of the burden on your spouse or significant other to make the changes necessary to improve the relationship? Can a more collaborative process be initiated? Are there more areas where you could take the initiative?
- **Identify opportunities for growth in the relationship and in your individual lives.** Creative activities nourish the chemistry of a close relationship. They enrich a relationship by helping both partners feel good about them-

selves and each other, and, consequently, to feel good about the marriage. Creative activities not only help maintain and repair a relationship, they influence even more the *growth* of a marriage or relationship. Fundamentally, they are pathways for discovering new aspects of ourselves and new aspects of those close to us. Creative activity with friends and family promote interaction, sharing, and communication.

TRACK I ACTIVITY PLAN: INDIVIDUAL INNER GROWTH

These activities focus on inner growth for you and for your partner, on an individual level and in relation to others.

- Explore new activities *separate from your partner* and *just by yourself.* For example, create a new home-based self-learning program on a topic that excites you and that you can build upon over time. Read and collect books and other materials that support your interest.
- Explore new activities *separate from your partner* and *involving others.* For example, take a class with others (not including your partner), especially one that excites you and that you can build upon, and where there is active interaction with the others. Or create a family tree or write a family history, ideally a project that has personal meaning for you and enables you to better understand yourself and your roots.
- Encourage and support your partner's inner growth through activities that are separate from you and solitary, as well as those that involve others.

TRACK II ACTIVITY PLAN: SHARED ACTIVITIES FOR GROWTH AS A COUPLE

These activities focus on creativity in your *relationship together,* first as a couple alone, and then as a couple in relation to others.

- Explore together new activities that are exciting for both of you and offer you something you can build upon over time, for example, a sport or recreational pastime, music, dancing, travel, theater, or sampling ethnic cuisines.
- Explore new activities that enable you, as a couple, to share meaningful time with old friends or to develop new ones to expand your circle of social relationship.

- Save something special for just you two. Some activities that you enjoy as a couple alone may also be fun to share with others, but find ways to develop facets of these activities in ways that are uniquely intimate for you and your partner.

Write a letter—and send it.

Autobiography: Learning from Your Own Life Stories

Reflection brings us closer to understanding, especially when it is our own life that we put under such thoughtful scrutiny. Autobiography begins with reflection, and in that simple mental exercise, we connect with our inner life and our inner source of creative energy. When you go further and share stories from your past, you share wisdom and experience with others and in that interaction enhance your own potential for new insights and self-discovery. Age and experience enable us to see and learn from patterns in our past, and our ability to do that grows and changes with age. You're never too young to reflect on your past, and you're never too old to take a fresh look at family fables. There are many ways to share your stories, including diary or journal-writing as a solitary pleasure, or more sociable forms of autobiographical expression.

Write a recipe and share it.

- Pick a form of life review that's easy for you, at least to get started. If you're comfortable writing, start with a private journal, letters to family members or friends inviting their memories of a time or person you recall, or sharing memories with younger family members or friends at milestones in their lives. If you're more at ease talking, tape or videotape your recollections in the same spirit of personal documentary.
- Start with a compelling memory of time, place, or people. Reflect on *key events* that created *turning points* in your life, or in how you viewed yourself. These might include discovering a talent, falling in love, losing a parent, getting the ultimate job, a conflict with someone special to you, achieving an important goal, suffering a major disappointment or experiencing something new and exciting.

Plant a flower.

See a movie or videotape about something that interests you, and discuss it with someone.

- Reflect on your experiences and inner growth during life's earlier developmental passages and life transitions, for instance: childhood, adolescence, young adult and middle-age years, and school days, college, military, marriage, career, and parenting.
- Examine influential relationships such as those with grandparents, parents, siblings, mentors, adversaries, spouse, and children. What made them important to you?

Foundations of Fact, Issues and Influences:

Whether you sit with your own thoughts or plan to share them with others, remembering details will help you get the most out of the autobiography experience, and make it more meaningful to others with whom you may share a story. It is in the detail of emotions and actions that you may eventually discover patterns that have special significance. Start with simple facts, and other details will come to mind. Include:

- Sensory impressions: colors, textures, smells, sound, and sight.
- Action: Who did what, where, and with or to whom?
- Emotions: How did you feel? Happy? Loving? Angry? Sad? Confused? Frightened? Powerful? Weak? Name your feelings and watch for cause-and-effect patterns between actions and emotions. Is there a pattern of anger and physical aggression in your life? A pattern of discomfort with social interaction? Is there a pattern of positive emotion with any particular activity or circumstances? Talking about feelings improves our coping skills: describe how you felt about different events, changes, people, and experiences in general.
- Conflicts and Crises: Describe these difficult moments in your life, the emotions and actions they triggered and how you resolved them.
- Highs and lows: Describe your hopes, fears, satisfactions, greatest disappointments, humorous experiences, angry experiences, what you love, what you hate, people and events that positively influenced you, people and events that nega-

tively affected you. Working in dichotomies like these—comparing and contrasting—is an effective technique for sharing the depth and breadth of your life experience.

- Family history: Describe your parents and grandparents (and great grandparents if possible), including their names, appearances, personalities, relationships with you and others, their work, what they accomplished, notable anecdotes. What is or was most special or memorable about them? How has your family most affected you? Did your relationship with your parents change over the years? Where were your parents and grandparents born? If they have died, how old were they and how did it happen? If you have pictures of them, collect them to accompany your story, whether it is in written form or simply told.
- Family context: Describe your siblings and details of the relationship you shared or share with each. How has the relationship stayed the same and how has it changed over time?
- Highlights: Describe periods of your life: For instance, when you think about your childhood, what do you believe was good and what was bad? What was family life like for you? What special events, dreams, hopes, fears, disappointments, accomplishments, and other memorable experiences stand out during this time? If you write about a disappointment or a mishap, how did it affect you, what did you learn from it? Did it influence the way you thought about or approached things from that point on? What stands out most during this period? Who influenced you most? Describe how.
- Self-image: How have you thought about yourself during different stages of your life; what images have you had about yourself? How have you thought about your body and your gender? How have these thoughts evolved or changed? What do you most like about yourself? What do you most dislike? What would you like to change? What do you do well? What are your special skills or talents?
- Attitudes and Beliefs: How have your life view, spiritual, political, and other attitudes changed or deepened over the decades?
- Friendships: Who were your closest friends in childhood, adolescence, young adulthood, middle age, later life? Which friendships continued? How did your friendships change? What significant events and conflicts occurred?
- Work: What was your first job, and how did you feel about it? How has your work life developed over the years?

- Love: What are your memories of romantic interests and sexual awakening? When did you first fall in love? What path did that relationship travel? How have your views of romantic love, sexuality, and intimate relationship developed over the years? If you have married, describe your marriage or relationships with significant others. How did they affect the way you thought about yourself, about others, and your life course? How have you felt about being married or about not being married?
- Death: What was your first experience centered on death? Who died? How did it affect you? What about other such experiences since? How do you think about death? How have such thoughts affected you? What would you like your obituary to say?

Ask yourself:

- Are there contemporary, historical, literary, or mythological figures with whom you identify? What qualities about them make you feel that connection?
- What were your biggest dreams, accomplishments, and satisfactions?
- What were your fears and biggest disappointments?
- What and when were your happiest times? Describe them and explain why they were the best.
- What were the funniest times and things you experienced?
- What and when were your most discouraging times?
- Are there secrets you have always wished you could tell? Any you want to share?
- Are there things you feel you still need or want to do?
- Are there other things you want to say or describe?
- Is there some way that you would like to sum up who you are, how you think, and how you feel about things?
- Is there advice you would like to leave people with, including important life lessons you've learned?

Begin simply by thinking consciously about these aspects of your life, perhaps when you take a walk or sit for a quiet time in the evening. You might go on to write your thoughts in letters to grandchildren or other younger friends and ask for stories of their own, enjoying the benefits of intergenerational creativity. You could enlist others to work with you to create brief snapshots of your life on paper; a page here and a page there add up. You may choose to make autobiography the central focus of your creative endeavors in the second half of life or in your postretirement period. Whether your autobiography work leads to published writings or film, a private diary or journal, a family scrapbook or simple, memorable conversation with family and friends, it is the process of meaningful reflection and sharing that is the greatest reward.

Visit someone you don't see often, or someone who is sick, and short on friends.

The Creativity Game

The goal of this game is to acquire 1000 Creativity Points, which permit you to give yourself a reward of your choosing. Be generous!

- Begin on the square labeled "START"
- Place a small object on the game board that can serve as a marker.
- Roll a die and move clockwise around the game board; you must roll the die at least once a day and carry out the command on the square you land on.
- Scoring: Earn 5 points each time you complete the command on the square you land on. If you land on or pass the "START" square, you collect a bonus 20 points; if you land

START → *Collect 20 Creativity Points*	**Visit a person**	**E-mail or write a letter**	**Visit a new place**	**Explore a new activity**
Describe a decade in your life	The Creativity Game			**Read an article or book**
Explore a new activity	**Record dreams or daydreams**	**Your choice**	**Record daily thoughts**	**See a movie or cultural event**

Visit someplace new, from a new lunch cafe to a new country, if foreign travel is possible.

on the "START" square, in addition to collecting 20 points, you take another turn. When you reach 1000 points, give yourself that special reward—a trip, a book, a day away—but the most exciting reward will be the sense of vitality, community, and self-esteem you'll gain through the activities themselves.

Game Pointers:

Whatever square you land on, try to carry out the command with a different twist, an added dimension, or a sense of flair.

- After you visit someone or some place special, write a descriptive journal entry about it, or sketch something from the experience.
- Take the opportunity to be creative and try something different.
- Feel free to draw upon your creativity by developing a new or expanded game board with squares of *your choosing*.

Creative Connections: More Ideas

Visit a hobby or crafts section at a bookstore

Another way to immerse yourself in possibilities and options is to go to spend an afternoon at your favorite bookstore. Even if you are not sure you want or are ready for a hobby, you should visit this section of the store anyway. There's an expression, "You don't know what you don't know." Maybe there's a hobby waiting for you after all?

I go to the bookstore on a regular basis, but I am always amazed at what I'll find. The last time I was there, I found a Readers' Digest book titled *Back to Basics: How to Learn and Enjoy Traditional American Skills*. As I read over the table of contents, I was intrigued by part five of the book on "Skills and Crafts for House and Homestead." The skills and crafts are listed to the left.

- ***Natural dyes***
- ***Spinning***
- ***Weaving***
- ***Hooked rugs***
- ***Braided rugs***
- ***Patchwork quilting***
- ***Rope and twine***
- ***Tanning and leatherwork***
- ***Woodworking***
- ***Broommaking***
- ***Scrimshaw***
- ***Household recipes***
- ***Metalworking***
- ***Stenciling***
- ***Flower drying and pressed flowers***
- ***Gourd craft***
- ***Soapmaking***
- ***Candlemaking***
- ***Basketry***

I was particularly interested in "Stenciling." Given my interest in inventing intergenerational board games that are intended to be both educational and artistic, the wheels in my head started turning about whether I could use stenciling to add to the artistic quality of my games.

I also wondered after reading more of this book whether I could get my wife interested in "Patchwork Quilting." I knew it would appeal to her sensibilities. I'd bring up the subject by saying something like, "Wouldn't it be great to have a patchwork quilt to add to the ambience of our old Victorian house?" Wendy, a highly regarded art therapist and also a talented sculptor, optioned out of the quilting idea but asked me instead for some pastel art equipment for her birthday. She wanted to "create warm pastel drawings that would add to the ambience of our old Victorian house."

Elderhostel

Lifelong learning is itself a creative venture, and can be approached in many different ways. *Elderhostel,* a nonprofit organization, provides learning opportunities for the fifty-five-and-older age group. It combines traditions of education and hosteling (inexpensive, informal lodgings) in a program designed exclusively for older adults.

Predict on paper what your situation will be like ten years from now. Save your prediction to check later for accuracy.

Elderhostel consists of a network of about two thousand educational and cultural sites. Its hosts include colleges and universities, conference centers, state and municipal parks, museums, theaters, and environmental/outdoor education centers among others. Programs are offered year-round throughout the United States and Canada and in over seventy countries overseas. Hence it can be an appealing way to learn and travel at the same time.

Most programs in the United States and Canada are one week long; programs overseas last one to four weeks and involve weeklong stays at institutions in different parts of one or several contiguous countries. Participants take up to three non-credit course while living at their host institution or in nearby commercial facilities. Nearly half of the programs house participants in nearby hotels and motels, while the rest are in a variety of accommodations from academic institutions to conference centers. U.S. programs focus on a wide range of liberal arts and sciences subjects, often drawing on unique local and regional features and resources. Programs in other countries have a strong cultural element, offering studies of the host country's history, literature, arts, culture, language, and natural environment. All the programs, at home and abroad, also include a variety of extracurricular activities, field trips, and cultural events.

Elderhostel strives to provide a stimulating environment for intellectual exchange and discovery. Prior formal education or knowledge of the subjects are not necessary to take advantage of Elderhostel's programs. While courses are designed to be challenging, there are no homework assignments, exams, grades, or credits. The informal classroom environment is designed to invite participation and discussion without pressure. Both couples and singles participate in Elderhostel programs. Participants from all walks of life share living quarters, meals, classes, and activities with their fellow hostelers, many forming lasting friendships as a result of their experiences together. (See also Elderhostel in Appendix D.)

Volunteer!

In previous chapters I described a correlation between increasing age and an increasing desire to share experiences and knowledge, either through storytelling or philanthropy. On one hand, volunteer work represents an important, enriching activity for one's social portfolio. On the other hand, volunteering offers myriad opportunities for social creativity.

You can volunteer for many things that are represented in each of the four categories of the social portfolio. Think about working with others in your community to launch a neighborhood watch group or volunteer to help with bloodmobiles for the American Red Cross. These two examples would fall into the Group/High Mobility category. On the other hand, answering phones with other volunteers during a PBS or National Public Radio fundraiser would fall into the Group/Low Mobility. Placing flyers for a political campaign could be an Individual/High Mobility activity, while writing letters to businesses or politicians for a cause would be an example of Individual/Low Mobility.

What many people fail to realize is that a volunteer experience can, at times, provide an opportunity for innovation in a manner not easily attainable at a regular job. My own volunteer experience is a perfect case. I have been volunteering half a day or more each week since 1971.

During this time, twenty-five years (1971–1996) were spent volunteering as a geriatric psychiatrist in a public housing building for more than two hundred older adults. The experience proved invaluable in my growth as a gerontologist and in developing innovative mental health service delivery techniques. Let me give you one example.

In private practice, psychiatrists do not get reimbursed for telephone follow-ups. They have little incentive with a crowded schedule to monitor the progress of their patients via the phone. But as a volunteer, working for free, I was not concerned with reimbursement. The building where I did my volunteer work had a small office for me with a phone. I would start my day by briefly checking in on ten to fifteen people via phone calls. If, during the conversation, I had the sense that things were not quite right, I would then ask the individual to come down to my office or, more typically, I would immediately take the elevator up to his or her apartment to see what was going on. If things on the phone were going well, I would call the next person. This approach proved to be very efficient and allowed me to treat many more people in a limited time span than would normally be possible in my regular work.

This experience also permitted me to have a remarkably rich twenty-five-year longitudinal perspective on the entire community of older persons living in that building. In fact, many of the ideas for successful research projects I have launched had their genesis from my volunteer experience. My work with Ms. Thompson, the blind, spirited ninety-five-year-old I described in Chapter 2, took place in that building. My early awareness of the potential and prevalence of creativity in later life as well as the phenomenon of unrecognized talented older artists hidden behind closed doors also came from this volunteer work. And of course, there was the wealth of wonderful relationships that these people and I developed and the very deep sense of gratitude I received.

There were also numerous touching acts of appreciation and fondness from the residents of the building. Two in particular stand out. On one occasion, the residents arranged a special party for me at which I received an "Outstanding Volunteer Services Certificate of Appreciation" from the District of Columbia, where the building was located. On another occasion, I was walking toward the building on my clinic day during a tornado watch, when, all of a sudden, an eighty-year-old woman I knew stuck her head out her window and bellowed, "Dr. Cohen, don't you know there's a tornado coming—get your ass in here, now!" Clearly, my patients have been watching out for my well-being as much as I have theirs.

You don't, however, have to commit to extensive hours or long years on a volunteer job. Start with something simple; you'll have lots of company. The 1991 Commonwealth Fund Productive Aging Survey identified the percentages of older persons volunteering at different ages (see table on next page). Note: Even in their early to mid-80s, more than one-fourth (28 percent) of older persons were still doing volunteer work. Though the amount of time older people (age fifty-five and older) in the Commonwealth Fund survey volunteered during the week varied considerably, the average was 6.3 hours weekly.

PERCENTAGES OF OLDER PERSONS VOLUNTEERING AT DIFFERENT AGES

Age	% Volunteering
55–59	31.0%
60–64	26.0
65–69	27.0
70–74	26.3
75–79	23.2
80–84	28.0
85 and older	9.4
TOTAL, AGE 55+	26.1

If you were to select a special and feasible surprise for a significant other, what would it be, and for whom? How about making it happen?

The 1991 Commonwealth Fund survey found that slightly more than one-fourth (26 percent) of Americans aged sixty-five and older provided assistance to a sick or disabled relative, friend, or neighbor during the previous week. It should be noted that the percentage of older persons providing help is double the percentage of Americans aged sixty-five and older who, in the 1989 National Long-Term Care Survey, reported they they themselves routinely received help from family, friends, and neighbors due to long-term care disabilities.

Forty percent of persons aged sixty-five and older with children had provided assistance of a nonfinancial nature to their children, grandchildren or great grandchildren during the previous week; eleven percent provided twenty or more hours of help. Seven percent of persons age seventy-five and older provided twenty or more hours of assistance to their children, grandchildren, or great grandchildren during the prior week. Moreover, persons age sixty-five and older were approximately three-and-a-half times more likely to give substantial financial help to children than to receive it. Clearly, portrayals of older persons as a national burden should be viewed in the shadow of portrayals of older adults as a national resource.

Strategies for getting involved in volunteering: In the United States, there are a wide number of local and national volunteer networks that one can contact to explore volunteer options and to start volunteering.

Area Agencies on Aging: Most communities across the country have a local office on aging or an Area Agency on Aging that provides information and referral services on programs relevant to older adults; these Area Agencies on Aging also typically coordinate various local volunteer programs and can put you in touch with national volunteer networks. The local phone directory should have the number for one of these offices or agencies. One could also contact Eldercare Locator at 1-800-677-1116 to find an Area Agency on Aging near you or near an aging relative living apart from you. (See also ElderPage in Appendix D.)

Corporation for National Service: Several long-standing and very successful volunteer programs targeted to older volunteers are included under the federally sponsored National Senior Service Corps (also known as Senior Corps), a component of the *Corporation for National Service.* These include:

- The Foster Grandparent Program, which offers older people an opportunity to develop close relationships with children who have special and exceptional needs.
- Retired and Senior Volunteer Program (RSVP), where participants work in schools, courts, libraries, day care centers, hospitals, and other community centers.
- Senior Companion Program, whose volunteers provide supportive services to older adults who have special health, education, or social needs in settings such as hospitals, social service agencies, or home health care agencies.

Write a rhyming poem about someone special—at least four lines. Feel free to be funny.

Create a dinner for a significant other or friends that is different from the usual way you would do it—different either in the food preparation, the setting selected, the attire worn, or in any other way that enters your imagination.

To obtain more information about these programs, contact the Corporation for National Service, in Washington, D.C., at 800-424-8867. (See also Senior Corps in Appendix D.) Another interesting federally sponsored volunteer program is SCORE (the Service Corps of Retired Executives), part of the U.S. Small Business Administration (SBA); SCORE volunteers provide technical assistance to small businesses (check the blue pages in your local phone directory for their number and see Small Business Administration in Appendix D). Other nonfederal opportunities targeted to retired executives are listed and described as follows:

- *National Executive Service Corporation.* This is a nationwide organization of volunteer executives who consult with nonprofit organizations for long-range planning, marketing, personnel management, budgeting, financing, and general operations.

Their headquarters is in New York City (212-529-6660), with affiliates in approximately forty cities across the country.

- *International Executive Service Corps.* Located in Hartford, Connecticut (203-967-6000), their volunteers receive expenses to help companies and communities in foreign countries. The focus of their consultations is broad, ranging from assistance in launching a new business to helping to solve a region's agricultural problems.
- *Volunteers in Overseas Cooperative Assistance (VOCA).* Located in Washington, D.C., this nonprofit organization provides expenses for various foreign consultations. The volunteer services of my Uncle Bud, described in Chapter 4, were supported by VOCA. They can be reached at 202-383-4961.

There are a range of other volunteer networks to tap into, and, in general, your Area Agency on Aging should be able to help you here. These other networks may have a special issue (e.g., with the Gray Panthers) or skill focus relevant to aging, they may be targeted to different racial or ethnic older population groups, or they may specialize in particular problems of older persons ranging from vision and hearing problems to osteoporosis and Alzheimer's disease.

It is worth the effort to explore what's available in terms of volunteer opportunities in your community or beyond. You may find that match that is just right for you. Even checking the Yellow Pages can be helpful, looking under "Volunteer Services" and/or "Social Service Organizations"; the Washington, D.C. Yellow Pages lists approximately 350 such organizations, the vast majority of which offer some form of volunteer service.

New Careers—Full-Time, Part-Time, and Temporary

Volunteering can be gratifying and creatively stimulating, but we should not forget the benefits of working, full- or part-time. In 1990, according to the U.S. Census, persons aged 55 and older represented 27 percent of the workforce. How has the overall labor participation changed since the 1960s?

LABOR FORCE PARTICIPATION RATES, 1960–2005

		1960	1975	1990	2005
MEN	aged 55 to 64	86.8%	75.6%	67.7%	67.9%
	aged 65 and older	33.1%	21.6%	16.4%	16.0%
WOMEN	aged 55 to 64	37.2%	40.9%	45.3%	54.3%
	aged 65 and older	10.8%	8.2%	8.7%	8.8%

Source: U.S. Bureau of Labor Statistics, 1989, 1992

Note that fewer people percentagewise are working now in their later years than they were nearly forty years ago. Yet it should also be noted that *retirees represent the fastest-growing segment of temporary help services.* Self-employment rates also rise with age. Older workers may be drawn to temporary or self-employment because of the more flexible schedules involved. Older persons are more likely to have accumulated business knowledge and contacts as well as financial savings that make starting their own business less risky for them than when they were younger. The U.S. Small Business Administration (SBA) can assist both through loans and technical help.

Thanks in part to these changes in the aging workforce, the attitudes toward older workers also has changed in the past thirty years. While ageist attitudes used to prevail in the office (e.g., "older people are less efficient and slower to learn new things"), now surveys indicate that executives view older employees as more conscientious and hard working than younger employees. Many managers believe older workers have stronger interpersonal communication skills and therefore deal more appropriately with customers. In addition, workers over the age of 65 tend to be quite healthy, tallying fewer sick days compared to workers aged forty-five to sixty-five. With the service industry predicted to grow nearly 30 percent in the next ten years, the climate for job placement among older workers has never been better.

Computer skills and SeniorNet. One of the most important new skills, especially for service-oriented work, is *using the computer.* Your local community college offers many introductory courses in this subject. You can also contact *SeniorNet,* a national nonprofit educational program founded to teach computer skills to older adults and to help form friendships within an online community; it is targeted to those age 55 and older.

SeniorNet teaching sites are located throughout the United States and are locally funded. They offer introductory classes for beginners and specialized classes in topics ranging from genealogy to financial management. *SeniorNet* also publishes a number of informational pamphlets of interest to older adults. *SeniorNet Online* is a national computer network that ties sites and members together, and can be used by any member with access to a computer and modem (see also SeniorNet in Appendix D).

Explore new careers. It's never too late to think about switching careers, even if you're retired and you haven't been working for some time. A good starting point is to go down to your local library's reference section and look at *The Occupational Outlook Handbook,* updated and published every two years by the U.S. Department of Labor. The book contains descriptions for approximately 250 jobs, covering 90 percent of all workers and most if not all major jobs in the U.S. Each job is discussed in terms of earnings,

Is there a museum or place of interest near where you live that you have never visited? How about exploring it?

training and educational needs, working conditions, skills required, advancement opportunities, projected growth, related jobs, and sources of additional information.

If you want professional advice, you might make an appointment with a career-planning counselor at one of your local community colleges or universities. The trusty Yellow Pages also lists sources for Career and Vocational Counseling where you can receive professional testing and advice for exploring new directions. A stop at the Career Planning section of a local major bookstore may also be helpful. A number of books offer self-assessment tests to help you discover areas of interest and capacity, while many others focus on different categories of work—providing you further lists just by examining the titles of different books.

In addition to reading the employment section of your daily newspaper, the Yellow Pages, once again, can help with its list of employment agencies—including those for temporary jobs. The Washington, D.C., Yellow Pages, for example, lists over 125 employment contractors for temporary help alone across a multitude of different occupations. Temporary positions have become very attractive to retirement-age workers, because they allow you to develop a varied and well-balanced social portfolio of work-related, recreational, and general social activities.

Temporary options are also becoming increasingly sophisticated. A good example is a temporary medical practice for physicians through Locum Tenums (national headquarters in Atlanta; 800-272-2707). Locum Tenums is Latin for "to hold the place for," where physician-temps "hold the place" for regular full-time doctors who have gone on vacation or left a full-time position. Schedules for doctors can be very flexible—from a weekend to three months, to a year, to longer. They get paid a daily rate based on their specialty in addition to travel (including local), lodging, and malpractice insurance. They are also helped with licensing issues if going to a state where they are not licensed. One-third of locum tenums doctors are retirement-age, one-third are middle-aged, and one-third are young (often just out of training).

PART II: SPECIAL PROJECTS

The TR-Bio (Therapeutic/Restorative Biography)
The Creativity Discovery Corps

The TR-Bio (Therapeutic/Restorative Biography)

When you create biographical materials for others—for instance, the chronically ill or disabled—you provide pleasure, social connections, and a visual reminder of their contribution and place in family and community. The TR-Bio uses a visual medium—a photo album, scrapbook, or videotape—to focus attention on the positive and meaningful details of an individual's life. Beyond the therapeutic benefits of the TR-Bio for the "featured" individual, the book or tape also enhances caregivers' understanding of the individual and thus strengthens the relationship. In the process of creating a TR-Bio you, too, come away enriched by the experience of examining one's life closely and helping someone in need connect with those who care.

TR-Bios can make a profound difference in the lives of chronically ill patients, especially those confined to nursing homes. TR-Bios create a patient profile and as a result improve communications between the patient and staff. Once staff members of a nursing home get to know the history of their patient, they usually are more effective caregivers.

I learned through the experience of my own father's deterioration with Alzheimer's Disease that TR-Bios are therapeutic for the ailing patient and families alike, because they provide a way for often frustrated family members to feel productive and helpful toward their loved one at times when the disease has made them feel for the most part helpless. The TR-Bio, in effect, is a form of *clinical roots*. When Alex Haley published his book *Roots,* which was then followed by a TV series based on the book, it became apparent how important a positive sense of heritage—or roots—is in building self-esteem and a feeling of well-being. TR-Bios apply this powerful influence of personal roots to a therapeutic or clinical situation where they add to the overall treatment program.

In addition to the obvious benefits for patient and family, the TR-Bio also appears to have positive effects on staff at nursing homes and assisted-living facilities. Because work in these environments can be stressful, turnover is usually high—especially among nursing assistants who tend to receive both limited training and limited pay. With little knowledge of the patient as a person, the staff often has a difficult time responding in a personal way. With the TR-Bio, however, staff members can get to know the special history of their patients' lives. Their image shifts to a more human level of understanding of these patients, and their jobs become more gratifying.

Note:

Because I originated the TR-Bio as a therapeutic tool for patients, and it holds special potential in healthcare settings, I use the word *patient* here to clearly identify the celebrated individual of the TR-Bio. But I encourage you to think of the TR-Bio as a special gift you might give to anyone to celebrate a milestone birthday, event, or their place in your family or community. One need not be ill or disabled to be greatly moved by such a tangible, affirming gift of recognition.

TR-BIO FORMATS

The Videocassette:

The TR-Bio can take many forms. For example, it can be in the form of a videocassette (see illustration on page 286). The use of music in the video can enhance the emotional impact of the images, including music that is associated with special memories or a past experience, such as a wedding or alma mater theme. In addition to music, commentary can help the patient recognize things and to aid the guide or companion with discussion. The image on the TV screen can, at times, be placed on *Pause* to extend discussion of a particularly engaging image.

The TR-Bio can also be created in the form of an audiocassette, scrapbook, or yearbook format as in the illustration on page 287.

One advantage of a videocassette format is that it takes advantage of the skills of the younger generations. From a process standpoint, intergenerational approaches build upon group interest and skill levels of today's adolescents and young adults by using computer, audiovisual, and other technology that younger generations are more familiar with, and at times more adept at manipulating. In other words, these young people play a key role in the production of the TR-Bios because of the expertise they possess in applying the required technology.

My study of the effects of TR-Bios involves high school and college-age students, many of whom have interests in oral history, journalism, film, and computer imagery. Who better to involve in getting and framing a history than those with these types of skills? Similarly, who better to involve in arranging the images than those with skills in film and computer imagery? Some of these students are motivated primarily by the spirit of volunteerism, but many also see this as an opportunity to practice and advance in their focus of study—be it journalism, film, or other fields of communication or arts—while at the same time making a socially meaningful contribution. They help patients and families while the patients and families allow them to sharpen their skills and gain valuable experience.

Seek out nurturing people and environments as encouragers and catalysts. Talk with a teacher, mentor, or friend. Take a walk in the woods, visit a playground or eat lunch in a setting that adds to the pleasure of your day.

TR-Bios Yearbook Format:

Another highly effective way to format the bio is modeled after the high school yearbook, as in the illustration that appears on page 287. The yearbook format facilitates the communication between the patient and young visitors. It provides ample visual material as well as a script, so to speak, to guide the visitor to ask questions and comment on the material. For example, a grandchild might open the TR-Bio Yearbook to a page with a picture of the grandparent at the grandchild's age. On the opposite page might be two columns, one suggesting possible questions if the patient has some capacity to answer, the other suggesting possible comments if the patient has limited capacity to respond but still displays some ability to comprehend. In doing so, this TR-Bio also illustrates how best to communicate with cognitively impaired patients who are easily frustrated, even those who have an inability to answer even simple questions. The book can be arranged as an attractive loose-leaf notebook to facilitate individualism and updating of Question/Comment pages.

TR-Bios Video Visits Format:

Like the longer video format, video visits are recorded on a camcorder to be viewed on television. But video visits consist of vignettes made by faraway family and friends who send the videotapes to the patient's home or nursing facility to share personal news and add their visual presence to the patient's day. Video visits represent a potentially important contribu-

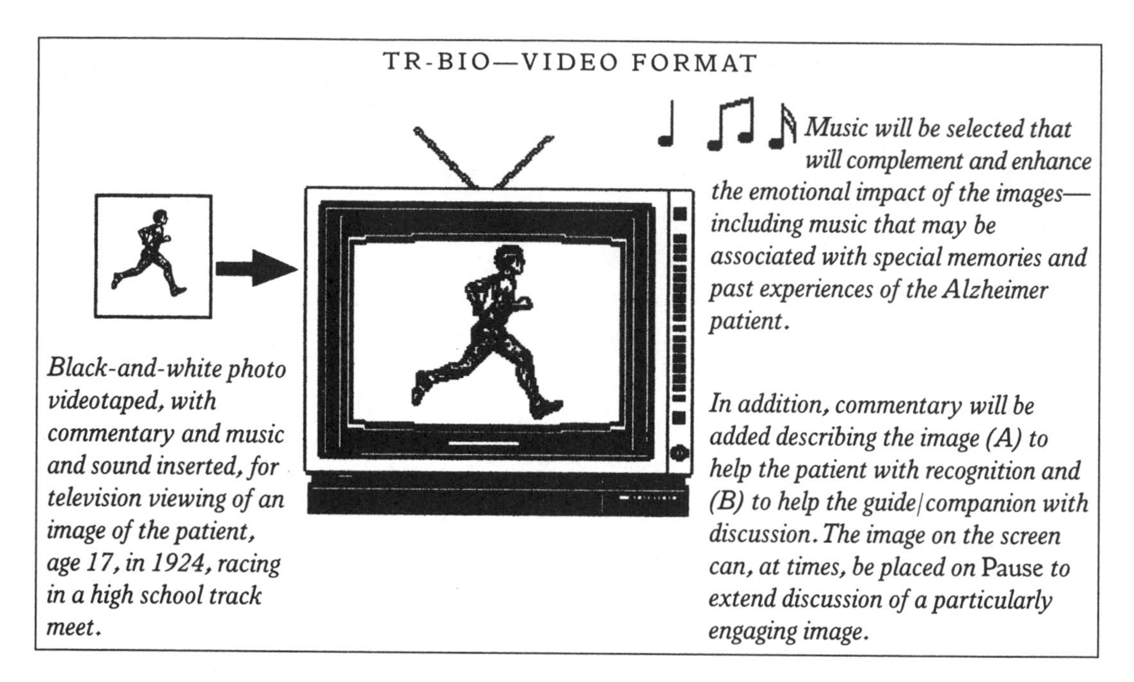

tion to quality time and quality of life for Alzheimer patients and others residing in such settings. They also complement the TR-Bio video format approach and, like that fuller video version, can tap the talents and energy of young people to assist in their production. Especially for a grandchild or other young family member who lives at a distance, this is a meaningful way to strengthen feelings of connectedness and caring to a faraway relative.

PRODUCING A TR-BIO

The strategies and techniques for creating a TR-Bio are ultimately a reflection of the creativity of the collaborating team. For example, a student of journalism or oral history and one in film or photography may team up to work with a family to obtain stories that reflect happy or interesting events over the course of the patient's life. Interviews with significant others may be videotaped and accompanied by commentary; if there were old videos or films (e.g., 16 mm) of the patient, these could also be incorporated; any associations that might enhance the memory of an event also could be incorporated, whether in the form of images, commentary, or even music.

Ultimately the goal of a TR-Bio, other than to be presented in the most personally engaging visual and auditory manner, is to attract patient interest and pleasure. Based on my understanding of research, most Alzheimer's patients who lack structure in their day-to-day lives gravitate toward unstructured, stressful activities that compound their already frustrating and agitated lives. TR-Bios provide a more structured and more pleasant context for them and their families. They enhance the quality of a family visit and allow for fruitful one-on-one visits, which Alzheimer's patients typically prefer over group activities as their condition gets worse. As illustrated below in the yearbook format, I encourage you to think about creating a *commentary* form of conversation as opposed to a conventional, but often frustrating, *question-and-answer* format.

Start a memoir where you look back at interesting episodes in your life, while adding any new ones that arise.

REMEMBER THEN, BACK WHEN

There are often times when a family sadly reminisces of a special time involving the loved one—what I call a "remember then, back when" phenomenon. The pathos surrounding a degenerative disease can build, particularly when linked with anguished looking back. These are sad and painful episodes, which I, too, experienced in thinking about my dad as his condition worsened. TR-Bios are extremely useful in resolving these feelings and addressing this phenomenon.

I wanted to develop a way of creating pleasant *present* memories for my family and for others, but my father's condition made that quite challenging. These thoughts led me to the develop "a-day-in-the-life" TR-Bio. Essentially, this technique captures a current event—birthdays, for instance—that leaves everybody feeling good.

TR-BIO—YEARBOOK FORMAT

QUESTIONS:	**COMMENTS:**
1. Granddad, what was it like being at that race?	1. Granddad, you were the same age then as I am now.
2. How did you do in that race?	2. We look alike.
3. Did you run after you graduated?	3. I also like to run, and am on my school team.

page 18

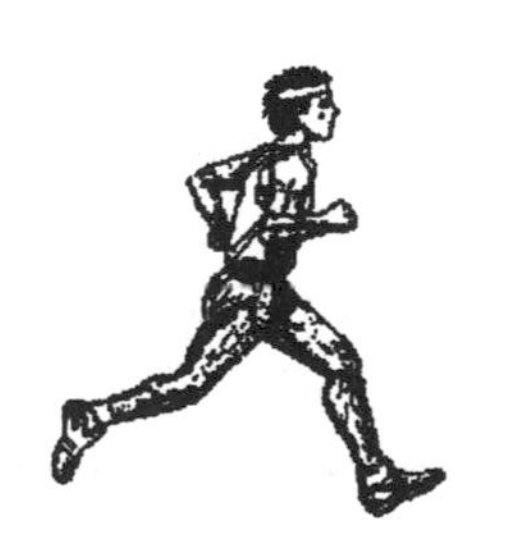

Granddaddy Arthur, at age 17, racing in a high school track meet in 1924.

page19

Spend some time in the library or on the Internet to find out as much as you can about the events of the year when you were born. Do the same for others in your family.

We held such an event for my father's eighty-sixth birthday. Not surprisingly, we titled it "Ben Cohen's Eighty-Sixth Birthday." My son Alex, just out of college, joined us to help in creating and filming the event for my father, who was then in a nursing home.

From his first weeks in the nursing home, we had started to create biographies about my father in yearbook and video formats. In fact, a short biography with my dad's picture on the cover was placed on the table next to his bed the day he entered the home. Numerous staff members read the biography and commented on both how impressed and flattered they were that such an effort had been made to help them get to know their patient.

My father liked to sit in the corridor outside his room to keep an eye on the world about him. For our "day-in-the-life" TR-Bio, this is where I planned to begin filming. As we appeared on the scene, we made quite a sight: I came carrying a tripod, my son Alex had the video camera, my wife Wendy the 35 mm camera, my mother brought the cake, my brother Franklin carried miscellaneous paraphernalia, and my little daughter Eliana, then two years old, proudly held the birthday balloon for her grandfather. Quite a scene, quite a crew. The nursing home corridor was abuzz with creative energy, as staff members and some ambulatory patients gathered, curious about the production hubbub. The activity itself placed my father in a different light; he had become the object of interest and stimulus of activity, all for the happiest of reasons.

The production team moved from the corridor to the activities room, where we held a party, then back to his personal room, where we showed my father the production on TV. He had more smiles on his face than we had seen in a long time. It was quite a day. A week later, when the family talked on the phone, everyone reminded him about the party he had had the week before. The TR-Bio had done its job, succeeding in providing us present-time pleasant memories, despite the realities of a devastating illness. It was, all in all, a wonderful day. The fact is, those fond memories became part of that same reality. On a later visit, Ben smiled as he reviewed his eighty-sixth birthday fresh on TV.

THE BEAUTY AND IRONY OF TR-BIOS

Once a TR-Bio is created, it can be used routinely to brighten a day, especially for Alzheimer's patients, because their extreme memory loss means that they may forget about the video or scrapbook from one day, or one hour, to the next, depending on how far the illness has progressed. In such situations, TR-Bios can be shared time and time again, without any sense of repetition for the ailing patient.

TR-BIO TECHNICAL NOTES

A TR-Bio scrapbook is a "low-impact" product, requiring only basic scrapbook materials. For video, so much sophisticated technology is now commonly available that it simply requires that you reach out to tap resources for equipment and volunteer assistance. If you have neither the equipment nor the expertise, call local schools and community agencies to recruit help. Often, young people are eager to help with such a project, and the schools, too, are on the lookout for ways to involve students in public service activities.

A CHALLENGE FOR THE BUSINESS AND CARING COMMUNITY

While TR-Bios can be created on a shoestring budget, they can also be produced under state-of-the-art conditions. The latter offer their own set of creative opportunities. For example, a fully equipped editing lab available on-site at a nursing home makes it all the more enticing for talented high school and college students to come to the nursing home and make high-quality TR-Bios. And, again, their youthful presence adds to the intergenerational ambiance of the predominantly geriatric setting.

The main costs for such labs are the start-up expenses. Once established, maintenance costs are relatively minimal. This is an opportunity for a local business to make a big difference with just a modest one-time contribution to provide funds to launch a lab. By so doing, it can join the collaborative process with the student volunteers in helping families and their community in creatively improving the quality of life for many suffering with Alzheimer's and other debilitating diseases.

As a community project, TR-Bios require two types of coordinators: (1) Coordinators to identify interested students; (2) Coordinators to supervise the student volunteers on location at a care facility (e.g., a nursing home) where Alzheimer's and other patients reside. The first category of coordination is already in place at high schools. Today, most high school students see it as obligatory to have a community service experience to get into college, and most high schools require such an experience. As a result, high schools have appointed coordinators to arrange volunteer experiences for their students. The TR-Bio process can easily tap into this existing coordination structure. Similarly colleges, in their efforts to be responsive to their communities, have established coordinator positions to facilitate student volunteerism.

The second category of coordination is also already in place. Today, most nursing homes, assisted-living facilities, continuing-care retirement communities, day programs, and other congregate care programs where Alzheimer's and other patients reside have paid activities coordinators who specialize in arranging and supervising a wide range of quality-of-life-enhancing experiences for residents at these facilities. TR-Bios could easily and desirably fit into these built-in activities programs, under their supervision.

The remaining costs are largely those of equipment. As discussed above, TR-Bios can be created on a shoestring budget, requiring little more than a video camera, which many families already have, and which most nursing homes, if encouraged, should certainly be able to provide. Local businesses should be approached, either through members of their boards of directors or directly through the community or public relations department, to help establish editing labs or supply equipment through private donations.

BIOGRAPHY AS THERAPY AND HISTORY

TR-Bios not only promote positive interaction and connectedness for the terminally ill patient, but also leave the family with a well-organized legacy of memories and family history that might otherwise have been lost. The TR-Bio can help the family work through the cognitive losses and eventual mortality of their loved one. They also are left with this unique biography, a poignant exit gift, so to speak, from the one whom they have lost. In this context, the TR-Bio illustrates how biography can be as important as biology in the overall approach to intervening in Alzheimer's and other degenerative and terminal diseases. At a family level, TR-Bios reflect the late-life poetry of William Carlos Williams: they contribute to an old age that can add as it takes away.

The Creativity Discovery Corps

You can make a lasting contribution to your community and enable others to do the same in years to come by creating a community-wide action plan for cultivating and celebrating creativity through a Creativity Discovery Corps. (See Chapter 7) This is public creativity—creativity with a "big *C*"—and it grows by encouraging creative contributions by all members of the community. This strengthens sense of community and enhances relationships through collaborative and intergenerational creativity and strengthens the older adult roles of keepers of culture and kin.

Take a young person out to lunch and catch up on the latest new phrases and hit tunes of the day that you might have missed.

To start a Creativity Discovery Corps of your own:

- Study the model for the original Creativity Discovery Corps presented in Chapter 7 for ideas.
- Identify the human and material resources available in your community.
- Define your own objectives for a similar program.
- Don't let setbacks shut you down. In any community, there is a need and the resources for a Creativity Discovery Corps. Start however small you must to make a go of it. Once established, the program will grow because it builds, strengthens, and affirms the best qualities of community.

The following profile of the Center on Aging, Health & Humanities Creativity Discovery Corps is offered as a guide to help other communities interested in replicating efforts or in establishing programs with related goals.

Dr. Barbara Soniat and I launched the Creativity Discovery Corps in 1997 as part of the Center on Aging, Health & Humanities, which I was directing at George Washington University (GW). Though formally under the GW Center, the Corps immediately established many partnerships with agencies, programs, and groups that became official cosponsors. The cosponsors included IONA Senior Services, a large community-based agency in Northwest Washington providing a wide diversity of professional and volunteer services to older persons; The

Washington, D.C., Area Geriatric Education Consortium, a federally funded coalition of all the major medical centers in Washington, D.C., providing continuing education and training focused on aging; the National Council for the Traditional Arts, Art Project Renaissance, a creative writing program for older persons; and a wide range of other programs ranging from residential care settings for older persons to academic programs at George Washington University, including the Art Therapy Program and the Program in American Studies, which houses the Oral History Program.

As you can see, the idea generated a tremendous amount of support from a variety of organizations and programs. Meanwhile the list of cosponsors continues to grow.

The Creativity Discovery Corps is an unfunded voluntary group, for which participating agencies have freed employee time to help carry out the work of the Corps. Other volunteers not affiliated with any particular agency simply give their time. Resources are essentially those contributed by the volunteer members with the help of a small outside monetary gift to the Corps. In the future we will apply for grants to cover the costs of a paid executive coordinator, at least part-time, and other expenses.

Because there is no outside funding, cosponsorship relationships become very important. IONA Senior Services, for example, has been an exemplary cosponsor, providing at no cost a small dedicated area for office and filing space; they have also contributed the use of a phone line and a computer and allow the Corps to use one of their conference rooms for its monthly meetings. IONA views the goals of the Corps as compatible with their overall mission.

Establishing a mission statement and objectives for the Creativity Discovery Corps. While taking organizational form, we began to prepare statements on our perspective, mission, and objectives.

Perspective: Creativity in later life has been greatly unrecognized—both its potential and its prevalence. When we become aware that age does not affect human potential, we change the way we prepare for our own future development, and also influence how society nurtures and benefits from its older human resources.

Mission: The mission of the Creativity Discovery Corps is fourfold:

1. To identify older persons whose creative work or ideas have been undiscovered and to provide visibility for their contributions;

2. To identify older persons whose creative work or ideas have not received adequate recognition and to provide added visibility for their contributions;

3. To identify and disseminate the best practices of programs, groups, and individuals in the community whose efforts create opportunities for older persons to explore, discover, and tap their human potential;

4. To provide opportunities for volunteers of all ages to be creative in their efforts to discover both unidentified older talent and innovative community catalysts fostering such talent.

Objectives: The intergenerational experience ensures that:

- Older persons may continue their creative growth
- We may celebrate and benefit from the achievements of these individuals, who often serve as *keepers of the culture*
- Negative stereotypes of aging may be dispelled
- More older persons can become role models for those at any age to explore creative potential

In short, the Creativity Discovery Corps targets the creative efforts of three groups: (1) creative older persons themselves; (2) programs that creatively foster the release of human potential in older individuals, and (3) volunteers who are creative in their efforts to promote both the visibility of talented older persons and the best practices of programs that help older persons to be creative.

Which older persons are candidates for the efforts of the Creativity Discovery Corps? There are three broad groups that capture most, though not all, of the candidates:

1. Those whose life history provides an unusual model for others; this category also includes those whose work, activities, or ideas have contributed to the preservation of their local or broader culture, like Ms. Jackie Griffith (see page 218), whose collection of artifacts and memorabilia has made an invaluable contribution in preserving and capturing African-American life in the nation's capital for most of the 20th century.

2. Those whose work, activities, or ideas reflect creativity in the domains of the expressive arts, including painting, sculpture, writing, poetry, music, and dance.

3. Those whose work, activities, or ideas reflect creativity in the domains of material culture, like the creation of a remarkable number of fashionable hats by Dorothy Lewis (see page 217).

How do you identify programs in the community that might offer special programming that promotes creativity in older individuals? A survey is a good way to start.

Document a day in your life. Take a camera with you and photograph events or scenes that offer a sense of a typical day in your life. After you get your prints back, put them in a scrapbook and write a story about each one. You have the option of creating a drama, a comedy, even an epic. Don't shy away from candor and good humor.

The surveys could be handed out at lectures on aging, where people connected to such programs might be attending. Checking with colleagues who work with older adults is helpful, asking them whether they have come across such programs; if so, send each potential program they identify a survey.

General features to include would be recruitment efforts aimed at attracting older participants and responsiveness to special needs experienced by some older individuals (e.g., providing transportation or outreach if necessary). Another general feature would be to ensure that those carrying out the program have had special training or experience in working with older persons.

Other questions for your checklist: Does it foster freedom, experimentation, spontaneity, innovation? Conversely, does it avoid patronizing programming (e.g., components or exercises that infantilize the older individual)? Does the program include an opportunity for feedback by participants and an evaluation process to help it meet its goals? (For more information on the Creativity Discovery Corps, see Appendix D—Center on Aging, Health & Humanities.)

Why I Prescribe Creativity as the Ultimate Natural "Supplement"

As a physician, a scientist, and a public policy advisor, I have often been asked why I chose to write a book about creativity rather than more traditional aspects of medicine, research, or politics. My answer comes from my experience in all three realms and from my belief that we each have an enormous and largely untapped source of healing energy that can better our lives in profound ways.

We live in a period during which the field of medicine has been making enormous leaps with wondrous new diagnostic procedures, powerful new drugs, and remarkable new surgical procedures. But these advances are largely aimed at treating disease or disorders, and the truth is that we can go only so far in altering the course of various disorders. In confronting these diseases and disabilities on a daily basis in my work, I have been challenged to look beyond my patients' clinical problems and limitations, to their everyday strengths and potential. This has taken me into the realm of creativity, even in the face of illness. Over the course of years, I have been struck by how the opportunity for an individual to draw upon inner resources and accomplish something new helped them cope with—and at times transcend—the effects of a disorder that prevented them from accomplishing what they were used to in a different area.

I have seen creative growth transform lives at every age and under vastly differing life circumstances. I have seen creative growth in terminally ill patients; the potential for joy in self-discovery and expression excludes no one. When we focus on this potential, we create a new synergy when coupled with attention to health problems, a synergy that advances our capacity to cope with illness and our ability to promote healthier aging. It is this wide-open human potential that I hope each of my patients and my readers can find and use to light their lives.

Also, I am moved by a sense of history and the power of human expectation. I feel we are at a new historic turning point in how we view aging, a turning point that is influencing our expectations and our sense of possibilities associated with advancing years. In addition to

Write daily in a journal. If you are not comfortable writing, then some other building process should be substituted, such as sewing, woodwork, etc. The regular, ongoing engagement in the activity provides a powerful concrete example of how much you yourself can influence your sense of satisfaction in everyday life. And it provides a genuine, reliable sense of accomplishment.

recognizing the ability to alter many health problems in later life, there is an emerging sense that beyond the problems are possibilities. This recognition is important, because it redefines our outlook on aging. It leads us to expect more from our lives and from each other as we shape our communities and social policy. It encourages us to begin now to plan for older age, not just in the financial sense that has been the traditional focus of "retirement years," but in the quality of our lives, including relationships, personal growth, and creative contribution. The timing has never been better. My hope is that the readers, too, recognize this historic change occurring in their midst and seize the moment to turn to this labor of love—awakening undeveloped potential.

We still face misconceptions and negative stereotypes about aging that produce doubts in others as well as in ourselves as to our ability to continue to experience creative potential and growth with aging. Then, too, there may be unresolved emotional conflicts that interfere with our exploring new territory, making us feel helpless or hopeless. Sometimes we get lazy, losing sight of the fact that what can be added with aging is worth the effort—no different than the obstacles and advantages surrounding effort at any age. All of these impediments are movable throughout the life cycle. It may take a little time, some new training, perhaps a bit of therapy, but it's all doable. And today's aging population group is the healthiest, best educated, and most resourceful ever.

Humor is liberating. Use it liberally. It loosens the muscles and frees the mind to make new connections.

Just recently I participated in a conference on creativity and aging and met a ninety-eight-year-old woman who was a retired legal secretary. An art exhibit that accompanied the conference featured some finely sculpted owls—all the work of this retired secretary now sculptor. All the more impressive was that she was sculpting despite visual impairment. She said she could feel the shapes and had such vivid images of the sights and sounds of barnyard owls from growing up as a young girl on a farm that their images were permanently implanted and virtually tangible in her mind, not unlike Beethoven experiencing beautiful sounds from within despite his external deafness in composing his Ninth Symphony.

I asked her when she first got involved with art. She said at age ninety-five. I asked her if she had done any artwork at all before then.

She said none, and didn't know why, whether it was not having the time or confidence—she wasn't sure. Then she sighed.

"What did I do with those ninety-five years?"

"I suspect you did a lot," I responded, "and what is so exciting is what you are doing now."

This is what the future holds for each of us: the potential for experience and insight to join with dreams and inspiration to create a richer, more satisfying life—beginning *now*.

Conclusion: Toward the Future

It is never too late to be what you might have been.

—GEORGE ELIOT

WHEN FEMINIST ACTIVIST GLORIA Steinem turned forty, someone remarked with thoughtless flattery that she didn't look her age. "This is," she retorted, "what forty looks like."

By defying the stereotypes and defining her age in terms of her own reality, Steinem was among the bellwether voices of our era to sound a new, more positive attitude toward aging. Forget traditional pressures to demur and follow a quieter, more compliant model of "aging gracefully." This new view of aging reflected an expectation of continued physical and intellectual vitality, continued creativity and contribution.

Today, as the ranks of those fifty and older is burgeoning with boomers, and retirement is just another word for career change, aging continues to be redefined. Science, medicine, and social advances provide a new and constantly changing landscape for aging. A dawning awareness of our inner lives and our untapped capacity for growth adds an even richer dimension to the picture.

What's next? What will fifty—or sixty, seventy, eighty, ninety and beyond—look like one hundred years from now? How about two hundred years from now, really just a few more generations down the road? I am often asked to speculate about the future and the influences that will shape the course of aging and the flow of creativity in later life with the progress of the twenty-first century. I see the future shaped by the push and pull of human desire, in this case the desperate push for longer life—more years—and the backward pull of negative stereotypes and shortsighted public policy reflecting our all-too-human fear of change and resistance to new ideas. As we move through the next century and beyond, the landscape for aging and creativity will be shaped by the way in which society balances its commitment to improve the quality of people's lives as it strives to increase the quantity of their years.

The tension inherent in this balancing act is not new to the twenty-first century, but in fact was the focus of an ancient Greek myth more than twenty-five centuries ago—the myth of Tithonos.

Tithonos, a mortal and the son of Laomedon, king of Troy, fell in love with Eos, goddess of dawn. Being immortal, Eos fretted that she would eventually outlive her lover, Tithonos, so she went to almighty Zeus, king of the gods of Mount Olympus, to plead for immortality for Tithonos. Zeus granted her wish, but alas, as the scores of years went by, Eos realized that she had neglected to also ask Zeus to bestow eternal youth upon Tithonos. Hence, to this day, Tithonos continues to grow older and older, and more and more frail. This twenty-five-century-old story captures one of the most critical ethical and scientific concerns in society and the field of aging in our struggle to assure that quality of life keeps pace with quantity.

This book has been all about what we can do to add to the quality of those years through the pursuit of creativity—with a big C or a little c. If we want to improve our aging bodies and minds, we don't have to wait for medical miracles or chase after the newest fad in antiaging products. You can take all the wonder pills and use all the creams that promise to alter the course of aging, and if they work at all, their effects will pale compared to that of a single continuing education course that stimulates your thinking and motivates you to try something new and interesting. Throughout the second half of life our psyches continue to develop in ways that improve our ability to gain access to our inner potential. This inner growth won't just happen on its own, but knowing that the potential is there can motivate us in powerful ways.

The Promise and Limits of the New Frontier: Research Affecting Aging in the Future

The change in attitude that allows us even to recognize there is creative potential in aging is a milestone for our culture. Remember that in the not very distant past the predominant view of aging was strictly one of diminishing health and opportunity. The biggest change that has occurred in society in relation to aging has not been a fundamental genetic discovery that enables scientists to alter the course of aging, but a fundamentally new recognition of the power we have to grow and transform our lives as we age.

I emphasize this not to diminish the promise of biological research. Rather, the glamour of these studies has been so great that it has distracted us from what is possible in the present, shining the light on tomorrow's hopes rather than today's deliverables. Remember, too, that the more than 50 percent increase in life expectancy in the twentieth century was not the result of genetic discoveries, but improved public health practices, sound health habits, and better medical care.

There remain those who insist that if we can just find that elusive gene that controls aging, we can manipulate it to buy ourselves a kind of eternal youth. But to expect that changing one gene would change the course of aging in humans is to expect that you can alter the music for one instrument in an orchestra and create a new symphony without disrupting the intricate beauty and timing of the original one. One gene may make a difference in a worm, but it does not follow that the same applies to men and women. Further, if one gene could make a big difference, we would expect that over the lengthy course of evolution someone would have had a gene mutation unleashing longer life. There is no evidence that there has been any exception to what presently appears to be an approximately 130-year upper limit to the human life span.

The greatest promise of genetic research lies in altering our susceptibility to certain diseases, and it is here that the research is most exciting and perhaps most imminent. If we can use gene therapy to mitigate or cure a disease that affects the quality of aging, then we enhance our life experience and creative potential. But, based on our understanding of genetics at this time, to genetically alter the aging process itself would require that we manipulate more than a hundred different genes, each responsible for some link in the process, and then modify these genes in a highly synchronized manner. This would be an extremely complicated feat, and not one likely to be accomplished anytime soon. Finally, it should be pointed out that our biological and genetic complexity is a good thing. It brings stability to the species. If it were so easy to break the lock on our genetic coding, then our species would be chaotic indeed. A constant battery of mutations would create a hodgepodge of physical and mental "versions" of a human, and would make it more difficult for our species to survive in the long run.

Quantity of Years versus Quality of Aging: The Ancient Role Models

The mythological Tithonos, whose story I shared, added only adversity in the form of frailty to his advancing years. His mythological counterpart Tiresias, whose story appeared in Chapter 6, found new potential and achievement in old age despite extreme adversity. Which story reflects your outlook? If we limit our view of the future to already outdated present-day stereotypes, then we steep in pessimism and limit our potential. But the history of futures has consistently been one of surprises, despite doubts and dire predictions by some of the most informed in their respective fields. Consider the following historic views of future events that turned out differently than was anticipated by experts:

Everything that can be invented has been invented.
—Charles H. Duell, Director of U.S. Patent Office, 1899

Sensible and responsible women do not want to vote.
—Grover Cleveland, 1905

Who the hell wants to hear actors talk?
—Harry M. Warner, Warner Bros Pictures, 1927

There is no likelihood man can ever tap the power of the atom.
—Robert Millikan, Nobel prize in physics, 1923

Heavier-than-air flying machines are impossible.
—Lord Kelvin, President, Royal Society, 1895

Ruth made a big mistake when he gave up pitching.
—Tris Speaker, 1921

The horse is here today, but the automobile is only a novelty—a fad.
—President of Michigan Savings Bank, advising against investing in the Ford Motor Company

Video won't be able to hold on to any market it captures after the first six months. People will soon get tired of staring at a plywood box every night.

—Daryl F. Zanuck, 20th Century Fox, commenting on television in 1946

What use could the company make of an electric toy?

—Western Union, when it turned down rights to the telephone in 1878

Hazel Henderson understood the phenomenon, commenting, "If we can recognize that change and uncertainty are basic principles, we can greet the future and the transformation we are undergoing with the understanding that *we do not know enough to be pessimistic*." Today's latest data reveal that as life expectancy has crept upward, the disability rate in later life has fallen, contrary to pessimistic predictions. While researchers work to unlock the secrets of aging, we need not rely on ancient myths for optimism; vibrant role models are all around us. We need not follow Tithonos' path of empty added years. We can find our inspiration for fruitful aging in Tiresias or the artist Titian or the many men and women whose stories fill the pages of this book.

Wanted: New Metaphors for Aging

Because expectations so powerfully shape our experience, we need to replace the outdated stereotypes and language of old age with new metaphors for aging. I personally find the story of artist Georgia O'Keeffe especially inspiring.

Various O'Keeffe biographers have described different anxieties she experienced, one of them being a fear of flying. As she grew more famous and as she had increasing demands to appear for shows and presentations around the world, her need to fly increased. One day, when she was in her late seventies, O'Keeffe gazed admiringly out the window of a plane at a formation of the clouds below. She recalled later that she suddenly realized at that moment that her fear of flying had disappeared. She was exhilarated. The experience provided a new direction for her art and the result was a huge exhibit—the biggest in her lifetime—consisting of ninety-six works. Among them was a series with paintings as large as 8 by 24 feet. The images in this series were inspired by the view from her airplane window; they were beautiful, semiabstract paintings of huge clouds in a blue sky. She titled them *Sky Above Clouds*. Old age was no "winter of life" for O'Keeffe; her art was not crippled by her age. Rather, her age, experience, and openness to new ideas allowed her to see the blue sky above the clouds. I believe that aging in the twenty-first century will increasingly show us the blue sky above clouds in the expression of human potential despite age-associated problems.

From Metaphors to Models: Centenarians as the Fastest-Growing Age Group

At the age of 104 retired teacher Sarah Delany collaborated with her 102-year-old sister, retired dentist Dr. Bessie Delany, to write *Having Our Say: The Delany Sisters' First 100 Years*. It was a wonderful example of the summing-up human potential phase facilitating autobiographical creative expression carried out collaboratively after one hundred. The book became a *New York Times* best-seller and a Broadway hit. In 1994, the sisters, at 105 and 103, published a sequel, as they drew upon the potential for creative expression associated with the encore human potential phase.

Two years later Bessie Delany died, and suddenly, for the first time in over a century, Sarah Delany felt alone. Among her creative coping strategies was, at the age of 107, another encore human potential phase product, writing the book *On My Own at 107*. Her struggle to adapt in new ways in order to stay healthy is reflected in the following excerpt from her book:

> The unthinkable happened. I felt like someone had cut off my arms. Somebody said, "There's probably nobody on Earth who has lived together for so long!"—the longest human relationship. And I'm thinking that may well be true. So, I'm charting new ground, Bessie.

George Abbott (1887–1995), the American director of theater and film, playwright, actor, and producer, was viewed as the dean of Broadway showmen. His career spanned more than eight decades and 120 productions. These productions included *Love 'em and Leave 'em*, 1925 (at age thirty-eight); *The Boys from Syracuse*, 1935 (at age forty-eight); *Damn Yankees*, 1955 (at age 68); *A Funny Thing Happened on the Way to the Forum*, 1962 (at age 75). The shows he was involved with accrued an awesome forty Tony Awards, including five for him.

At age 101 (1989), he directed a new musical, *Frankie*, for which he also wrote the book; *Frankie* was a two-act musical remake of *Frankenstein*, taking place in Westchester County, New York. Shortly before he died, he collaborated on a Broadway revival of

Damn Yankees, at the age of 107, reflecting a final encore human potential phase creative accomplishment.

Centenarians are the fastest-growing age group. In 1900 only one in 100,000 Americans were one hundred years old or older. By the year 2000, that number had grown tenfold or more, with at least one in 10,000 Americans reaching one hundred. Scientists estimate that by the year 2050, this number could increase another ten or even twentyfold. We have as many as 50,000 centenarians in America today, and by the middle of the twenty-first century there could be as many as 1 million. And, everyone who will be one hundred then is alive today.

The impact of this growing age group is without precedent; only time will tell how they will shape our literature, music, science, politics, our families, and our communities. Whatever else they do with their numbers and experience, though, their larger presence resets the clock on our expectations of a future. That, in turn, profoundly influences how we plan and fantasize about what's to come and what can be expected in our later years. Research indicates that centenarians are enjoying increasingly good health longer than was possible historically. To the extent that these men and women are modeling extreme old age with vitality, our sense of what is possible in later life is elevated even more. All of this contributes to a psychological feedback loop that can motivate us to start planning for our future even earlier than before, knowing that the health, education, work, and lifestyle choices we make earlier in life may significantly improve the quality of our increasingly long lives.

The Creative Challenge for Society: Create a New Landscape for Aging in the Twenty-first Century

If we view our aging adults as a national resource of talent and creativity, then the challenge for our society is to cultivate that resource and tap it for the common good. In terms of public policy and in many other ways on the whole, society has not yet risen to a sense of challenge or responsibility to maximize the benefits of this enormous and growing national resource. Societies strive to be creative in how they develop educational and recreational opportunities for children and young adults, in how they plan for further residential and business development in their communities, in how they provide for public health and safety, and so forth. But they have not brought to bear the same creativity in looking at the needs and contributions of middle age and older populations—even less so from an intergenerational perspective.

Despite the sluggish pace of change in government and public policy, many local communities and the consumer-driven marketplace are blazing the trail of change into this new landscape for aging. The Creativity Discovery Corps discussed in Chapter 7 and other similar programs illustrate a creative response on the part of a community to foster and benefit from the human potential of older persons. Residential lifestyle options are blossoming, reflecting a fundamental diversification and expansion underway in the settings where older persons reside. These creative options include innovations in independent living, the rapid growth of very diverse retirement communities, assisted-living facilities, continuing-care retirement communities, and naturally occurring retirement communities in neighborhoods or buildings that simply attract a large number of retirement-age individuals. When residential and vacation communities attract retirees as well as affluent singles, couples, and families with children, we see a new form of the traditional multigenerational community, and with it the benefits of intergenerational creativity.

But research has been thin and planning inadequate to understand how they affect the inner and outer lives of older persons and their relationships with their families and other age groups in general. Among the questions in need of greater discussion at all levels of society are:

- What can society at all levels—policy makers, local community planners, and families alike—do to defuse further the numerous myths and stereotypes about aging and the potential for creative contributions independent of age?
- What can society at all levels do to promote further opportunities for those in the second half of life to explore their potential—both for their own benefit and for that of their communities?
- What can society do at all levels to promote further innovative and rewarding forms of intergenerational interaction—in living arrangements, work, social activities, education, and recreation?

The landscape is changing dramatically, and in many ways for the better, but we don't as a society have a sense of the territory or what to do with it in order to support meaningful change and plans for the future.

The growing new awareness of human potential in the second half of life and the recognition of rising change in lifestyles with aging should be a wake-up call for society to seize the moment and proactively bring creativity to the community planning table. Never before in numbers, diversity, or capacity have older individuals presented society with such an opportunity to nurture and draw upon a great new national resource.

More than ever before, creative planning from a full life cycle perspective is likely to pay off not only in improved quality of life for persons in the second half of life, but in greater cohesiveness for families and communities. We need to pay attention to the enormous potential of our aging population and to better understand the unique issues and opportunities that exist in the increasingly diverse settings where they spend their everyday lives in the new landscape for aging. We have a major new national resource in our midst. And as President Franklin Delano Roosevelt keenly pointed out, "No country, however rich, can afford the waste of its human resources."

The Universal Value of the Creativity in Aging

The most important finding about creativity with aging is its essential universality. For instance, everybody dreams. When we study dreams, or even just talk about them, we see the richness, complexity, and mystery they hold; we catch a glimpse of the creative powers of the dynamic unconscious. Our dreams illustrate our inherent creative potential, complex and mysterious, but also rich and real.

The universality of creativity with aging is also illustrated in the many everyday profound experiences that younger persons experience around older ones. Let me illustrate with two examples, the first one little *c* public, the second one little *c* personal.

Recently, a big media story in the Washington, D.C., area involved a talented sophomore college basketball player indicating that he was going to accept an offer by one of the National Basketball Association teams to turn pro. There had been much speculation about what he was going to do. For a long time he denied that he would go pro before finishing college. The local media played up this promise, emphasizing his importance to his college team and fellow players, the importance of a commitment, and that of completing one's education. There was an unabashed use of guilt to influence him to stay. Then the sophomore, after a great season, announced he was indeed going pro. The media punished him with an endless rehash of his earlier promise. Then an interview took place in which one of the sports reporters confronted him and asked him directly to explain how he came to his decision, why he changed his mind. His answer almost immediately ended the media harangue.

He explained that he had thought long and hard about the choice, which was a difficult one because of all the reasons that the media had outlined. But then he had discussed it with his grandmother, who, after a careful review of all the pros and cons, advised him that it was a tough decision, but that it was in his best interest to accept the offer now; she said he could always go back to school later. He said he greatly valued his grandmother's advice. End of discussion. The ongoing media harangue ceased instantly. The abrupt stop of the media assault made a strong statement about the creative influence an older person can have on important decisions and public reactions. This was creativity with a little c exerting a powerful punch.

The second example arose with the death of my father. At his funeral I read a eulogy that I had written about him. Although I have given numerous talks, this was my most difficult to get through. To prepare the eulogy I had gone through his thick navy scrapbook, cover to cover, Among the things that struck me were the discharge papers he received from the national guard, in which he served after leaving the navy. Looking at his scrapbook was a very profound experience for me; my father was the same age then as my son Alex at the time I wrote the eulogy. On my father's discharge form was a section—the only one in bold type—titled "Character." Next to that heading was a word, spelled out in capitalized letters: *EXCELLENT*. It was true. Even in his painful experience of Alzheimer's disease, my father never lost his character. It showed through in abundance and was part of his creative legacy.

Stories like these remind us of the creative dignity that older persons bring to their families and their communities. Again, it is creativity with a little *c*, but creativity that lives long in memory, influence, and effect on a family's sense of identity. It is this social creativity that is often one of the most powerful benefits of growing older. My hope—indeed my prediction—is that this profound sense of human dignity and appreciation for life that so often occurs in our encounters with those at an advanced age will one day, with the increased numbers of the very old, successfully draw us from our tendencies toward hate, killing, and war, toward a more enlightened age of human relations. It is my belief that the growing social creativity, the grace and the spirit of the old, combined with their wider presence as a growing population group, will bring more character, more integrity, to our society.

A Creative Age for Each of Us, a New Age for Humanity

We are at a most exciting time in history—a time unparalleled in the long trail of human existence—when the advances in public health, nutrition, overall health habits, medical technology, and science have expanded our opportunity for greater years and greater experience. Generations before us had neither the time nor the technology to explore the wonders of older living the way we do now. We are entering a new era of social living, with population growth exploding in the fifty-plus population, expected to double from 1990 to 2030, and with new opportunities afforded to older people to express themselves and fulfill their creative needs.

The walls of ageism are being torn down, brick by brick, with each example of an older person accomplishing, contributing, enjoying, changing, growing, *creating* new facets of life. We can look for inspiration to the widely recognized creativity of people like Georgia O'Keeffe or George Burns. We can look closer to home, in our communities, where new contributions and friendships result from intergenerational creativity. Finally, we can look inward, and, like many of the men and women in this book, find in ourselves the capacity for creative growth and expression that can uplift our lives and inspire others. Truly, this is a creative age, for humanity and for each of us, whether we are fully retired, on the verge of retirement, or still in the prime of our young adult life. Our willingness to embrace the challenge and the opportunity will define the legacy that each of us builds, and the gift that each of us gives, in every season of our lives.

APPENDIX A

Why Do We Age? Biology's Creative Mystery

WHILE SOME OF THE information that follows was presented in the chapters of the book, it is revisited here in more detail for readers who enjoy more background.

Why Do Living Things Age?

To ask why living things age is to pose two questions: (1) What is the purpose of aging? In other words, are there advantages to aging that outweigh its disadvantages? What would be the consequences of not aging? (2) What are the mechanisms, the biological processes, that make us age, and what factors influence this process? The short of it is that we do not have a definitive answer to either question. As for biological explanations of aging, experts have elaborated on more than a dozen, ten of which I present here. All of them have inherent flaws. I have been tracking the biological theories since 1971, when I formally entered the field of gerontology, and have never encountered a mystery that even comes close to matching this one. It is so cleverly and creatively crafted that this alone may be the main reason I have remained in the field for nearly three decades.

As for the purpose of aging, scientists cannot agree about whether it is adaptive or nonadaptive. That is, whether aging is necessary for the survival of the species. Some scientists argue that if animals did not age and die, there would be overcrowding and eventually a shortage of food and other essentials to go around (adaptive). On the other hand, those who believe aging is not essential believe that many animals fail to live to old age owing to the rigors of their environment. Hence, they don't need aging to control their numbers (nonadaptive).

Of course, with humans, the story is different. It is easier to see how aging is an adaptive or survival response. The following fairy tale, reconstructed by the psychiatric researcher Allan Chinen, illustrates this point of view:

> Once upon a time, a great king went hunting with his comrades. They stopped for lunch at the summit of a hill. The king lamented the thought of his own death, and how he would lose his royal possessions. His nobles also bemoaned the thought of their deaths. One among them laughed, however. The king ignored the laughter and went on to wish for immortality. His lords chimed in in agreement, but the last noble laughed again. The lords demanded to know the reason for their comrade's laughter, but he would not explain. Finally, the king himself demanded the reason. The lord acquiesced and said he was thinking about what it would be like if they all lived forever. In that case, the First King would still be alive, and the Great Sage, and all the other heroes of history. Compared to them, the King would only be a clerk, and they, only peasants! That thought made him laugh. After a tense moment, the king raised his drinking glass and penalized the other nobles two draughts of wine each for encouraging his royal vanity.

Like the myth of Tithonus, which was discussed in the Conclusion, this fairy tale reminds us of the social complexities brought about by immortality. It makes the adaptive point of view much easier to understand in man, yet it is another matter for mice and other animals, big and small. They all age.

Not All Living Things Age

Mice and men age for adaptive or nonadaptive reasons, but not all living things age alike, certainly not in duration. For that matter, not all living things age. The variation is remarkable, from under twenty-four hours for the common mayfly to over 2400 years for the giant sequoia in the western United States. Aging is not apparent among more primitive species. In fact, growth does not appear to stop. Various fish (including sharks and sturgeon) and amphibians (alligators), certain tortoises, and sponges all exhibit these unusual characteristics of adding years, but not aging in the conventional sense.

Among those species that do not appear to age, death is more closely associated with increased risks related to time and environment, as opposed to aging and compromising internal biological changes. The longer a fish lives, for example, the greater risk it runs of being caught by a fisherman. These species are more the exception than the rule, however. With most living things aging is apparent, and in pursuing the reasons for the aging process, scientists have arrived at a host of theories.

Biological Theories of Aging

Gerontologist Leonard Hayflick, an active major contributor to our understanding of underlying mechanisms of aging, believes that aging theories fall into two broad groups: "Those that presume a preexisting master plan, and those based on random events." In other words, we age because we are programmed that way or because of outside factors. As we follow the different pathways proposed by different theories, we become increasingly aware of the extraordinary mystery of aging; it is a veritable whodunit with all the suspects and confusing clues that one finds in any great mystery. The magnitude of the mystery, the great curiosity about it, the glamour that would be associated with cracking it, and the universal interest in aging—since it so profoundly affects each of us—help explain why gerontology has become such a popular field. Let's look at a number of the respective theories about aging.

THE GENETIC PROGRAMMING THEORY

The attention given to the field of genetics has never been greater. Not surprisingly—right or wrong—we are attributing more human physical and behavioral traits to genetics. One of the leading theories on aging is that the process of aging is genetically programmed, genetically built in. After all, why should house mice consistently have around three years as their upper limit of longevity, while humans can live to be over 100? The remarkable consistency in the life span of a species suggests that there is a unique genetic coding for each species. With humans, for example, excluding Biblical references to people like Methuselah, nobody has ever been documented to have aged beyond 130 years. This points to remarkable stability within our biological system, again suggesting a built-in mechanism that determines the upper limits of our life span.

But aging is not the same as life span. An organism can show few significant signs of what is referred to as aging or senescence (changes associated with growing old), but still not exceed the life span. Indeed the goal of modern geriatrics is to allow people to achieve a "rectangular curve" of functioning where they function at essentially the same level until just before the end. In effect, the goal is "dying with our boots on." Historically, people have viewed aging as a process of gradual decline in multiple, if not all, areas of functioning; a normal curve illustrates this. But history has changed owing to improved public health practices, better general medical and geriatric care, and more informed personal health habits (e.g., improvements in diet and exercise along with reduction in smoking, excessive drinking, and other toxic factors). Hence, these factors are helping to shape the rectangular curve.

While a strong case can be made for the role of genetics, the nature of that role is not resolved. Genetics may influence the limits of our longevity, but it may not play as strong a role in influencing the quality of our path. This is not to say that genetics has little influence on the cause or course of aging. Rather, there seems to be more variability in how we might age as opposed to when we must end. For example, in the United States, life expectancy was less than fifty years in 1900. Life expectancy is defined by the average number of years (average longevity) of a given population group at a given point in history; it differs from life span—the upper limit of human age—which has not changed since the beginning of humankind. By 1990 in America, life expectancy had passed seventy-five years. This change, greater than a 50 percent increase in average longevity during the same century, was not caused by an internal genetic alteration, but instead to external environmental factors such as healthier practices and habits. Nurture influenced aging in the twentieth century more heavily than nature.

Genetic programming at the cellular level. Leonard Hayflick's research on cells was groundbreaking for the field of aging. Cells are studied by removing a small cluster—from someplace on the body like skin—and placing it into what is called a "cell culture." The culture consists of a special nutrient mix in a specially designed laboratory glassware container that enables the cells to continue living. In culture, typical cells are found to grow, divide, and increase in number. Until Hayflick's research, scientists thought that cells in culture could divide indefinitely. What Hayflick discovered, though, was something remarkable: After a certain number of divisions (in humans, approximately fifty), cells stop dividing. He found that cells slowly lose their capacity to function, stop dividing, and die. He concluded that the same phenomenon of aging occurs in humans as occurred in the individual cells. Hayflick emphasizes, though, that he does not believe that people age or die because their cells stop dividing. He believes the mystery force that causes aging in turn causes cells to stop dividing.

Studies like Hayflick's bring us closer to a more fundamental understanding of the mechanisms that influence the process of aging. Let's look further to where science has taken us. Hayflick's findings of cellular division raised the specter of some kind of biological clock at work. Scientists immediately began searching for it. The search led researchers to the tips of chromosomes found in the nucleus of the cell.

Chromosomes house genes—tens of thousands of them. At the tips of chromosomes are structures known as *telomeres,* which consist of DNA, but themselves do not give out genetic instructions. Curiously, each time a cell divides, the size of the old and new cells remains the same, but the length of the telomere in the new set of chromosomes is reduced. The telomere seems to be used up in the process of cell division.

Cells that do not exhibit shrinking telomeres are called immortal cells. They are also better known as cancer cells. These immortal cells produce an enzyme called *telomerase* that allows the regeneration of shrinking telomeres or the production of new ones. Scientists who observed this pattern artificially synthesized telomerase and applied it to normal cells. The result was increased cell longevity—a breakthrough in the field of aging, but in no way a technique that has a reverse-aging effect.

The more immediate questions of this finding apply for scientists in the field of cancer research. Will artificial telomerase induce cancer in a normal cell? Will findings from research on aging offer new approaches to altering telomerase activity in cancer cells? The telomere story illustrates a further opportunity provided by research on aging: to provide a new window on how we examine the human condition or health or illness independent of age. Studies of telomeres by gerontologists, on the one hand, can lead to new clues about aging associated with cells that stop dividing. At the same time, such research could lead to new avenues of cancer treatment, which would benefit all age groups. If we understand what makes normal cells stop dividing, we might come to understand how to intervene with those cells that divide abnormally.

When I was at the National Institute on Aging, defending the Institute's budget during Congressional testimony, I would occasionally be asked whether we as a society should be concerned about putting more money into research on aging. Might it affect money available for the study of problems of other age groups? I would often respond with the telomere story because it so poignantly shows how research on aging can benefit all age groups. The point was not lost at the hearings.

Meanwhile, the telomere story is still unfolding. For example, what inhibits telomerase in cells that stop dividing, and what allows them to rejuvenate or reproduce in immortal cells? Researchers are still investigating that question, the results of which may lead to breakthroughs in more than one field of health and medicine.

THEORIES ABOUT HORMONES AS CLOCKS OF AGING

"Death" hormones or hormonal clocks have been a strong focus of investigation since the late nineteenth century. These hormones are thought to increase longevity and/or improve the manifestations of aging. Phenomena like puberty and menopause are clock-like events; they have long raised the suspicion that the endocrine system produces hormones that determine this biological clock. When and how long we develop age-related changes are determined by these mystery hormones.

It is suspected that the state of the brain's neurons has a role in aging, and so, too, do the parts of the brain involved in hormonal activity, our neuroendocrine system. Puberty and menopause, for example, are directed by neuroendocrine events. But there are discrepancies when making these connections. Menopause occurs only in women, not men. Not all species that age possess neuroendocrine systems complex enough to influence the aging process. Finally, no one has found the smoking gun that clearly links the neuroendocrine system or identifies any purported death hormone with all age changes that scientists have discovered.

THE IMMUNE SYSTEM—ANOTHER BIOLOGICAL CLOCK THEORY

Given how fundamental immunity is to both the survival and quality of life of most living things, we see how change in immune function can obviously have significant consequences. Under the immunologic theory of aging, negative changes occur with deleterious effects building up over time. Responses of the immune system become less efficient, leading to increased vulnerability to infection and general breakdown.

As with other theories on aging, there are connections as well as discrepancies with the immune system theory. For example, research from the mind-body field—studying effects of the mind on the body—has identified a range of effects of psychological state on immune functioning. These effects seem to be mediated through the neuroendocrine system. Hence, the neuroendocrine system at times appears dominant over the immune system. Also, as in the case of the neuroendocrine system, various organisms that age have immune systems that appear too primitive to affect the nature and diversity of changes associated with aging.

ENTROPY, EXHAUSTION, AND WEAR-AND-TEAR THEORIES

One of the oldest theories of aging has been elaborated in at least three different ways—the "entropy" or "exhaustion" theory or the "wear-and-tear" theory. Not uncommonly, theories in one scientific field influence the formulation of theories in other fields. Hence prevailing theories in physics—particularly if they are highly significant or boldly innovative—might influence how concurrent theories are conceptualized in the fields of biology or psychology. The nineteenth century's impressive Second Law of Thermodynamics exerted such an impact. It contends that over time energy becomes increasingly unavailable to perform work or to maintain order—a quality described as entropy. Entropy explains the tendency for a physical system to run down or to move to a state of disorder caused by energy loss.

Late nineteenth- and early-twentieth-century theories on aging proposed similar explanations. Like a windup clock or a battery-operated device or a machine with a fixed energy reserve, the aging individual supposedly experienced a gradual exhaustion of capacity and efficiency over time. But there are problems with this theory. For example, regular work and exercise, which consume considerable energy, keep the individual in better shape, often increasing the interval between periods of exhaustion and allowing the person to look the better for wear.

CALORIC AND CROSS-LINKAGE THEORIES

Heavy caloric intake has been hypothesized to contribute to the aging process by leading to the buildup of harmful by-products that interfere with normal cell function. Heavy caloric diets cause abnormal biochemical cross-linkages among cells, impairing proper cell activity. For example, cross-linking could "clog" glandular cells, impeding the release of hormones and other essential cell products. In addition, caloric restriction in lower animals (mice, for example) can increase longevity—indeed life span. Critics of this theory emphasize the absence of any direct evidence showing that cross-linking is either essential or sufficient to explain the changes observed with aging.

THE FREE RADICAL THEORY

Not to be confused with political mavericks, "free radicals" refer to mischievous molecules that many believe cause biological mayhem. Free radicals are unstable molecules because they consist of an atom or groups of atoms that carry an unpaired electron. Electrons seek to pair. Hence, when free radicals interact with stable molecules they compete for one of the other molecule's electrons, thereby destabilizing the robbed molecule. According to the free radical theory of aging, this destabilization causes cellular damage, which gradually builds up over time and results in progressive deterioration in normal cell functioning and age-associated changes.

Antioxidant compounds, like vitamin E, keep free radical reactions in check. Antioxidants get their name from their ability to prevent oxygen from combining with vulnerable molecules to form damage-inducing free radicals known as *oxy-radicals.* Based on these claims, antioxidants have been used by individuals to try to retard the aging process.

Doubters of the free radical theory point to the lack of clear findings that antioxidants retard aging itself, as opposed to certain age-associated diseases. They also raise the possibility that many free radical reactions may not be deleterious—that cell products formed from these reactions may be harmless waste substances, themselves the focus of a dismissed theory on aging.

Genetic Mutation or Error Theory

DNA is nothing more than the genetic command center of a cell that tells it what to do and what proteins to produce. Hence, a radiation-induced mutation in the DNA could result in faulty instructions being given to the cell, such as a wrong protein being produced. Errors of this nature could build up to the point of compromised cell division or other impairment. Over time, this impairment in different cell types or organ systems across the body might then translate into what we know as aging.

The production of altered proteins could also trigger an autoimmune response. The organism may view the new protein as a foreign invader even though it is a part of its own cell. The immune system might weaken the cell to combat this invader, causing the cell to destabilize or be destroyed. As inviting as this theory sounds, critics point out that cells also contain the ability to repair DNA damage, mitigating the accumulated effects of mutations and errors. Even more important, cells can be specifically examined for the buildup of deleterious genetic effects. When examined, they fail to show the magnitude of changes or faulty proteins that one would expect to account for the range and depth of age-associated changes in the individual as a whole.

CONCLUSIONS ABOUT THEORIES OF AGING

Clearly there is no shortage of theories to explain the mystery of why we age. Each offers its own clues. Each theory appears to have a smoking gun that implicates it as a suspect in causing or contributing to the aging process. But each has one or more inconsistencies that keep us from fingering it as the ultimate culprit.

As alluded to earlier, it is difficult to determine whether a finding reflects cause or effect. Does the buildup of free radicals cause aging, or is it an effect? Do decrements in immune system activity influence aging, or does aging influence changes—a deconstruction of the immune system?

The number of ways these theories intersect with one another is both confusing and intriguing. Many do not appear to be mutually exclusive. For example, hormonal changes are suspected to play a role in aging; cross-linkages can interfere with endocrine system efficiency in the production or release of hormones. Free radicals are implicated in causing faulty protein formation, which can trigger an autoimmune response where the body doesn't recognize the protein as its own and attacks it; this is analogous to adverse events in the genetic mutation theory where resulting errors induce autoimmune responses. Genetic mutations can generate free radicals. Free radicals can induce cross-linkages. Cross-linkages can affect wear and tear or disorder. Is there a master mechanism of aging? We do not yet have an answer. Despite the glimmers of insight offered by continuing research, the more we understand, the more we understand the complexity of the mystery.

APPENDIX B

Historical Quests to Reverse the Effects of Aging

THIS APPENDIX BUILDS UPON the brief discussion in Chapter 9 of historical efforts to reverse aging or age-associated changes in the body and brain.

Throughout the world and throughout history, humans have tried to find a way to achieve longevity. That special pill, that magic potion or elixir, or that one procedure that promises longer life has been the subject of endless pursuit, the reason for vast amounts of wealth and countless lives to be spent in vain. It has been the subject of fortune as well as folly, the hopeful as well as the macabre. Typically, this quest to extend life has been associated with a linked triad of goals that includes the quest for creativity—enhancing the aging body, brain, and libido. As will become clear in this appendix, the search for a quick fix to the problems associated with aging (mainly death) are not unique to this century. The quest for solutions has a long, robust, and at times ignominious history.

These approaches have relied heavily on (1) ingestible and injectable substances and (2) bodily manipulations or surgical interventions. There are sometimes comical, sometimes tragic ways in which people have attempted to regain their youth.

Let's begin with ancient approaches and move forward to modern times.

Ingesting Animal Viscera for Vigor

The earliest recorded regimens for reversing aging are found in the *Ebers papyrus,* an Egyptian compilation of medical advice dating from around 1550 to 1800 B.C., representing one of the oldest known medical works. Noted for the vast number of remedies it offered—more than seven hundred—this famous scroll described interventions ranging from the treatment of crocodile bites to the extermination of house scorpions. Its recommendations on aging included recipes for ingesting the internal organs of young animals. The new youthful viscera would impart renewed vigor to the patient's own aging parts.

Mind-Enhancing Medicinal

From around 800 B.C. to 1000 A.D., medicine in India matured to an early golden age. Out of that productive period came the work of the great Hindu physician Sushruta and his medical treatise *Sushruta Samhita,* which elaborated on more than one thousand diseases and over seven hundred medicinals—the latter mainly derived from indigenous plants. One of these prescriptions included soma, a mountain plant likely valued for its exhilarating, mind-stretching, probably hallucinogenic effect. It is one of the earliest reported drugs prescribed to alter mental functioning caused by aging.

Fountains of Youth

Also around 700 B.C. Hindus attempted to find the restorative waters of the Pool of Youth. Stories of the Hindu Pool of Youth are associated with the legend of Cyavana, the aged and venerable priest, to whom Sukanya, the king's young daughter, was given in marriage. Increasingly distressed by their age difference, Cyavana sought the Pool of Youth, discovered it, bathed in it, and emerged youthful, handsome, and adorned with glittering jewelry.

Over two thousand years later Cranach the Elder painted the Fons Juventutis (the fountain of youth), while his contemporary, Juan Ponce de Leon, began his legendary sixteenth-century search for the same magical water source. While Ponce de Leon failed to locate the mythical fountain, he did discover Florida, whose warm waters have attracted retirement living for hundreds of thousands of people.

The early Europeans were also attracted to "healing waters," such as the hot springs at Bath, England, which were used by the Celts and then the Romans approximately two thousand years ago. These special sites in Bath remain a tourist attraction today. There is also a fascination with healthful mineral water, whether in the pools at health spas or in the bottles at supermarkets.

The Rejuvenating Power of a Virgin's Breath

Just as there has long been fascination with finding rejuvenating waters, there has been similar attraction to capturing a virgin's breath. The ancient Greeks and Romans in particular believed in the restorative powers of the virgin. The technique itself came to be known as "gerokomy," the stem (gero) of the word reflecting the focus on old age. The practice continued into the eighteenth century, where all over Europe people knew the prescription of the renowned Dutch physician and professor of medicine Hermann Boerhaave. According to Boerhaave, an old man should sleep between two virginal young women to regain health and vitality.

In the Bible (1 Kings, 1:2), it is written about the aging King David: "Let them seek out for my lord the king a young virgin, and let her stand before the king, and let her be an attendant on him; and let her lie in thy bosom, that my lord the king may become warm."

The interest in the power of breath and breathing continues today. In yoga, for example, awareness of one's breath and patterns of breathing play an integral role in many relaxation and meditation exercises. Like other forms of relaxation techniques, yoga is intended to improve quality of life, if not improve one's longevity.

From Alchemy to Snake Oil

One of the more familiar examples of antiaging techniques is that of the magic elixir or potion that promised renewed vigor and essence of youth. These pursuits fit into the category of alchemy. The central focus on alchemy lies with transmutation, transmuting or changing one form, substance, or condition into another. Alchemists historically attempted to transform sickness into health, poverty into wealth, uncertainty into foresight, tedium into talent, common metals into gold, old age into youth, languid desire into eroticism, and mortality into immortality. Two of the most vigorous attempts in alchemy were the conversion of common metals into gold and the quest for immortality. And though the practice of alchemy dates back thousands of years, there has been no documented success of either one.

The earliest attempt to achieve immortality through ingestible substances appears to go back to China in the fourth century B.C. A magical substance or potion is alluded to around that time. The actual term *elixir,* however, may first have been used only around the seventh century A.D., when alchemy was reported to have been introduced to Europe by the Arabs. The Arab name for miracle substances was "al iksir," which likely evolved into English as "elixir."

For the Chinese of the first century B.C., the most potent elixir was considered to be a solution containing flecks of gold. The Chinese also believed they could eat and drink their way to immortality by using gold utensils. The catch, though, was that the gold had to be transmuted from mercury in order to have transforming properties. The Chinese emperors who abided by this notion were unwittingly *shortening* their lives with mercury poisoning. It was not until the nineteenth century that scientists concluded that gold cannot be synthetically produced.

Around the seventh century A.D., China's most famous book on alchemy, *Tan Chin Yao Ch'eh* (*Great Secrets of Alchemy*), was published. This was around the same time that interest in alchemy was growing in Europe. This ancient Chinese text codified the recipes for potent elixirs. These included mercury, the salts of mercury, sulfur, and arsenic. Given the list of harmful ingredients in these mixes, it is not surprising that the practice of alchemy often resulted in curious fatalities.

One of alchemy's greatest proponents was the noted English Franciscan philosopher, scientist, and thirteenth-century scholar, Roger Bacon. He experimented with optics and knew how to make gunpowder and had speculative ideas about lighter-than-air flying machines, eyeglasses, microscopes, and telescopes. Bacon believed that owing to immorality and poor personal hygiene mankind lost the capacity for longevity that the Bible talked about before the Flood. Noah, for example, grandson of Methuselah—age 969, according to the Bible—lived, according to the same source, to approximately 950 years of age. Bacon cited numerous examples of individuals who experienced marked extensions of longevity and other changes after ingesting wondrous secret potions. One of his stories was about a man who after drinking a mysterious drug soon felt "renewed in mind and body beyond measure." Bacon himself never discovered a magical elixir, though he did live to nearly 80—an advanced age indeed for the late 1200s.

Around age sixty-five, Bacon was forced to serve time in prison by his fellow Franciscans because of certain "suspected novelties" (his excessive beliefs in alchemy and astrology and his attacks on his critics) in his teachings and writing. He continued writing productively after his release until his death.

Despite its misguided and often harmful remedies, alchemy can be credited for serving as the basis for modern chemistry and pharmacology. But even as alchemy faded in popularity, a new generation of potion pushers emerged to fill the void with their panaceas of dubious mixtures and snake oils.

Present-Day Wonder Drug Claims

Those of us in the late twentieth century have witnessed a panoply of purported wonder drugs. Many of these continue the long tradition of promising extended life and improved mental functioning and libido. The twentieth-century trendsetter was Gerovital, a substance found to be virtually indistinguishable from procaine hydrochloride (the anesthetic with the trade name Novocain). It was promoted in the 1950s by the late Professor Ana Aslan, a Romanian physician working at the Institute of Geriatrics in Bucharest. The compound was soon slightly modified to differentiate it from the anesthetic, and renamed Gerovital-H3. Its claims ranged from altering the course of aging to improving skin texture to bettering memory. Large numbers of individuals, convinced of the drug's many restorative features, flew to Bucharest to visit Dr. Aslan's institute. It was not until the 1970s, after more than thirty years of zealous prescribing, that definitive studies, supported by the National Institute of Mental Health in the

United States, showed that Gerovital's claims were false. At best, the drug was found to have mild antidepressant qualities.

Among the latest successors to Gerovital are human growth hormone, melatonin, and DHEA.

CONTRAPTIONS AND DEVICES

Cryonics and the cryo-capsule. The Cryonics Society became active in the 1960s. Its goal was to freeze people immediately upon dying—and, if legally permissible, just before dying—to preserve them for a time in the future when medical breakthroughs would restore their health and longevity. The term *cryonics* comes from the Greek *kryos,* or "icy cold." According to an early ad placed by the society, its goal was to achieve "biological immortality—a life of youthful vigor untempered by physical limitations." Its motto summarized the plan: "Freeze-Wait-Re-animate."

During the cryogenic process, a person was fit into a large cylinder called a cryo-capsule after having been placed in a state of deep freeze with liquid nitrogen. To an extent the concept was a modern-day counterpart to the mummification of the ancient Egyptians, who were placed in well-furnished tombs to ensure a smooth transition to the afterlife.

If the cost of the cryo-capsule was too prohibitive, a lower-budget alternative allowed one to preserve just the brain. Cryogenic proponents believed that science would become advanced enough to reconnect one's brain to a transplanted body. A basic problem with the procedure, however, was how to deep-freeze cells—especially brain tissue—without damaging them. The Cryonics Society outlined procedures to accomplish this task, but independent laboratories have emphasized that no matter how advanced the cryogenic equipment or process, tissue damage will result from extreme cold temperatures. To further tarnish the reputation of the cryogenics movement, some families and estates have filed lawsuits against these cryogenics laboratories for allowing bodies to "thaw" owing to mechanical error.

The concept of cryonics was just the latest version of the "Sleeping Beauty" theme (The French writer Charles Perrault was sixty-nine when in 1697 he wrote his version of the folk tale "The Sleeping Beauty"); variations on the theme go back to the myths of the ancient Greeks. In Greek mythology Endymion was placed in an eternal sleep by Zeus; the benefits of this uninterrupted slumber were a preservation of his good looks and immortality.

The Integratron. The Integratron was another immortality device invented in the 1960s by George W. Van Tassel, the former safety inspector for Howard Hughes. The

Integratron was promoted as a rejuvenation machine whose intricate formulae were allegedly conveyed to Van Tassel by a UFO rider. Thirty-eight feet high and fifty-three feet in diameter, it resembled an old-fashioned observatory. Sixteen laminated Douglas fir arches formed its dome, fitted together without a single nail, screw, bolt, or metal fixture of any kind. Van Tassel's inspiration was financed primarily from contributions to the Ministry of Universal Wisdom, Inc., a nonprofit religious-scientific enterprise run by his family.

Within the dome, a huge diesel-fueled turbine generated up to 100,000,000 volts of electricity. Prospective rejuvenates would simply stroll in a 270-degree arc under the armatures to "recharge their batteries" and emerge from the Integratron healthier, younger, and handsomer. It was quite a dream but it failed to intersect with reality.

Injections and Grafts of Blood, Glands, and Gonads

In the fifteenth century, the injection of fluids became increasingly popular as a form of rejuvenation. The injection of blood, in particular, was considered one of the more effective fluids for this procedure. Pope Innocent VIII, for example, wanted to increase his longevity, so he arranged to have a coterie of young men provide him with their blood. He died almost immediately from the procedure, most likely from incompatible blood types.

By the nineteenth century the type of injections broadened in scope, and one of the more popular was the processed sex glands of young animals. On the one hand, this approach mirrored strategies two thousand years earlier when seekers ingested fragments of animal organs containing such hormones. On the other hand, this hormone technique and others that shortly followed it anticipated the fascination with hormone treatments that reemerged in the late twentieth century.

One of the most noted providers of the rejuvenating injections was famous French physiologist and Harvard Professor Charles-Edouard Brown-Séquard. In 1889 scientists assembled to listen to the renowned seventy-two-year-old describe how he had injected himself in the arms and legs with filtered extracts from crushed testicles of young dogs and guinea pigs. The results, he emphasized to them, were remarkable. Not only did medical tests indicate renewed muscle strength, but the physiology professor reported he had regained the vigor and intellectual stamina of his youth. He had a renewed capacity to work in his laboratory long into the night, even the ability to run up staircases. But best of all, just hours earlier he passed the culminating test. "Today," he told his distinguished audience, "I was able to pay a visit to my young wife."

The key to longevity, Brown-Séquard asserted, lay in correcting hormonal balance by infusing minced gonads and maintaining carefully calibrated semen reserves. His presentation caused a sensation and a stampede of eager Frenchmen to partake of his pioneering technique. He constructed a complicated machine that pulped and filtered bull testes to produce his claimed rejuvenating fluid. A Parisian newspaper initiated a fund for an Institute of Rejuvenation to improve access to the "Methode Séquardienne." Meanwhile, the scientific community reacted mercilessly, ridiculing Brown-Séquard's celebrated results as senile delusions. The critics held the day. No one recovered lost youth and potency from Séquardienne treatments. Whatever positive manifestations had been described were attributed to the effect of positive expectations—what we now understand as the placebo effect. The 6-foot, 4-inch professor suffered severely in scientific stature. His career fell apart, his young wife deserted him. Soon after this downfall, he left Paris and died of a stroke less than five years following his fateful lecture.

FROM INJECTIONS TO GRAFTS

During the early part of the twentieth century, the flamboyant Russian-born surgeon Serge Voronoff moved from injecting testicle extract to grafting testicles themselves into the scrotums of aging men. From his chateau overlooking the Italian Riviera, Voronoff is reported to have carried out over two thousand such operations. Unfortunately, he neglected advice from colleagues who urged that his donors be bulls. Instead, Voronoff used monkey testicles for his grafts. He asserted that since man is a primate, the procedure would be more successful by using other primates (e.g., monkeys or apes) as donors. He predominantly used monkeys, failing to realize that they are much more likely than bulls to transmit venereal disease to man because of their biological proximity as primates. In addition to numerous problems with the immunologic rejection of the grafts, many of his high-paying subjects also contracted syphilis.

But Voronoff was not alone in developing this technique. Others adopted it with enthusiastic clients over a period of more than twenty-five years, largely between the two world wars.

BACK TO INJECTIONS

While Brown-Séquard and Voronoff viewed sex hormones alone as accounting for loss of youth and vigor, a contemporary Swiss surgeon and endocrine expert, Paul Niehans, put forth the notion that the cell degeneration was a central factor in aging. Basically, he believed that by replenishing deteriorating cell groups with young cells of the same type, bodily decline could be reversed or at least prevented. Niehans began to develop his general approach during the 1930s, going on to refine it over the next three decades. It came to be called Cell Therapy, or CT.

Niehans used minced preparations of organs from sheep, which were selected as a species because of their apparent resistance to disease and low incidence of allergic reactions in humans. To ensure the effectiveness of the foreign cells, usually fetal tissue, he would make the dissections just minutes before injections into the patient's buttocks. Fetal cells greatly minimized adverse immune responses in the patient because fetal tissue typically does not trigger immunologic reactions. Also, Niehans contended that the chemistry of embryonic cells from fetuses exerted a more potent impact than that of older cells. However, for injections of testes, ovary, adrenals, pituitary, and parathyroid, mature animals had to be used because these organs are not sufficiently developed in fetuses.

Unlike with Voronoff, Niehans's technique—in his hands—appeared relatively safe. This was not the case with others who attempted to emulate his work. Hundreds of people died at the hands of others. But Niehans was very careful, and his work most likely endured far beyond Voronoff's because of his safety record. Cell therapy is, in fact, still conducted in different sites in Europe today, though it is illegal in the United States. Though safer than the techniques of Voronoff, cell therapy today is generally considered ineffective by the scientific community. Any positive CT results have been attributed to the placebo effect.

Often what propels interest in a new technique is a story that is told or published about someone who appears to have had a positive response to the intervention and speaks highly if not ecstatically about its effects. In Niehans's case he had the great fortune of having a highly visible and respected public figure seek his help—Pope Pius XII. Presenting with a range of disturbing symptoms, the Pope appeared to be on a steady downward course. He seemed to respond dramatically to Niehans's cell therapy, his clinical course reversing in a positive uphill direction, and his satisfaction with the procedure registering high on the enthusiasm scale. The resultant publicity catapulted Niehans into enduring notoriety and considerable wealth within a few months.

One lesson taken from the Voronoff and Niehans stories is that a procedure can remain in use—indeed with enthusiastic reception—for a long time, regardless of its efficacy. With Niehans's story, like that of Ana Aslan's with Gerovital, it is perhaps more understandable that its popularity was sustained. At the very least, it did not bring as many bad side effects. But Voronoff's story is more difficult and disturbing to understand. How could such freak shows (Voronoff's and others performing related techniques) with their macabre techniques and grotesque consequences endure for so long? The lesson here is that one cannot assume that because some approach seems to have long-lasting popularity that it works or that it is not egregious.

Claims About Different Geographical Settings and Lifestyles

For years media stories have identified groups of individuals across the globe as being well over a hundred years old, attributing their advanced longevity to special features about where and how they lived. Some groups receiving attention include the Los Viejos ("the very old") in the small Andes village of Vilcamba in Ecuador, the Hunzukuts of the Karakoram Range in Kashmir, and the Abkhazians of the Republic of Georgia.

However, these reports of extra-long lives have turned out to be grossly misleading. A series of studies conducted on these different groups showed that the inhabitants of the various sites simply had not told the truth about their ages. Self-reports of very old age, in each case, had been greatly exaggerated. Russian scientists, for example, determined that the oldest resident in the Republic of Georgia was only ninety-six.

Why did the locals stretch the truth? Well, for one thing, it was terrific for generating tourism and elevating local revenues. It also brought prestige to many who inflated their age and notoriety to their communities. Human nature ended up not being defied by an altered biology of aging and record life spans, but instead exhibited through the behavior of good old vested self-interest.

CALORIC RESTRICTION

For hundreds of years, people have tried to link the role of diet with longevity. For example, the sixteenth-century treatise Castel of Helthe, famous for its time as a popular regimen of health, contained important dietary advice for older readers. The work was written in 1534 by Sir Thomas Elyot, a member of Sir Thomas More's circle and noted for his breadth of knowledge in literature, philosophy, and medicine. Elyot's admonitions to aging people included a prudent diet: "Always remember that aged men should eat often; and but little every time, for it fareth by them as it doth by a lamp, the light whereof is almost extinct, which by pouring oil and little is kept long burning, but with much oil poured in at once, it is put out."

Of all the approaches attempted and studied in warm-blooded animals, only *caloric restriction* has been shown to increase life span. In the laboratory, caloric restriction consists of nutritionally balanced undernutrition, or undernutrition with neither malnutrition nor starvation. Most of these experiments have been performed on mice and rats whose very limited life span make such research feasible. With the higher mammals, such studies are more difficult to conduct because of the duration of time required. Nonetheless, they are now being attempted in nonhuman primates (i.e., monkeys), but there is still not enough information available to reach firm conclusions. To date there are no experiments of this nature being conducted with humans, though one prominent gerontologist, Roy Walford of the University of California–Los Angeles, has been examining himself on a calorically restricted diet since 1987. But one subject does not a study make, and unless Walford ends up living beyond 125 to 130 years, we will be able to conclude little or nothing from his significant efforts.

Nonetheless, since the 1930s, research has consistently demonstrated that lower animals, on reduced-calorie diets at the 30 to 40 percent level, experience not only increased longevity, but reduced incidences of cancer and many other serious diseases throughout the systems of the body.

Why caloric restriction should exert these effects is not understood. Some reports suggest that restricting calories curtails collagen cross-linking—a phenomenon discussed earlier as a possible mechanism of aging. The work of another gerontologist, Edward Masoro, points to the role of reduced intake of energy as having a physiologic effect of slowing down the process of aging. Interestingly, Masoro's explanation resembles the recommendation of Sir Thomas Elyot four centuries earlier expressed through his metaphor of pouring less oil into the lamp.

Clearly all the research on nutrition has pointed to the healthful role of a good diet and the deleterious role of a bad diet—the latter usually explained as a factor of eating too much, ingesting the wrong things (e.g., too much fat), and becoming obese, which in turn adds risk factors for heart disease, diabetes, and other disorders. In contrast, a healthy diet is viewed as reducing risk factors that could cause earlier onset or aggravated courses of various illnesses, thereby reducing both longevity and the quality of one's life.

Proponents of caloric restriction argue that the procedure does much more than reduce the frequency of disease. Still, it remains to be proven that it can have the same effect on man as on mice, who have one-fiftieth the life span of humans. There is also a very practical obstacle: Achieving a 30 to 40 percent caloric reduction in the diets of most people would leave them hungrier and craving foods, even though they would not be malnourished. Hence, there is a significant quality-of-life issue that makes it less feasible for large groups of men and women.

In addition to these arguments against caloric restriction, there is also one more serious question that concerns our ongoing learning, intellectual growth, and creativity with aging. This is that the brain uses much more energy than any other part of the body. Consider that oxygen is critical for the body's metabolism and that glucose is the primary energy source for animal cells to metabolize. Consider, too, that glucose—the intake of which is significantly reduced in calorically restricted diets—is the primary oxidizable substrate in the central nervous system (the brain and the spinal cord) and that rates of glucose metabolism are highest in the thinking parts of the brain. Then consider that while the brain represents about only 2 percent of adult body mass, it consumes nearly 25 percent of the total oxygen needed by the whole body. In other words, the manifestations and the ramifications of energy dynamics are greatest in the brain.

To the extent that part of the mechanism of caloric restriction is via energy reduction, what are the long-term ramifications of this for the performance of the aging human brain in the face of added years? Keep in mind that the human brain is much more complex than the mouse brain, so mental effects on mice are not necessarily applicable to humans. Long-term side effects are an important consideration with any intervention that requires long-term administration. Certainly they should be of concern here, considering the lesser reserves of the brain. One needs only to consider the field of prenatal health to put perspective on the value of adequate nutrition. The full development of the central nervous system in a baby needs more than just adequate nutrition. It needs a healthy, well-balanced, liberal—hardly restrained—diet. To this extent, calorically restricted diets provide just adequate nutrition.

Moreover, the work of geriatric researcher Reuben Andres in the internationally regarded Baltimore Longitudinal Study on Aging conducted under the auspices of the U.S. National Institute on Aging added new information about the relationship of weight to longevity. Contrary to popular belief that thin is better, Andres and colleagues found death rates among the middle-aged to be lowest not in the leanest but among those ranging from the middle-weight group to those 20 percent heavier than the middle group in the original life insurance height/weight tables established around 1960. They found further that the extremely thin or the extremely overweight live shorter lives than the average. In short, with humans, the jury is still out about caloric restriction at the level used in experimental laboratory animals.

DIETARY SUPPLEMENTS

More and more people these days are adding daily supplements of vitamins and minerals to their regimen of exercise and a healthy diet. Yet there is little scientific evidence to support most of the claims about supplements. These daily tablets may be beneficial to some people, but there is still some debate in the medical field about the benefits of these supplements on *all* people. In fact, large doses of supplements may disturb the body's natural equilibrium of nutrients, sometimes even permanently damaging organs. Too much vitamin A, for example, can cause headaches, nausea, diarrhea, and even liver or bone damage. Too much vitamin D, on the other hand, can cause kidney damage and even death.

A major summary of findings on life extension attempts using vitamins and minerals with antioxidant and other supposed antiaging effects was published in the prestigious *New England Journal of Medicine*. Its authors, gerontologists Edward Schneider, M.D., and John Reed, Ph.D., wrote: "Although the possible antineoplastic and antiaging effects of vitamins A, C, E and the mineral selenium deserve further investigation, the available evidence at this time does not support recommending diet supplementation with these vitamins or selenium for either life extension or prevention of cancer. It is of interest that studies of vitamin consumption by a highly selected group of people (pooled readers of *Prevention* magazine) over age sixty-five found no dose-response relationship between mortality and the levels of vitamin supplementation. In this same study, increased mortality was observed in people who consumed very high levels of vitamin E—more than 1,000 I.U. per day. Although this last observation may reflect the attraction for less healthy persons to large doses of vitamins, it may also reflect some vitamin toxicity. Thus, caution is advised before the ingestion of large doses of these vitamins or selenium is considered."

So who benefits from dietary supplements? Some people—a number of older persons in particular—do not get the vitamins and minerals they need from their daily diets. Digestive problems, chewing difficulties, and side effects of certain drugs can interfere with good nutrition. People with these problems may need and benefit from specific dietary supplements. They should consult their doctors. Dietary supplements may also be needed to correct nutrient deficiencies diagnosed in individuals with or at risk for various disorders. For example, those at high risk for developing osteoporosis—a condition causing thin, brittle bones—are often advised by their physicians to take calcium supplements; a number of menopausal women are in this category. Those recovering from surgery or an illness, including colds, may also need or benefit from certain supplements. Dieters, heavy drinkers, and others whose diseases or health habits alter their balance of vitamins and minerals may require supplements as well.

Findings and contradictions from studies. The problems lie not just with snake-oil peddlers. Scientific studies themselves have been contradictory and result in further confusion in the field of research on aging. The media, for example, published the results of a major study suggesting that antioxidants that combat free radicals have been found to retard aging. The power of such reports builds upon theories (as above) that address our current understanding of the role of free radicals in our body. But a few months later another major study came out where the impact of antioxidants on the body was found to be minimal and produced negative side effects.

Nature doesn't produce pills. Another part of the problem is that people believe that if "they are natural substances, what's wrong with taking them?" The answer is simple: Though various vitamins and minerals are natural, the natural way in which we take them is not via pills. We get our vitamin C from nature via fruits such as oranges. We get our vitamin A via vegetables such as carrots. We get our vitamin E via varied sources such as vegetable oil, egg yolk, leafy vegetables, and legumes. We don't get these vitamins from nature via pills. Nature doesn't produce pills; man does. This doesn't mean that pills are bad. It's just that they aren't natural as claimed or might not be achieving the natural effects that we desire. When we eat a carrot for vitamin A, the carrot contains more than just vitamin A. It contains other constituents that may well interact with the vitamin A and/or help deliver it to the cells of our body in a more healthful and efficient way than via vitamin A alone. This is why the most enthusiastic new nutritional recommendations are not dietary supplements but food groups—at least five servings daily of fruits and vegetables. Remember, too, that when the Bible reported Methuselah and some of his progeny living beyond nine hundred years, vitamins and other dietary supplements were not available.

The Latest Recommendations for You to Swallow

We are now witnessing a new generation of miracle drugs being pushed as panaceas. They build upon a double heritage: (1) the long tradition of magical elixirs and (2) hormone treatments via various routes going back centuries. Many of the new drugs are hormones. Since they are found in pill form the side-show quality that accompanied hormone treatments in the past is reduced. The mode differs with modern hormone interventions, but the promises of outcomes are similar to prior guarantees. This especially applies to the drugs melatonin, DHEA, and human growth hormone (hGH).

The promoters of these drugs are similar in that they all lack restraint in making claims about the effectiveness of them. We have come to learn of these drugs in special terms, such as *The Melatonin Miracle* or *The Super Hormone Promise* for DHEA. An author advocating the properties of melatonin claims that it "extends life," "enhances sexual vitality," "restores normal sleep patterns," and "maintains youthful health and vigor." With respect to DHEA, the author of *The Definitive Book on DHEA* claims that it will help you "grow younger," "revitalize your sex life," "enhance memory" (the age-old triad). The best that can be said about these hormones is that to date nobody has shown scientifically that they are effective, except possibly some benefit from melatonin in treating jet lag.

What do findings from research reveal about all the promises pertaining to hormone supplements? They may best be summarized in a report from the U.S. National Institute on Aging: "Certain hormone supplements have received a lot of attention lately, including DHEA (dehydroepiandrosterone), human growth hormone (hGH), melatonin, and testosterone. Unproven claims that taking these supplements can make people feel young again or that they can prevent aging have been appearing in the news. . . . The fact is that no one has yet shown that supplements of these hormones add years to people's lives. And while some supplements provide health benefits for people with genuine deficiencies of certain hormones, they also can cause harmful side effects."

The National Institute on Aging reports two serious flaws with most of the wild claims about these hormones: (1) the claims are unfounded, and (2) the claims neglect to mention side effects, which can be quite serious. Side effects of melatonin, for example, include "confusion, drowsiness, and headaches the next morning. Animal studies suggest that melatonin may cause blood vessels to constrict, a condition that could be dangerous for people with high blood pressure or other cardiovascular problems." As for DHEA, the NIA reports that this hormone may cause liver damage, even when taken briefly, and that it may cause high levels of estrogen or testosterone in some people, which puts a person at greater risk for breast cancer and prostate cancer, respectively.

The use of estrogen is a special case, where its application has not been promoted to reverse aging, but rather to help with certain age-associated problems such as osteoporosis and heart disease in women. One's physican should be consulted to review benefits and risks of taking estrogen, and for whom its prescription is most appropriate.

MELATONIN'S AND DHEA'S EFFECTS ON MENTAL PERFORMANCE

Research shows that rather than enhancing mental functioning, melatonin actually causes a slowing down of the ability to process information by the brain's centers of higher intellectual performance. Research on DHEA similarly finds no beneficial effect on any psychological or intellectual measure.

GINKGO BILOBA

Perhaps the most interesting results to date on mental functioning are with ginkgo biloba extract from the leaves of the ginkgo tree. Some people claim that ginkgo enhances mental alertness and performance. However, studies are inconclusive. Observable positive effects on humans have been equivocal; in these studies when observable mental effects are described, they might best be characterized as subtle as opposed to substantial, and transient in contrast to enduring. Other studies show no significant effects on cognitive function in healthy humans. For example, in a well-designed study comparing ginkgo biloba to a placebo, no clear differences were found in comparisons of attention, reaction time, and memory.

To best put such questionable or equivocal results in perspective—whether with ginkgo biloba or other purported mind-enhancing drugs—one need only compare their results with those from taking a continuing education course on some subject important to you. No contest, and you'll wonder why you waited so long to explore tried-and-true learning and behavioral approaches rather than popping a pill.

THE MAGIC BULLETS ARE BLANKS

Despite claims to the contrary, all the purported magic bullets prescribed to extend life and reverse the effects of aging have been blanks. They have been fired with great leaps of faith, where hope has been elevated to belief and speculation to conviction. In cases that have produced seemingly positive results, critics have been able to attribute these results to powerful placebo effects or outright distortion. Facts and findings take a back-seat to hype and zeal. These examples remind you of the baseball player about whom it was said "although he can't hit, neither can he field."

Lessons from Theories of Aging and Attempts at Life Extension

The discussion of these theories and the history of these attempts to prolong life illustrate what a mystery aging remains. The science of aging is advancing rapidly, but with its progress the mystery of aging has actually deepened. Leads have become more diverse and require ever more specialized knowledge. There is no magic bullet to stop aging, and none lies just around the corner. For the moment one should not deplete creative energies with the false hope or a desperate quest for a miracle pill or potion. Get it out of your system! Instead, focus your aims on what is feasible, tried, and true. Redirect your energy into exploring, discovering, and tapping your own real inner strengths rather than fictional external distractions. The chapters of this book provide you with strategies to do just this. The strategies don't promise magical results, but they can help you to jump-start your potential for a better aging experience. Be warned by history. Beware of purported shortcuts. Be ready to follow a more realistic path to achieving your goals and realizing your own creativity in the second half of life.

APPENDIX C

Creating an Autobiography: My Personal Approach

IN THIS APPENDIX, I describe a few techniques for creating your autobiography that I have applied in the development of my own. I will include sections from my own autobiography to illustrate my examples. I use four interacting steps:

1. Pick a period of your life and outline personal experiences, memories, and other facts about that time that reflect your life.
2. Identify any photography or personal memorabilia (such as a newspaper clipping) of that period that could be used to illustrate your life.

3. Get a book out of the library that chronicles key developments of any given year. There are books that do this going back at least until the year 1900 (for example, David Brownstone and Irene Franc's *Timelines of the 20th Century*). The process often jogs your memory or provides an "aha!" experience in which you realize that certain historical events or cultural factors influenced you in significant ways. By identifying them, you have a chance to incorporate them into your autobiography.
4. Take out library books (e.g., the Time-Life Series: *This Fabulous Century—1870–1970*) or magazines (e.g., *Life*) in search of interesting photos of your specific time. You might make high-quality color photocopies of these images and paste them into your text, thereby expanding the flavor of the day you are writing about. Or if you have a computer with a scanner, you can scan the images and pull them into your copy where you want them. (This step is advisable only for personal use; if you make multiple copies and "self-publish" your work you must then request the publisher's permission to use the photo(s), which can make your costs mount.)

If you do not have a scanner, but you have a fax machine, remember that your fax is, in effect, a lower-level scanner. You can fax the images to your computer if it has a fax/modem. Once the images are stored in your computer, you can manipulate the images and place them wherever you like in the text. A 600-dot-per-inch (dpi) laser printer will produce newspaper quality or better images.

To illustrate these four steps, I will share a section of my autobiography from 1961. Note: I will use two personal photographs along with two historical photos—one of President John F. Kennedy at his 1961 presidential inauguration, the other of astronaut Buzz Aldrin saluting the American flag on the moon at the end of the decade. I will also incorporate into the text six historical events in 1961 that I felt influenced me. These six events were the following:

1. The inauguration of John F. Kennedy in Washington, D.C., in 1961. People were calling it Camelot.
2. The Peace Corps was established.
3. American aid to Vietnam was expanded, with increased involvement of American "advisers."

4. Yuri Gagarin from the Soviet Union became the first human to orbit the earth on a 1.8-hour flight in *Vostok 1.* That event fully launched the space age and the space race, with President Kennedy later that year promising to land humans on the moon within a decade.
5. The drug thalidomide was recognized as causing severe birth defects.
6. New York Yankees outfielder Roger Maris hit sixty-one home runs that year, breaking Babe Ruth's 1927 record.

My Autobiography—*during part of 1961*

1961

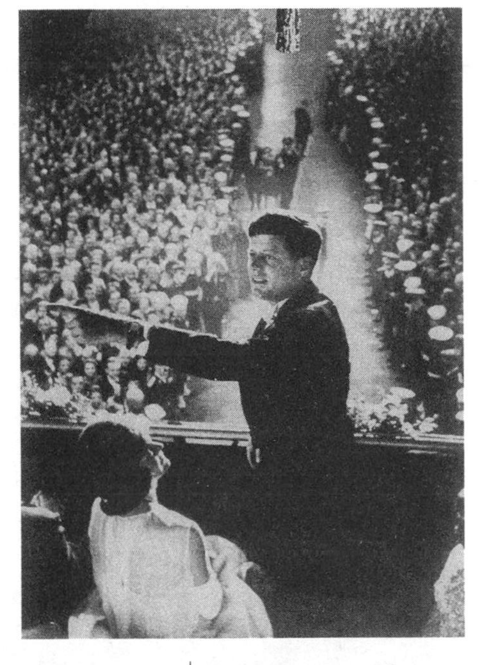

To guests at one of five inaugural balls, the dashing new President exclaimed, "I don't know a better way to spend an evening.

PAUL SCHUTZER/ LIFE MAGAZINE © TIME INC.

In 1961, with the inauguration of John F. Kennedy, people were calling the new administration Camelot. For me, too, at age sixteen, the year was like Camelot. Well, not quite. But it was still a very good year. For the country it was a year of contrasts. On the one hand, the Peace Corps was established, but also American aid to Vietnam was expanded, with increased involvement of American "advisers." Also in 1961, Yuri Gagarin from the Soviet Union became the first human to orbit the earth on a 1.8-hour flight in *Vostok 1.* That event fully launched the space age and the space race, with President Kennedy later that year promising to land humans on the moon within a decade. I can remember the public's increasing attention to science education in America, driven by the fear and obsession that we were falling behind the Soviet Union.

What followed was an extraordinary new educational focus on the sciences, and as I recall, a major public media campaign to elevate the image of scientists. It seemed that every other movie I went to had a scientist appear in some problem-solving if not heroic role.

All of this was certainly influencing my own thoughts and pursuits of science, but they still had to do a bit of catch-up to my interest in sports, especially baseball. In 1961, Roger Maris hit sixty-one homers, breaking Babe Ruth's 1927 record. While I started to daydream about science, I dreamed even more about baseball.

In the town where I lived, we had street baseball teams, and I played second base for a street team named the Center Street Sluggers. While Roger Maris had slugged three score and one balls over the fence that year, I longed to hit just one homer. I never did. Part of the problem was that I was rather overweight. Okay, I was a fat boy then, very overweight—by forty to fifty pounds! The football coach took a second look at me (I'm sure he was thinking I might serve a function on the team's front line). I was getting increasingly interested in the girls, but they did not dare take a second look at me. With the girls on my mind, I spent the next three years getting my weight down to where it should have been, at which time my prospects improved.

As a footnote, during the time of my successful diet, my mother lamented that my "drastic diet" probably was the reason that I stopped growing (vertically). She kept telling me that if only I hadn't cut back so much on what I was eating, I could have been six feet tall. Still, to this day (she's eighty-six, I'm fifty-five), she wonders whether if I had eaten more, I could have been taller. One thing for sure, her being such a good cook, with great-looking dinner plates, didn't make the diet any easier.

Meanwhile, in the absence of setting new records at the baseball plate, I was catching the fever in the air about science. I was certainly affected by society's growing romance with science, stirred by the start of the space age, and the year before had already become attracted to oceanographic research. The new scientist-as-hero milieu further catalyzed my interest in scientific research as a junior in high school. Living on the south shore of Massachusetts, I ventured to the Woods Hole Oceanographic Institute an hour away on Cape Cod in search of a guide. One of the scientists there agreed to mentor me, and I would make periodic trips down to meet with him. That I had just turned sixteen and had gotten my driver's license added to the adventure. How could my father say no to my driving his car? After all, it was for his son's education and science project.

On my trips to Woods Hole I would stop to eat at a little diner there. The waitress appeared to be in her seventies and acted rather grandmotherly to me. One day, while I was sitting at the counter, she stared at me and said that I reminded her of someone else in his younger days who used to frequent the diner. Curious, I asked her who that might be. "Jonas Salk," she replied. I was stunned. Needless to say, she made

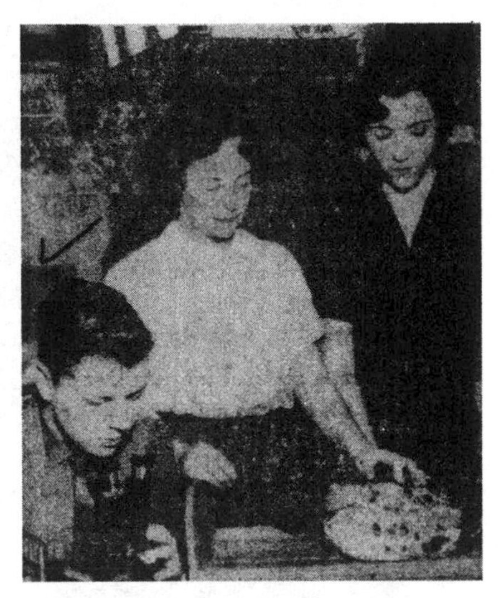

my day. No comment could have been more inspiring to this dreaming young science student.

The school newspaper, caught up in the scientific fever of the times, was always in search of local science stories, and I would on occasion find myself in their print. That, too, motivated me to excel even more in science. Interestingly, my science project was on *aging*, the area that later became my career. It was a project where I studied age and growth relationships in fish. I had refined a previously abandoned method to determine the fish's age using the otolith bone found in the inner ear of the fish.

New tools allowed me to crack the bone more cleanly than in the past, permitting me to more effectively count the rings inside the bone—the rings that corresponded to the fish's age. The project actually used a focus on age to answer broader questions about the health of the fish and its habitat. By establishing norms about the size and corresponding age of fish, one could postulate that the habitat was not healthy if fish sizes were smaller than this norm. The project, in effect, used a focus on age to assess ecology. I came to realize later that, conceptually, my focus on age was one that facilitated new knowledge in other areas. The programs on aging that I would head later at NIH took a double focus: one on older adults, the other where attention to aging could lead to new clues about health and illness independent of age. My science project had planted the seed for the latter approach.

Members of Randolph High's Oceanographic Laboratory measure one of the first robins they found. This one happens to be a sea robin, and he's well-frozen. At the microscope is Gene Cohen. Left to right are Sally Dean and Jean McNeil.

My 1961 science project ended up winning a first prize at the Massachusetts State Science Fair held at MIT, and I became a finalist at the National/International Science Fair. My excitement rose another notch when I was interviewed about my project on Boston's PBS television station, WGBH. This success had a profound influence on me and my self-confidence.

My success and excitement with science fairs fed my growing enthusiasm for medicine, which I increasingly saw as my career path. The Jonas Salk scenario often revisited my daydreams. But events of 1961 made me aware that not all was glamorous in medicine, that it was

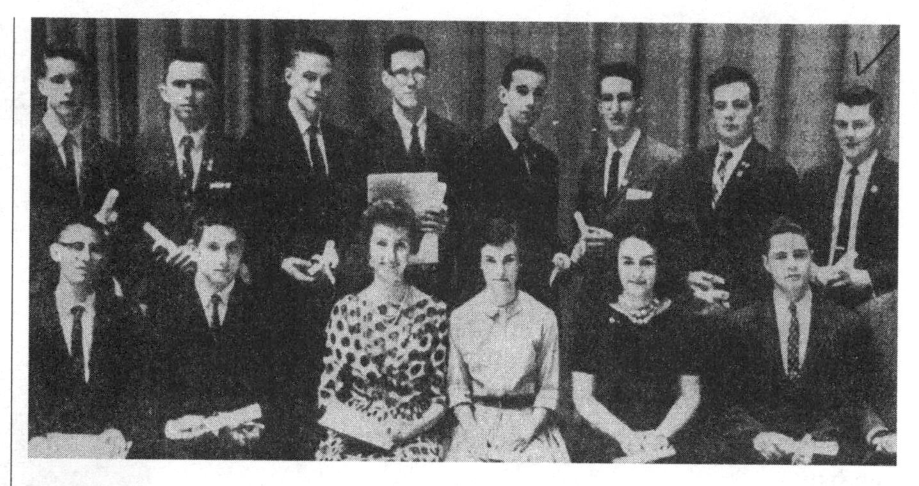

From *The Boston Globe*, May 2, 1961: "These 16 youngsters won first-place honors at Massachusetts State Science Fair."
COURTESY *THE BOSTON GLOBE*

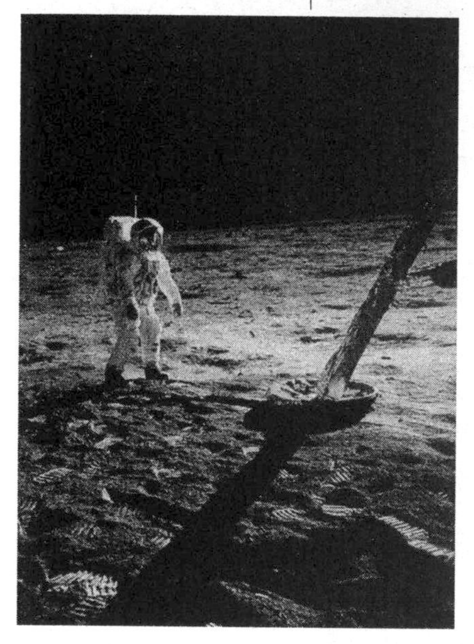

Buzz Aldrin on the lunar surface.
COURTESY NASA, PHOTOGRAPHED BY NEIL ARMSTRONG

not just a field of adventure, but also one of risks. That was the year when the drug Thalidomide was recognized as causing severe birth defects characterized by gross malformations. Tragically, the baby brother of one my friends was one of those babies. The Thalidomide story has always provided an important backdrop of caution in my memory, especially working in a field where the quest for breakthrough experimental drugs runs strong.

All in all, 1961 was a very good year for me, and a great way to start the decade of the turbulent sixties. The decade ended with men landing on the moon, and, for me, getting ready to graduate from medical school. As Neil Armstrong's foot first touched the surface of the moon, he exclaimed, "That's one small step for [a] man, one giant leap for mankind." At that time I was considering additional schooling beyond my M.D. I thought to myself of my med school experience, "One small step taken, the giant leap still to come."

The Family Newspaper Approach

The approach above allows one to assemble one's autobiography in a stepwise gradual pace, focusing on a given year or specific period in one's life. A further plus with this approach is that initially the time frames do not have to be in order—you can write about any period and then piece them together. Another similar technique is the family newspaper, which allows considerable flexibility with a different format. You can focus on a particular time or even a specific event (e.g., your sixteenth or sixty-fifth birthday, your first day of college, your wedding day, etc.) or a related set of events as illustrated in the following news feature from the "Cohen Chronicles" about my son Alex as a young boy.

The newspaper format also provides another context for both creative design and use of images that go beyond the content of the story. One can be very imaginative in the design of a newspaper logo and the use of photographs to illustrate stories. This layout also allows a combination of personal information and historical facts in much the same way as in the earlier example; the difference is that the newspaper format is used instead of an illustrated text layout. See the page that follows from the *Gene Cohen Times*. Since this example largely takes place in the 1960s, it is labeled Volume 3; I was born in 1944, so a focus on the 1940s would be Volume 1, the 1950s Volume 2, etc.

Constructing a family newspaper provides another great opportunity for a creative collaboration that can involve several generations of family members. Putting out any newspaper is a team effort. Your own autobiographical newspaper need be no exception. Begin by talking in general about a given period with your children and grandchildren, testing the waters, so to speak, to assess what might interest them most. Then involve them like good reporters in coming up with good source material.

If you were focusing on the 1960s, see what areas and issues the younger ones seem interested in, and try to build your story around those. In my case, my son Alex, who recently graduated from college, was curious about my hairstyle in college. I wove the *Gene Cohen Times* around the theme of hair, though this theme doesn't become apparent until the story builds. Think about involving the family in the process of designing the layout of the columns.

COHEN CHRONICLES

SPECIAL REVIEW ISSUE

Vol. 1
No. 1

Famous Kid Stories

1/1/99
page 1

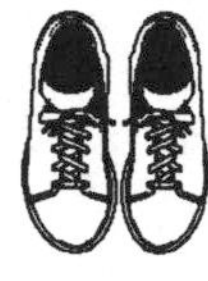

Alex and Shoes. Until he was about six, my son, Alex, seemed obsessed with shoes. If a store window contained shoes, then you couldn't even think about passing it without stopping. Shoes, sneakers, and slippers alike were all part of the obsession. Three stories in particular illustrate Alex's special attraction to shoes as a little boy—a relationship ranging from observant powers to unique demands. The setting for the first story was the Christmas party at my office at NIH in 1975 (Alex was two and a half); the second was on the street several blocks from our house in 1978 (Alex was five), while the third was his bedroom on the first night of Hanukkah 1979 (Alex was six).

The Christmas Party at Work, 1975. The Center on Aging at the National Institute of Mental Health was launched in 1975 and held its first Christmas party that December. Since several of the staff, including me, had young children, we decided to invite them to the party. Someone suggested that it would be great to have Santa there. As head of the Center, I was nominated to be Santa. Getting into the role, I obtained a Santa costume for the event. When the big day arrived, the kids all understood that Santa was coming, and kept asking for him. At the critical moment, I indicated that I would look for him and retreated to my office.

A few minutes later, out came Santa; the kids were ecstatic. My son, Alex, forgot about me at this point, focusing all his attention on Santa. An hour later, Santa said goodbye. He said he would leave by the window in the back office (mine). He went into my office, and about five minutes later I came out saying that Santa's sleigh had come up to the window, that he hopped in, and drove away. The story made complete sense to all the little people. About an hour later, when I was taking Alex home, he looked down at my feet, and exclaimed, "You know, Dad, you have the same shoes as Santa!"

Several Blocks from Our House, 1978. One day in September 1978 while I was working at home a police car pulled up in front of the house with flashing lights and the brief sound of its siren. Out came a policeman, accompanied by a little boy whom I quickly recognized as my five-year-old son, Alex. I was puzzled and worried. I ran out, only to find Alex with a big smile and a lollipop and the policeman praising him as a very responsible and observant young man. The story that unfolded was that Alex was in the front yard of his babysitter's house when an elderly woman walking by was suddenly knocked to the ground and had her purse stolen by a mugger. The mugger then dashed away, at which point Alex ran to the woman, helped her up, and asked her if she was OK. He then yelled for the babysitter, who immediately called the police.

When the police came, they interviewed the elderly woman and Alex. The policeman who accompanied Alex home marveled that Alex had given the most detailed description of a robber's shoes and laces that he had ever encountered during his seventeen years on the force.

Alex's Bedroom, Hanukkah 1979. When Alex was six, he made his most challenging request to me. For Hanukkah, he wanted two very special presents—a bunkbed and a multicolored pair of slippers we had seen recently in the window of a shoe store. Moreover, he wanted to wake up on the first day of Hanukkah in the top bunk of the bunkbed, wearing his multicolored slippers. What could I say? I said, "I'll see what I can do."

I was determined to pull off this dream, but had high anxiety about whether I could be successful or not. I thought, though, wouldn't it be wonderful, for at least once in life, to have a most special dream that was fulfilled? It would be such a lesson that one could dream big, and perhaps it just might come true.

When the first night of Hanukkah arrived I had carefully hidden the big boxes containing the bunkbed and the little box containing the slippers. Alex was so excited in anticipation that the bunkbed would magically appear the next morning with him awakening on top of it that he didn't finally fall asleep until after 11 P.M. I knew I would have a long night, especially since I was not the most handy person at assembling such large items.

At 2 A.M. I finished assembling the bed. Then the supreme test began. Could I move Alex and everything else without awakening him? In the third most crucial step, I moved Alex to another room and got rid of the bed he had been in, replacing it in its spot with the brand-new bunkbed. Then the second most key step—placing Alex's new multicolored slippers on his feet; he was still asleep. Sweating and hyperventilating a bit, I set the most critical step in motion—lifting Alex to the top bunk of the bunkbed. Just as I ever so gently laid him down, he turned over, mumbled something unintelligible, but miraculously remained asleep. Thank goodness at that age kids sleep as if they are in a coma. It was now 3 A.M. I was totally exhausted, dripping wet with sweat, and soon fell asleep.

At 6:30 A.M. I was startled awake with a shrill shriek of delight. Though I was a basket case, I knew my little boy's dream had come true.

GENE COHEN TIMES

DECADES IN REVIEW

Vol. 3
No. 1

The 1960s

The Astronauts. With President JFK's promise to put an astronaut on the moon by the end of the decade, the imagination of the nation caught fire. Soon, a crew of hand-picked test pilots—short-haired and clean-cut young men—emerged as America's new space-age heroes.

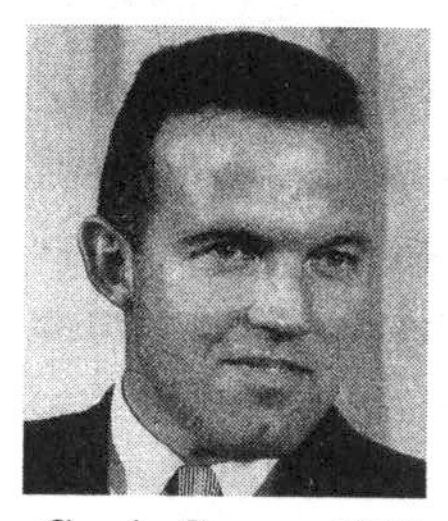

Gordo Cooper, 1963

COURTESY WALTER BENNETT/TIME MAGAZINE

Project *Mercury* became the first stage to reaching the moon. Six men were selected to fly alone in a series of missions aimed at testing the ability of the men and the capacity of the spacecraft to tolerate sub-orbital and orbital flight. On the last flight of the *Mercury* stage, astronaut L. Gordon (Gordo) Cooper Jr., sent back the first TV pictures from space.

Back on Earth, I was a college freshman in quite a new atmosphere, for me, at Harvard. I had arrived at the ivory tower, as they say, having come from a largely blue-collar community. While Gordo Cooper wanted to soar into space, my challenge was to keep my feet on the ground while immersed in all those head-in-the-clouds discussions that come so natural to cocky eighteen-year-old college freshmen. One thing I did have in common with astronaut Cooper, though, was my short-haired clean-cut look.

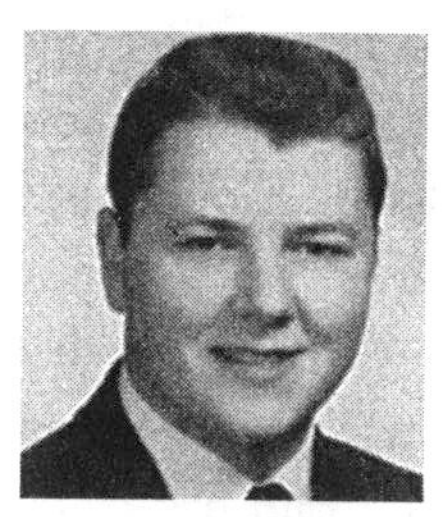

Gene Cohen, 1962

The Militants. By the late 1960s, hairstyles along with behavior had changed. The militants arrived on the cultural scene; one of the most flamboyant was Jerry Rubin. Rubin was a University of California dropout who, along with fellow militant Abbie Hoffman, helped form the Youth International Party—whose members were better known as "Yippies."

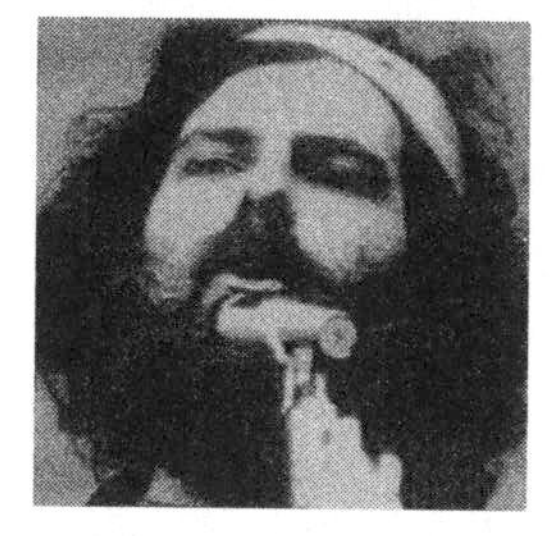

Jerry Rubin, 1968

KEN REGAN, *CAMERA 5 INC.*

My hairstyle changed, too, but not until the early 1970s. Unlike Jerry Rubin, I wore a tie.

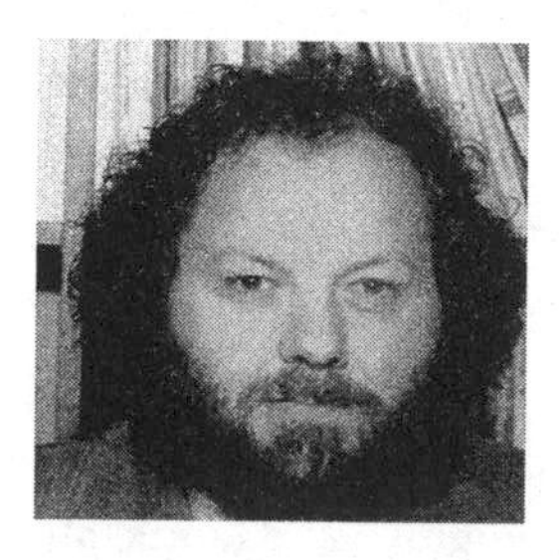

Gene Cohen, 1973

APPENDIX D

Internet and Other Resources

AARP
601 E Street, N.W.
Washington, DC 20049
800-424-3410
www.aarp.org

AARP, with a membership in excess of thirty million people age fifty and older, is a major leader in addressing the interests and issues of older people. The organization offers many services and a wealth of information on diverse aspects of aging.

Alliance for Aging Research
2021 K Street, N.W., Suite 305
Washington, DC 20006
202-293-2856
www.agingresearch.org

The Alliance for Aging Research is America's leading citizen advocacy organization for promoting research in human aging and working to ensure healthy longevity for all Americans.

American Association of Geriatric Psychiatry (AAGP)
7910 Woodmont Avenue
Bethesda, MD 20814
301-654-7850
www.aagpgpa.org

A national professional society dedicated to improving the mental health and well-being of older people. Informational materials are available to both professionals and the public.

American Geriatrics Society (AGS)
350 Fifth Avenue, Suite 801
New York, NY 10018
212-308-1414
www.americangeriatrics.org

A national professional society dedicated to improving the general health and well-being of older people. Informational materials are available to both professionals and the public.

American Society on Aging (ASA)
833 Market Street, Suite 511
San Francisco, CA 94103
415-974-9600
www.asaging.org

The ASA is a national nonprofit membership organization that informs the public and health professionals about issues affecting the quality of life for older people and promotes innovative approaches to meet these needs.

Center on Aging, Health & Humanities
The Creativity Discovery Corps
George Washington University
2175 K Street, N.W., Suite 810
Washington, DC 20037
202-467-2226
www.gwumc.edu/cahh

Programs headed by Gene D. Cohen, M.D., Ph.D. at George Washington University that include a special focus on studying and promoting creativity and aging.

Directory of Web Sites on Aging
Administration on Aging
330 Independence Avenue, S.W.
Washington, DC 20201
800-677-1116
www.aoa.dhhs.gov/aoa/webres/craig.htm

Provides a wide diversity of useful Web sites addressing issues of aging, including academic research sites, organization sites, sites by state, international sites, and sites by subject and topic.

Elderhostel
75 Federal Street
Boston, MA 02110–1941
877-426-8056
www.elderhostel.org

About itself, Elderhostel says, "Elderhostel is a nonprofit organization providing educational adventures all over the world to adults age fifty-five and over. Study the literature of Jane Austen in the White Mountains of New Hampshire or travel to Greece to explore the spectacular art and architecture of its ancient civilization, or conduct field research in Belize to save the endangered dolphin population. Elderhostel is for people on the move who believe learning is a lifelong process."

ElderPage: Information for Older Persons and Families
Administration on Aging
330 Independence Avenue, S.W.
Washington, DC 20201
202-619-7501
www.aoa.dhhs.gov/elderpage.html#wal

Provides a wealth of useful information, from Eldercare Locator, which helps one contact local agencies that can help obtain services, to an extensive resource directory for older people, and the National Institute on Aging (NIA) Age Pages, which provide valuable information on many issues and problems older people deal with.

GENCO, International
P.O. Box 66
Kensington, MD 20895–0066
301-946-6446
www.GENCO-GAMES.com

Gene D. Cohen's creativity company focusing on the development of intergenerational, educational, artistic board games that provide mental exercises for aging.

Generations United
440 First Street, N.W., Suite 310
Washington, DC 20001–2085
202-662-4283
www.gu.org/gul.html

At this Web site you can obtain information on a list of intergenerational coalitions, links to sites with an intergenerational theme, intergenerational programming, and other intergenerational-related resources.

Gerontological Society of America (GSA)
1030 Fifteenth Street, N.W., Suite 250
Washington DC 20005–1503
202-842-1275
www.geron.org

The GSA is a national nonprofit professional society promoting the scientific study of aging in the biological, behavioral, and social sciences. It has a humanities and arts committee with a strong focus on creativity and aging.

International Federation on Aging (IFA)
425 Viger Avenue, West Suite 520
Montréal, Québec H2Z 1×2 CANADA
514-396-3358
www.ifa-fiv.org

The IFA helps link more than one hundred associations as well as interested individuals representing or serving older people in approximately fifty nations around the world.

International Longevity Center (ILC)
60 East 86th Street
New York, NY 10028
212-288-1468
www.ilcusa.org

The ILC is dedicated to the study of longevity internationally, improving the availability of data as well as the identification of programs and approaches to improving the quality of one's added years.

International Psychogeriatric Association (IPA)
550 Frontage Road, Suite 2820
Northfield, IL 60093
847-784-1701
www.ipa-online.org

An international professional society dedicated to improving the mental health and well-being of older people. Informational materials are available to both professionals and the public.

National Aging Information Center
Administration on Aging
330 Independence Avenue, S.W.
Washington, DC 20201
202-619-0724
www.aoa.dhhs.gov/naic

Includes a range of information, from publications on aging, to a calender of coming events on aging, to statistical reports on aging.

National Council on the Aging (NCOA)
409 Third Street, S.W., Suite 200
Washington, DC 20024
202-479-1200
www.ncoa.org

NCOA is an association of organizations and individuals dedicated to promoting the self-determination, well-being, and continuing contributions of older perople through service, education, and advocacy. Its members include professionals and volunteers, service providers, consumer groups, businesses, government agencies, religious groups, and voluntary organizations.

National Institute on Aging (NIA)
Public Information Office
9000 Rockville Pike, Bldg. 31, Room 5C27
Bethesda, MD 20892
301-496-1752
www.nih.gov/nia

NIA is the federal research program most involved in supporting studies of aging. In addition to providing information on research findings, much practical information is offered through the Institute's diverse publications—especially their Age Pages.

Old-Time Radio
(note: no address or phone number available.)
www.old-time.com

About itself, Old-Time Radio says, "If you are interested in radio programs from radio's 'golden age,' this is the site for you. It is filled with many entertaining and educational topics for fans of nostalgic old-time radio shows."

Older Jokes for Older Folks
Writers Consortium
5443 Stag Mt. Road
Weed, CA 96094
916-938-3163
www.seniors-site.com/funstuff/jokes97.html
This site provides jokes, just as it promises.

Senior Corps
1201 New York Avenue, N.W.
Washington, DC 20525
800-424-8867
www.cns.gov/senior/index.html

Through the National Senior Service Corps, nearly half a million Americans age fifty-five and older share their time and talents to help their communities. Its component programs include the Foster Grandparent Program, RSVP (Retired Seniors Volunteer Program), and Senior Companion program.

SeniorNet
121 Second Street, 7th floor
San Francisco, CA 94105
415-4990
www.seniornet.org

About itself, SeniorNet says, "SeniorNet's mission is to provide older adults education for and access to computer technology to enhance their lives and enable them to share their knowledge and wisdom. The nonprofit SeniorNet teaches seniors (age fifty plus) to use computers and the Internet at over 140 Learning Centers nationwide."

Small Business Administration (SBA)
1110 Vermont Avenue, N.W., Suite 900
P.O. Box 34500
Washington, DC 20043–4500
800-827-5722
www.sba.gov

The U.S. Small Business Administration provides financial, technical, and management assistance to help Americans start, run, and grow their businesses. With a portfolio of more than $45 billion, SBA is the nation's largest single backer of small businesses. In 1998, SBA offered management and technical assistance to more than one million small-business owners.

SPRY Foundation
10 G Street, N.E., Suite 600
Washington, DC 20002
202-216-0401
www.spry.org/MISSION.htm

The National Committee to Preserve Social Security and Medicare established the SPRY Foundation in 1991 as an independent 501 (c) (3) nonprofit organization. The SPRY Foundation's mission is to conduct and coordinate research and education efforts that seek ways to assist mature adults both in planning and achieving a healthy, financially secure, and satisfying future. SPRY also disseminates information and raises public awareness about such efforts to achieve its vision.

Third Age
Third Age Media
585 Howard Street, First Floor
San Francisco, CA 94105–3001
www.thirdage.com

About itself Third Age says, "In creating ThirdAge.com, we wanted to make a trusted place for all of us, a place where your choices and your contributions help shape a home on the Web for our generation. We have succeeded wildly. ThirdAge is a vibrant, exciting place where you can always come to find friends and tools and resources to help you design your own Third Age. And what an age it is!"

U.S. Census Bureau
Information on Aging
U.S. Department of Commerce
U.S. Census Bureau
Washington, DC 20233
301-457-4100
www.census.gov/population/www/socdemo/age.html

Provides very well done, brief, and in-depth data reports on both boomers and older adults.

U.S. Senate Special Committee on Aging
Senator Chuck Grassley, Chairman
G31 Dirksen Senate Office Building
Washington, DC 20510–6400
202-224-5364
www.senate.gov/~aging/jurisdic.htm

The Special Committee on Aging has served as a focal point in the Senate for discussion and debate on matters relating to older Americans. Often, the committee will submit its findings and recommendations for legislation to the Senate. In addition, the committee publishes materials of assistance to those interested in public policies that relate to the elderly.

Virtual Internet Guide
(note: no address or phone number available.)
www.dreamscape.com/frankvad/internet.html

This site offers "virtual" Internet guides to acquaint surfers to all avenues on the Internet and World Wide Web.

Bibliography

BOOKS ON CREATIVITY IN GENERAL

Arieti, S. *Creativity: The Magic Synthesis*. New York: Basic Books, 1976.

Brockman, J., ed. *Creativity*. New York: Touchstone, 1993.

Cohen, D. *Creativity: What Is it?* New York: M. Evans, 1977.

Csikszentmihalyi, M. *Creativity*. New York: HarperCollins, 1996.

Fritz, R. *Creating*. New York: Fawcett Columbine, 1991.

Gardner, H. *Creating Minds*. New York: Basic Books, 1993.

Ghiselin, B., ed. *The Creative Process*. New York: Mentor, 1952

Goleman, D., P. Kaufman, and M. Ray. *The Creative Spirit*. New York: Dutton, 1992.

Johnston, C. M. *The Creative Imperative*. Berkeley, Calif: Celestial Arts, 1986.

May, R. *The Courage to Create*. New York: Bantam Books, 1975.

Runco, M. A. and S. Pritzker, eds. *Encyclopedia of Creativity*. New York: Academic Press, 1999.

BOOKS EXPLORING POTENTIAL OR CAPACITIES WITH AGING

Adams-Price, C. E., ed. *Creativity and Successful Aging: Theoretical and Empirical Approaches*. New York: Springer Publishing Co., 1998.

Baltes, P. B., and M. M. Baltes. *Successful Aging: Perspectives from the Behavioral Sciences*. New York: Cambridge University Press, 1990.

Bass, S. A., ed. *Older and Active: How Americans over 55 Are Contributing to Society*. New Haven: Yale University Press, 1995.

Benson, H., with M. Stark. *Timeless Healing: The Power and Biology of Belief*. New York: Simon & Schuster, 1997.

Billig, N. *Growing Older and Wiser*. New York: Lexington Books, 1993

Birren, J. E., and D. E. Deutchman. *Guiding Autobiography Groups for Older Adults: Exploring the Fabric of Life*. Baltimore: Johns Hopkins University Press, 1991.

———, and L. Feldman. *Where to Go from Here: Discovering Your Own Life's Wisdom in the Second Half of Your Life*. New York: Simon & Schuster, 1997.

Cole, T. R., D. D. Van Tassel, and R. Kastenbaum, eds. *Handbook of the Humanities and Aging*. New York: Springer Publishing Co., 1992.

———, and M. G. Winkler, eds. *The Oxford Book of Aging: Reflections on the Journey of Life*. New York: Oxford University Press, 1994.

Dychtwald, K. *Healthy Aging*. Gaithersburg, Md.: Aspen Publishers, 1999.

Mahoney, D., and R. Restak. *The Longevity Strategy*. New York: John Wiley & Sons, 1998.

Restak, R. M. *Older and Wiser*. New York: Simon & Schuster, 1997.

Rowe, J. W., and R. L. Kahn. *Successful Aging*. New York: Pantheon, 1998.

POPULAR BOOKS ON THE COURSE AND POSITIVE ASPECTS OF AGING

Brontë, L. *The Longevity Factor*. New York: HarperCollins, 1993.

Carter, J. *The Virtues of Aging*. New York: Ballantine Books, 1998.

Downs, H. *Fifty to Forever*. Nashville, Tenn.: Thomas Nelson, 1994.

Delany, S., and E. Delany, with A. H. Hearth. *Having Our Say: The Delany Sisters' First 100 Years*. New York: Dell Books, 1996.

Friedan, B. *The Fountain of Age*. New York: Touchstone, 1994.

Gill, B. *Late Bloomers*. New York: Artisan, 1996.

Jacobs, R. *Be an Outrageous Older Woman.* New York: Harperperennial Library, 1997.

Lindeman, B. *Be an Outrageous Older Man.* Manchester, Conn.: Knowledge, Ideas & Trends, 1998.

Rijmes, J., K. N. Brandt, and S. Niederman. *Living Treasures.* Santa Fe, N.H.: Western Edge Press, 1997.

Sheehy, G. *New Passages.* New York: Ballantine Books, 1996.

Yolen, J. *Gray Heroes: Elder Tales from Around the World.* New York: Penguin Putnam, 1999.

BOOKS AND MONOGRAPHS ON ADULT PSYCHOLOGICAL DEVELOPMENT AND PERSONALITY

Colarusso, C. A., and R. A. Nemiroff, eds. *Adult Development,* New York: Plenum Press, 1981.

Erikson, E. *Identity and the Life Cycle.* New York: International Universities Press, Inc., 1959.

Levinson, D. *The Seasons of a Man's Life.* New York: Ballantine Books, 1986.

McRae, R. R., and P. T. Costa Jr. *Personality in Adulthood.* New York: Guilford Press, 1990.

Nemiroff, R. A. and C. A. Colarusso. *The Race Against Time.* New York: Plenum Press, 1985.

Pollock, G. H., and S. I. Greenspan. *Late Adulthood.* Vol. 6, *The Course of Life.* New York: International Universities Press, 1993.

———. *Completing the Journey* Vol. 7, lbid., 1999.

Vaillant, G. E. *Adaptation to Life.* Boston: Little Brown, 1977.

Wheelis, A. *The Quest for Identity.* New York: W. W. Norton, 1958.

BOOKS WITH GENERAL OVERVIEWS OF AGING

Binstock, R. H, L. K. George, V. W. Marshall, J. H. Schulz, and G. C. Myers, eds. *Handbook of Aging and the Social Sciences.* New York: Academic Press, 1995.

Birren, J. E., V. W. Marshall, T. R. Cole, and A. Svanborg, eds. *Encyclopedia of Gerontology: Age, Aging, and the Aged.* New York: Academic Press, 1996.

———, K. W. Schaie, and R. P. Abeles, eds. *Handbook of the Psychology of Aging.* New York: Academic Press, 1996.

Hayflick, L. *How and Why We Age.* New York: Ballantine Books, 1994.

Maddox, G. L., R. C. Atchley, and J. G. Evans, eds. *The Encyclopedia of Aging: A Comprehensive Resource in Gerontology and Geriatrics.* New York: Springer Publishing Company, 1996.

Schneider, E. L., J. W. Rowe, T. E. Johnson, and N. Holbrook, eds. *Handbook of the Biology of Aging.* New York: Academic Press, 1996.

BOOKS WITH OVERVIEWS OF THE AGING BRAIN AND MIND

Birren, J. E., R. B. Sloane, and G. D. Cohen, eds. *Handbook of Mental Health and Aging*. New York: Academic Press, 1992.

Butler, R. N., M. I. Lewis, and T. Sunderland, eds. *Aging and Mental Health: Positive Psychosocial and Biomedical Approaches*. Needham Heights, Mass.: Allyn & Bacon, 1998.

Coffey, C. E., and J. L. Cummings, eds. *Textbook of Geriatric Neuropsychiatry*. Washington, D.C.: American Psychiatric Press, 1994.

Cohen, G. *The Brain in Human Aging*. New York: Springer Publishing Company, 1988.

BOOKS ON CENTENARIANS

Cutler, C. L. *How We Made It to 100: Wisdom from the Super Old*. Rockfall, Conn.: Rockfall Press, 1978.

Perls, T. T., M. H. Silver, with J. F. Lauerman. *Living to 100: Lessons in Living to Your Maximum Potential at Any Age*. New York: Basic Books, 1999.

Poon, L. W., ed. *The Georgia Centenarian Study*. Amityville, N.Y.: Baywood, 1992.

BOOKS AND JOURNAL ARTICLES ON OLDER POPULATION DATA TRENDS

Fries, J. F. "Aging, Natural Death, and the Compression of Morbidity." *New England Journal of Medicine* 303, no. 3 (1980): 130–135.

Manton, K. G., L. Corder, and E. Stallard. "Chronic Disability Trends in Elderly United States Populations: 1982–1994." *Proceedings of the National Academy of Sciences*, USA 94, no. 6 (1997): 2593–98.

Olshansky, S. J., B. A. Carnes, and C. K. Cassel. "The Aging of the Human Species." *Scientific American* 268, no. 4 (1993): 46–52.

Suzman, R. M., T. Harris, E. C. Hadley, M. G. Kovar, and R. Weindruch. "The Robust Oldest Old: Optimistic Perspectives for Increasing Healthy Life Expectancy." In *The Oldest Old*, edited by R. Suzman, D. Willis, and K. G. Manton, 341–58. New York: Oxford University Press, 1992.

Vaupel, J. W., J. R. Carey, K. Christensen, T. E. Johnson, A. I. Yashin, N. V. Holm, I. A. Iachine, V. Kannisto, A. A. Khazaeli, P. Liedo, V. D. Longo, Y. Zeng, K. G. Manton, and J. W. Curtsinger. "Biomedical Trajectories of Longevity." *Science* 280 (1998): 855–60.

OTHER SOURCES CITED OR EXPANDING ON INFORMATION THROUGHOUT THIS BOOK

Introduction

Butler, R. N. *Why Survive? Being Old in America*. New York: Harper & Row, 1975.

de Beauvoir, S. *The Coming of Age*. New York: Warner Books, 1978.

Hayflick, L. "Some Animals Age, Some Do Not." In *How And Why We Age,* by L. Hayflick, 19–33. New York: Ballantine Books, 1994.

U.S. Bureau of the Census. Current Population Reports, Special Studies. pp. 23–190, *65 + in the United States*. U.S. Government Printing Office, Washington, DC, 1996.

Chapter 1. The Flames of Creativity

Diamond, J. "The Great Leap Forward," *Discover* 10 (1989): 50–60.

Levenson, J. L., J. S. McDaniel, M. G. Moran, and A. Stoudemire. "Psychological Factors Affecting Medical Conditions," in *Textbook of Psychiatry,* 3rd ed., eds. R. E. Hales, S. C. Yudofsky, and J. A. Talbott, 635–61. Washington, D.C.: American Psychiatric Press, 1999.

Maier, S. F., L. R. Watkins, and M. Fleshner. "Psychoneuroimmunology. The Interface Between Behavior, Brain, and Immunity," *American Psychologist* 49, no. 12 (1994): 1004–1017.

Pert, C., H. E. Dreher, and R. Ruff. "The Psychosomatic Network: Foundations of Mind-Body Medicine," *Alternative Therapies* 4, no. 4 (1998): 30–41.

Tricerri, A., A. R. Errani, M. Vangeli, L. Guidi, I. Pavese, L. Antico, and C. Bartololini. "Neuroimmunomodulation and Psychoneuroendocrinology: Recent Findings in Adults and Aged," *Panminerva Medicine* 37, no. 2 (1995): 77–83.

Chapter 2. Biology and Mystery

Achterberg, J. *Imagery in Healing*. Boston: New Science Library, 1995.

Diamond, M. C. "An Optimistic View of the Aging Brian," in *Mental Health and Aging,* ed. M. A. Smyer, 59–63. New York: Springer Publishing Co., 1993.

Katzman, R. "Can Late Life Social or Leisure Activities Delay the Onset of Dementia?," *Journal of the American Geriatrics Society* 43, no. 5 (1995): 583–84.

Miller, B. L., J. Cummings, F. Mishkin, et al. "Emergence of Artistic Talent in Frontotemporal Dementia," *Neurology* 51, no. 4 (1998): 978–82.

Neylan, T. C., C. F. Reynolds, and D. Kupfer. "Neuropsychiatric Aspects of Sleep and Sleep Disorders," in *Textbook of Neuropsychiatry,* 3rd ed., eds. S. C. Yudofsky and R. E. Hales, 583–606. Washington, D.C.: American Psychiatric Press, 1997.

Reeves, G. E., M. S. Graziano, and C. G. Gross. "Neurogenesis in the Neocortex of Adult Primates," *Science* 286, no. 5439 (1999): 548–552.

Reynolds, C.F., A. Dew, T. H. Monk, and C. C. Hoch. "Sleep Disorder in Late Life: A Biopsychosocial Model for Understanding Pathogenesis and Intervention," in Textbook of Geriatric Neuropsychiatry, eds. C. E. Coffey and J. L. Cummings, 323–31. Washington, D.C.: American Psychiatric Press, 1994.

Chapter 3. Transition and Transformation

Antonini, F. M. and S. Magnolfi. "Successful Aging and Artistic Creativity," *Aging Clinical Experimental Research* 4, no. 2 (1992):93–101.

Arnheim, R. "On the Late Style," in *New Essays on the Psychology of Art,* by R. Arnheim, 113–120. Berkeley: The University of California Press, 1986.

Cohen, G. D. "Human Potential Phases in the Second Half of Life: Mental Health Theory Development." *The American Journal of Geriatric Psychiatry* 7, no. 1 (1999): 1–7.

Flood, D. G. and P. D. Coleman. "Hippocampal Plasticity in Normal Aging and Decreased Plasticity in Alzheimer's Disease," *Progress in Brain Research* 83 (1990): 435–443.

Chapter 4. The "When" of Creativity

Hartigan, L. R., ed. *Made With Passion: The Hemphill Folk Art Collection.* Washington, D.C.: Smithsonian Institution Press, 1990.

Livingston, J. and J. Beardsley, eds. *Black Folk Art in America.* Jackson, Mississippi: University of Mississippi Press, 1982.

McLeish, J. A. B. *The Ulyssean Adult.* New York: McGraw-Hill Ryerson Limited, 1976.

Chapter 5. Creative Growth and Expression in the Context of Relationship

Brody, E. *Women in the Middle: Their Parent Care Years.* New York: Springer, 1990.

Cohen, G. D. "Marriage and Divorce in Later Life." *The American Journal of Geriatric Psychiatry,* 7 no. 3 (1999): 185–187.

Myers, M. F. *How's Your Marriage?* Washington, D.C.: American Psychiatric Press, Inc., 1998.

Chapter 6. Creativity in Response to Adversity

Elderfield, J. *Henri Matisse: A Retrospective.* New York: The Museum of Modern Art, 1992.

Glass, T. A., C. M. deLeon, R. A. Marottoli, and L. F. Berkman. "Population Based Study of Social and Productive Activities as Predictors of Survival Among Elderly Americans," *The British Medical Journal* 319 (1999): 478–483.

Kaller, J. *Grandma Moses: The Artist Behind the Myth.* Secaucus, N.J.: Wellfleet Press, 1989.

Shavit, Y. "Stress-Induced Modulation in Animals: Opiates and Endogenous Opioid Peptides," in *Psychoneuroimmunology II,* eds. R. Adler, D. L. Felton, and N. Cohen, New York: Academic Press, 1991.

Chapter 7. Creativity and Community

Bengtson, V. L., N. E. Cutler, D. J. Mangen, and V. W. Marshall. "Generations, Cohorts, and Relations Between Age Groups." In *Handbook of Aging and the Social Sciences, Second Edition,* eds. R. H. Binstock and E. Shanus, 304–338. New York: Van Nostrand Reinhold, 1985.

Cohen G. D. "Intergenerationalism: A New 'ism' with Positive Mental Health and Social Policy Potential." *The American Journal of Geriatric Psychiatry* 3 (1995): 1–5.

Cohen, G. D. "Journalistic Elder Abuse: It's Time to Get Rid of Fictions, Get Down to Facts." *The Gerontologist* 34 (1994): 399–401.

Cole, T. and M. Winkler. "The Old Grandfather and the Grandson." In *The Oxford Book of Aging,* eds. T. Cole and M. Winkler, 114. New York: Oxford University Press, 1994.

Cole, T. and M. Winkler. "The Mountain of Abandoned Old People." In *The Oxford Book of Aging,* eds. T. Cole and M. Winkler, 116–117. New York: Oxford University Press, 1994.

Gatz, M., V. L. Bengtson, and M. J. Blum. "Caregiving Families." In *Handbook of the Psychology of Aging, Third Edition,* eds. J. E. Birren and K. W. Schaie, 404–426. New York: Academic Press, 1990.

Gist, J. *Entitlements and the Federal Budget Deficit: Setting the Record Straight.* Washington, D.C.: AARP Public Policy Institute, 1992.

Sussman, M. B. The Family Life of Old People." In *Handbook of Aging and the Social Sciences, Second Edition,* eds. R. H. Binstock and E. Shanus, 415–449. New York: Van Nostrand Reinhold, 1985.

Chapter 8. Identity and Autobiography

Birren, J. E. and D. E. Deutchman. *Guiding Autobiography Groups for Older Adults.* Baltimore: Johns Hopkins University Press, 1991.

Butler, R. N. "The Life Review: An Interpretation of Reminiscence in the Aged." *Psychiatry* 26 (1963): 65–76.

Chapter 9. Creativity in Everyday Life

Cohen, G. D. "Mental Health Promotion in Later Life: The Case for the Social Portfolio." *The American Journal of Geriatric Psychiatry* 3 (1995): 277–279.

Conclusion: Toward the Future

Robinson, R. *Georgia O'Keeffe.* Hanover, N.H.: University Press of New England, 1989.

Sacher, G. A. "Evolution of Longevity and Survival Characteristics in Mammals." In *The Genetics of Aging,* ed. E. L. Schneider, 151–167. New York: Plenum, 1978.

Schneider, E. L. "Theories of Aging: A Perspective." In *Modern Biological Theories of Aging,* eds. H. R. Warner, R. N. Butler, R. L. Sprott, and E. L. Schneider, 1–4. New York: Raven Press, 1987.

Appendix A. Why Do We Age? Biology's Creative Mystery

Hayflick, L. "Why Do We Age?" 187–262. In *How and Why We Age* by L. Hayflick. New York: Ballantine Books, 1994.

Kirkwood, T. *Time of Our Lives*. New York: Oxford University Press, 1999.

Warner, H. R., R. N. Butler, R. L. Sprott, and E. L. Schneider, eds. *Modern Biological Theories of Aging*. New York: Raven Press, 1987.

Weiss, R. "Aging—New Answers to Old Questions." *National Geographic* 192, no. 5 (1997): 2–31.

Appendix B. Historical Quests to Reverse the Effects of Aging

Busse, E. W. "The Myth, History, and Science of Aging." In *Textbook of Geriatric Psychiatry, Second Edition,* eds. E. W. Busse and D. G. Blazer, 3–24. Washington, D.C.: American Psychiatric Press, Inc., 1996.

Editors of Time-Life Books. *Search for Immortality, Mysteries of the Unknown Series*. Alexandria, VA: Time-Life Books, 1992.

Hayflick, L. "Slowing Aging and Increasing Life Span." 263–310. In *How and Why We Age* by L. Hayflick. New York: Ballantine Books, 1994.

Kirkwood, T. *Time of Our Lives*. New York: Oxford University Press, 1999.

McGrady, Jr., P. M. *The Youth Doctors*. New York: Coward-McCann, Inc., 1968.

Appendix C. Creating an Autobiography: My Personal Approach

Brownstone, D. and I. Franck. *Timelines of the 20th Century*. Boston: Little, Brown and Company, 1996.

Index

Page numbers in italics refer to sidebars and illustrations.

R

S

T